Paediatric Infectious Diseases

Yhu-Chering Huang
Ping-Ing Lee • Po-Yen Chen
Editors

Paediatric Infectious Diseases

A practical guide and cases

Springer

Editors
Yhu-Chering Huang
Pediatrics
Chang Gung Memorial Hospital,
Chang Gung University
Taoyuan, Taiwan

Ping-Ing Lee
Pediatrics
National Taiwan University Children's
Hospital, National Taiwan University
Taipei, Taiwan

Po-Yen Chen
Pediatrics
Taichung Veterans General Hospital,
National Chung Hsing University
Taichung City, Taiwan

ISBN 978-981-19-7275-1 ISBN 978-981-19-7276-8 (eBook)
https://doi.org/10.1007/978-981-19-7276-8

This Springer imprint is published by the registered company Springer Nature Singapore Pte Ltd.
The registered company address is: 152 Beach Road, #21-01/04 Gateway East, Singapore 189721, Singapore

Preface

Infectious diseases are among the most common diseases making children seek medical care. Most pathogens of infectious diseases in pediatric patients are viruses and the illness is usually self-limited. However, certain infectious diseases may be severe and even fatal. Pediatric patients are also characterized by uncertain subjective symptoms and obscure objective signs that may delay making a correct diagnosis. An early recognition of serious infections that need special management is crucial for managing pediatric patients with symptoms and signs of infection. Being pediatric infectious disease specialists for more than 30 years, we have encountered many such conditions. To share our experiences with all readers, we collected and chose 50 cases from our careers of clinical practice and drafted them in this book, hoping to assist all physicians who are taking care of pediatric patients.

We thank all the contributors who were committed to drafting manuscripts in this book. Without these commitments, we cannot complete this work. Lastly, we would like to show our greatest gratitude to all patients who have inspired us in the appropriate management of children with infectious diseases. Here, with these sharing experiences, we deeply hope that more and more clinicians can learn from you, making all children in the world more and more healthy.

Taoyuan, Taiwan — Yhu-Chering Huang
Taipei, Taiwan — Ping-Ing Lee
Taichung, Taiwan — Po-Yen Chen

Contents

Part I

Neonatal Infection

Case 1. A 6-Day-Old Female Newborn with Fever and Decreased Appetite and Activity: Enteroviral Infection in Neonates

Yhu-Chering Huang

Keywords

Enterovirus · Neonates · Intravenous immunoglobulin · Myocarditis · Coagulopathy

Key Points

- Not uncommon and difficult to be differentiated from bacterial sepsis.
- Echovirus and coxsackievirus B are the most common serotypes associated with neonatal sepsis.
- Manifestations range from mild to severe and life-threatening diseases, including hepatic necrosis with coagulopathy, and myocarditis.
- A high index of suspicion, followed by RT-PCR, is the key to an early diagnosis.
- Early intravenous immunoglobulin treatment may help in reducing morbidity and mortality for severe diseases.

Case Report

A 6-day-old female neonate was admitted to the neonatal unit due to fever and decreased appetite and activity for one day. The baby was born at the gestational age of 37 weeks with a birth weight of 2820 g via cesarean section due to maternal fever and fetal distress. The Apgar score was nine and ten points at the one-minute and 5-min checks, respectively. The mother developed fever one day before delivery. On admission, the baby appeared lethargic and vital signs were body temperature 37.20 °C, pulse rate 162/min, respiratory rate 42/min, and blood pressure 69/58 mmHg. Icteric skin discoloration, mottling skin with a capillary refilling time of three seconds, and mild hepatomegaly were noted. Other physical examinations as well as neurologic assessments were essentially negative. Initial laboratory data showed leukocytosis (WBC 23,900/μL, immature neutrophils 17%, segmented 42%, lymphocytes 27.5%, monocytes 8%, eosinophil 3%), thrombocytopenia (platelet 20,000/μL), and hemoglobin (Hb) 18.8 g/dL. Blood biochemistry data showed sugar 80 mg/dL, blood urea nitrogen (BUN) 20 mg/dL, creatinine 0.2 mg/dL, bilirubin (direct/total) 1.0/12.2 mg/dL, aspartate transaminase (AST) 481 U/L, alanine transaminase (ALT) 57 U/L, sodium 131 mEq/L, potassium 6.5 mEq/L, chloride 107 mEq/L, and C-reactive protein (CRP) 3.08 mg/L (normal, <5 mg/L). Arterial blood gas showed metabolic acidosis (pH 7.290, HCO_3 14.1 mm/L). Under the impression of severe viral sepsis, intravenous immune globulin (IVIG) (400 mg/kg/day) was administered for five days. Blood components, if needed,

Y.-C. Huang (✉)
Pediatrics, Chang Gung Memorial Hospital, Chang Gung University, Taoyuan, Taiwan
e-mail: ychuang@cgmh.org.tw

Y.-C. Huang et al. (eds.), *Paediatric Infectious Diseases*,
https://doi.org/10.1007/978-981-19-7276-8_1

were transfused for several occasions. On hospital day 3, the baby developed tachypnea, hypotension and desaturation, and petechiae and ecchymosis over limbs were noted. Laboratory data showed anemia (Hb 6.6 g/dL), prolonged prothrombin time (international normalized ratio [INR], 2.77 [normal 0.8–1.2]), activated partial thromboplastin time (aPTT, 80 s), elevated AST (1906 U/L) and ALT (477 U/L), and elevated creatine kinase (CK)-MB form (111.8 ng/mL, normal 0.6–6.3 ng/mL) and troponin-I (67.9 ng/mL, normal <0.04 ng/mL). An endotracheal tube was inserted, and an inotropic agent (dopamine) was administered. Cardiac ultrasound, performed on hospital day 4, revealed decreased ejection fraction (EF) to 47% (normal, >70%). Viral isolation from both throat swabs and rectal swabs revealed positivity for coxsackievirus (CV) B3 on hospital day 5. General edema and intractable hypotension were noted. On hospital day 6, extracorporeal membrane oxygenation (ECMO) was applied to the baby. The condition was stabilized gradually, and coagulopathy, cardiac enzymes, and transaminase improved. ECMO was removed on hospital day 18. Renal function deteriorated to acute renal failure with oliguria, and continuous ambulatory peritoneal dialysis commenced on day 19 and stopped on day 39. Endotracheal tube was extubated on day 29. However, impaired cardiac function did not return to normal with a sustained low EF of <50%. The baby was discharged on day 57 with a final diagnosis of neonatal CVB3 sepsis with myocarditis and multiorgan failure. Follow-up cardiac ultrasound one month after discharge showed a dilated chamber size with poor left ventricular performance. With the sequelae of cardiomyopathy, she passed away at the age of 12 years.

Discussion

Enteroviruses (EVs) are RNA viruses. EVs were formerly classified into enteric cytopathic human orphan (Echo) viruses, coxsackievirus A, coxsackievirus B (CVB) viruses, polioviruses, and newly identified serotypes. Recently, a new classification was developed based on genome sequencing and EVs are now subgrouped into human enterovirus (HEV)-A, HEV-B, HEV-C, and HEV-D.

The circulating serotype of EVs varies over time and location and may change year by year. Clinicians should be alert to the local epidemiology of EV activity. EVs infections are common in neonates. Data from the National Enterovirus Surveillance System of the USA between 1983 and 2003 showed that of approximately 26,000 enteroviruses detected, neonates accounted for 11.4% of those of known age. Enterovirus is a frequent etiologic agent identified for nonspecific febrile illness in young infants, accounting for 47%–63% of cases requiring hospitalization to exclude bacterial sepsis. The incidence of neonatal enteroviral infection is related to the serotypes of circulating EVs (frequently due to CVB group and echoviruses) in the community.

Enteroviruses are transmitted predominantly via fecal–oral and respiratory routes. Infections in the newborn may be acquired vertically before, during, or after delivery. After delivery, the acquisition may be via breast milk, horizontally from family members, or nosocomial transmission in nurseries and neonatal units. The predominant timing of transmission is intrapartum, at the time of delivery through contact with maternal blood, stool, amniotic fluid, or vaginal or cervical secretions. Nosocomial outbreaks in neonatal units and nurseries have frequently been reported and the index cases were usually from newborns that had been vertically infected. The attack rate for infants at risk is estimated to range from 22% to 53%.

Neonatal enteroviral infections may manifest from asymptomatic, non-specific febrile illness, aseptic meningitis to severe fatal multi-system disease. Clinical manifestations in neonates, such as fever, poor feeding, lethargy, respiratory distress, and cardiovascular collapse, are difficult to differentiate from those of bacterial sepsis. Severe, life-threatening complications in neonates include hepatic necrosis with coagulopathy and myocarditis. Once occurred, these manifestations usually present during the first two weeks of life, mostly in the first week of life. In a study from Taiwan, approximately 30% of 146 hospitalized young infants <3 months of age with EV infection presented with severe diseases. Prematurity, maternal history of illness, and early age of onset (≦7 days) were risk factors for hepatic necrosis with coagulopathy. Signs of myocarditis usually include respiratory distress, tachycardia, cardiomegaly, arrhythmias, and ECG signs of myocardial injury and some cases may develop circulatory collapse rapidly. Mortality may be as high as 30–50%. As the illustrated case, survivors may develop dilated cardiomyopathy and ventricular aneurysms. Factors affecting severity and outcome include virus serotype, mode of transmission, and presence or absence of passively acquired, serotype-specific maternal antibodies. Echoviruses and CVB are the most common serotypes associated with neonatal sepsis. Early onset of disease in the first week of life were associated with absence of serotype-specific transplacentally acquired neutralizing antibody to the infecting serotype in the neonate and resultant severe neonatal disease.

Clinically, the diagnosis of neonatal EV infection is difficult without the help of laboratory tests to exclude bacterial or other viral sepsis. A high index of suspicion is the key to an early diagnosis. During the EV season, EV infection should be first considered in a neonate or young infant with fever and/or sepsis-like illness. Then, diagnostic virologic methods for the detection of enterovirus should be applied immediately. Viral culture is a conventional diagnostic method, but is time-consuming. Reverse-transcriptase polymerase chain reaction (RT-PCR) provides a rapid diagnostic tool to confirm EV infection. The specimens can be blood, serum, cerebrospinal fluid, oropharyngeal swab, rectal swab, urine, or stool. Higher viral loads in blood detected by real-time RT-PCR are associated with a more severe disease. Early diagnosis and prediction of disease severity is possible in severe neonatal EV infection.

Most enterovirus infections are self-limited, no specific therapy is needed, and care is essentially supportive. However, for life-threatening infections, administration of intravenous immunoglobulin (IVIG) may be considered due to the high mortality. The effect of IVIG therapy on severe neonatal EV infection varied in different studies. In a retrospective analysis of 67 cases of culture-confirmed neonatal enterovirus infection with severe hepatitis and coagulopathy, we found that early IVIG therapy was independently associated with survival. We think the timing of IVIG administration is crucial, and early IVIG may be beneficial for survival in severe cases. In addition, we found that serum AST levels in most cases usually peaked within three days of illness onset. Hence, we suggest that frequent sampling for monitoring serum AST levels within three days of illness onset may provide opportunities to detect potentially severe cases of neonatal enterovirus disease earlier.

Currently, there are no antivirals licensed for the treatment of EV infection. The antiviral drug pleconaril is a capsid inhibitor that prevents the virus from attaching to cellular receptors. Pocapavir, also known as Scheme 48973 and V-073, is a potent, selective anti-enteroviral agent only available as an emergency investigational drug. The drug is a capsid inhibitor administered orally and is highly protein-bound and excreted exclusively in feces. As some neonates with severe enteroviral myocarditis may rapidly progress to cardiovascular collapse, which may be refractory to conventional medical treatment, extracorporeal membrane oxygenation (ECMO) may have a role in these patients.

An awareness of the clinical syndromes, recognition of the risk factors and monitoring parameters associated with severe cases, plus the use of real-time RT-PCR for measuring viral load in blood may help clinicians diagnose severe cases of enteroviral infection in neonates in a timely manner. Prompt aggressive treatment, including early intravenous immunoglobulin administration, may help reduce morbidity and mortality. Enterovirus infections in neonates are common and should be routinely considered in the differential diagnosis of febrile neonates, particularly during the enterovirus season.

Further Reading

Abzug MJ. Nonpolio enteroviruses. In Nelson's Textbook of Pediatrics. 20th ed. Philadelphia, PA: Elsevier. 2016:1561-8.e1.

Chuang YY, Huang YC. Enteroviral infection in neonates. J Microbiol Immunol Infect 2019;52:851–7.

Lin TY, Kao HT, Hsieh SH, Huang YC, Chiu CH, Chou YH, et al. Neonatal enterovirus infections: emphasis on risk factors for severe and fatal infections. Pediatr Infect Dis J 2003;22:889–94.

Souverbielle CT, Feister J, Leber A, Salamon D, Mejias A, Ramilo O, et al. Multiple sites PCR testing for enteroviruses in young febrile infants. Lancet Infect Dis 2019;19;239–240

de Jong EP, van den Beuken MGA, van Elzakker EPM, Wolthers KC, Sprij AJ, Lopriore E, et al. Epidemiology of sepsis-like illness in young infants. Pediatr Infect Dis J 2018;37:113–8.

Civardi E., Tzialla, C, Baldanti, F, Strocchio, L, Manzoni, P, Stronati M. Viral outbreaks in neonatal intensive care units: What we do not know. Am J Infect Control 2013;41:854–6.

Yen MH, Tsao KC, Huang YC, Huang CG, Huang YL, Lin RY, et al. Viral Load in blood is correlated with disease severity of neonatal coxsackievirus B3 infection: early diagnosis and predicting disease severity is possible in severe neonatal enterovirus Infection. Clin Infect Dis 2007; 44:e78–e81.

Yen MH, Huang YC, Chen MC, Liu CC, Chiu NC, Lin RY, et al. Effect of intravenous immunoglobulin for neonates with severe enteroviral infections with emphasis on the timing of administration. J Clin Virol 2015;64:92–6.

Abzug MJ, Michaels MG, Wald E, Jacobs RF, Romero JR, Sánchez PJ, et al. A randomized, double-blind, placebo-controlled trial of pleconaril for the treatment of neonates with enterovirus sepsis. J Pediatr Infect Dis Soc 2016;5:53–62.

Cortina G, Best D, Deisenberg M, Chiletti R, Butt W. Extracorporeal membrane oxygenation for neonatal collapse caused by enterovirus myocarditis. Arch Dis Child Fetal Neonatal Ed 2018; 103:F370–F376.

Case 2. 17-Day-Old Female Baby with Fever and Decreased Appetite and Activity: Herpes Simplex Virus Infection in Neonates and Children

Yu-Yu Chuang and Yhu-Chering Huang

Keywords

Herpes simplex virus · Encephalitis
Neonates

Key Points

- Herpes simplex virus (HSV) causes a variety of clinical manifestations, ranging from mild to life threatening.
- Neonatal herpes simplex encephalitis can be subtle on presentation and difficult to identify promptly.
- Polymerase chain reaction (PCR) assay is the diagnostic method of choice for HSV encephalitis or central nervous system involvement.
- Neonatal herpes simplex encephalitis is associated with a high mortality and significant neurologic disability among survivors, and timely initiation of antiviral therapy is imperative, as outcome depends on treatment.

Y.-Y. Chuang (✉)
St. Mary's Hospital, Luodong, Yilan, Taiwan

Y.-C. Huang
Pediatrics, Chang Gung Memorial Hospital, Chang Gung University, Taoyuan, Taiwan

Case Report

A 17-day-old baby girl was admitted to the neonatal unit due to fever and decreased appetite and activity for one day. She was born at the gestational age of 38 weeks with a birth weight of 3100 g via normal spontaneous delivery. The Apgar score was nine and ten points at the 1-min and 5-min checks, respectively. On admission, the baby appeared lethargic, and vital signs were body temperature 36.90 °C, pulse rate 166 beats/min, respiratory rate 56 breaths/min, and blood pressure 72/50 mmHg. Physical examinations showed no bulging fontanelle and no oral or skin lesions or conjunctivitis. Heart, lung, and abdomen were normal. Initial laboratory data showed white blood cell (WBC) count 17,100/μL, segmented 42%, lymphocytes 39%, monocytes 18%, platelet 673,000/μL, and hemoglobin (Hb) 14 g/dL. Blood biochemistry data showed blood urea nitrogen (BUN) 12 mg/dL, creatinine 0.32 mg/dL, bilirubin (direct/total) 0.4/4.5 mg/dL, aspartate transaminase (AST) 45 U/L, sodium 136 mEq/L, potassium 5.1 mEq/L, chloride 102 mEq/L and C-reactive protein (CRP) < 0.2 mg/L (normal, <5 mg/L). Urinalysis showed pH 8.5, leucocyte +++, nitrite negative, bacteria positive, red blood cell (RBC) 12/μL, and WBC 369/μL. The initial diagnosis was neonatal fever, suspected urinary tract infection, and empiric antibiotics with ampicillin and gentamicin.

On hospital day 3, her fever persisted, and she developed seizures. Urine culture showed *Escherichia coli*, 10^4 colony-forming units/mL.

Y.-C. Huang et al. (eds.), *Paediatric Infectious Diseases*,
https://doi.org/10.1007/978-981-19-7276-8_2

Follow-up blood tests showed normal WBC and CRP levels and hyponatremia 125 mEq/L. Cerebrospinal fluid (CSF) studies showed protein 84.4 mg/dL, sugar 43 mg/dL, lactate 12.3 mg/dL, WBC 23/μL, neutrophil 1%, lymphocyte 32%, monocytes 64%, negative for bacterial culture. We discontinued her feedings due to severe abdominal distension and antibiotics upgraded to ampicillin, cefotaxime, and metronidazole. Her condition deteriorated with altered consciousness, shock, and intubation. Brain computed tomography (CT) scan showed diffuse hypodensity of the left cerebral hemisphere and left subcortical white matter. Electrical encephalogram (EEG) showed focal epileptiform discharges over bilateral parietal areas.

Consultation with the infectious diseases specialist on hospital day 7 and the CSF specimen for herpes simplex virus (HSV) polymerase chain reaction (PCR) examination was suggested and subsequently showed positive (324.9 copies/mL) on hospital day 10. Brain magnetic resonance imaging (MRI) showed encephalitis or meningoencephalitis involving the deep gray nuclei (mainly thalami), corpus callosum, and cerebral cortical/subcortical regions and diffuse brain swelling. Follow-up blood tests showed Hb 10.3 g/dL and thrombocytopenia (platelet counts 53,000/μL). Biochemistries showed acute hepatitis without cholestasis, bilirubin (direct/total) 0.2/0.3 mg/dL, AST 1213 U/L, alanine transaminase (ALT) 400 U/L, gamma glutamyl transpeptidase (γ-GT) 413 U/L, sodium 145 mEq/L, and CRP 3.49 mg/L. Abdominal echo revealed hepatomegaly and no ascites. The anticonvulsant drug phenobarbital was changed to levetiracetam. Fundoscopy showed multiple necrosis on the retina (Fig. 1), and bilateral and intravitreal antiviral agents were used. Bone marrow examination showed neutropenia and thrombocytopenia. On the second week of hospitalization, blood for HSV PCR was positive (10521.2 copies/mL), and intravenous acyclovir was given. The patient regained her consciousness, but opisthotonus and poor suck-swallow coordination reflex were noted. Follow-up brain CT scan in the third week of hospitalization showed diffuse encephalomalacia (Fig. 2). Follow-up CSF studies showed protein 595.8 mg/dL, sugar 17 mg/dL, lactate 21.8 mg/dL, WBC 156 μL, neutrophil 0%, lymphocyte 90%, monocytes 6%, and CSF HSV PCR was still positive (144349.7 copies/mL). Eye HSV PCR was positive (14414.3 copies/mL). After 2 weeks of treatment, a third follow-up CSF study showed protein 666.6 mg/dL, sugar 23 mg/dL, lactate 13.4 mg/dL, WBC 21 μL, neutrophil 0%, lymphocyte 58%, monocytes 40%, and CSF HSV PCR was still positive (402.7 copies/mL). Maternal and newborn serology showed HSV-1 IgG positivity. HSV-1 IgM and HSV-2 IgG were negative. The final diagnosis was neonatal herpes simplex virus meningoencephalitis with severe leukomalacia and disseminated herpes simplex virus infection with central nervous system (CNS), eyes, bone marrow, and liver involvement.

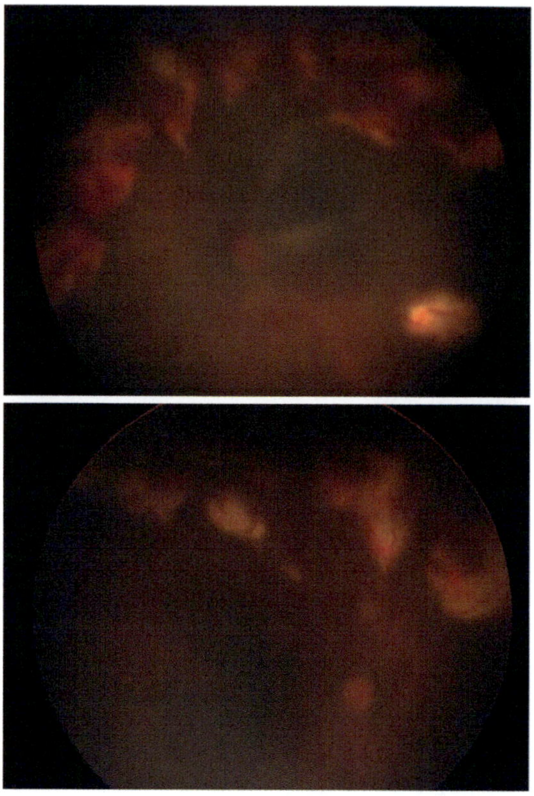

Fig. 1 Eye fundi showed multiple necrosis on retina of both eyes on day 14 (upper) and improvement after intravitreal acyclovir treatment (lower)

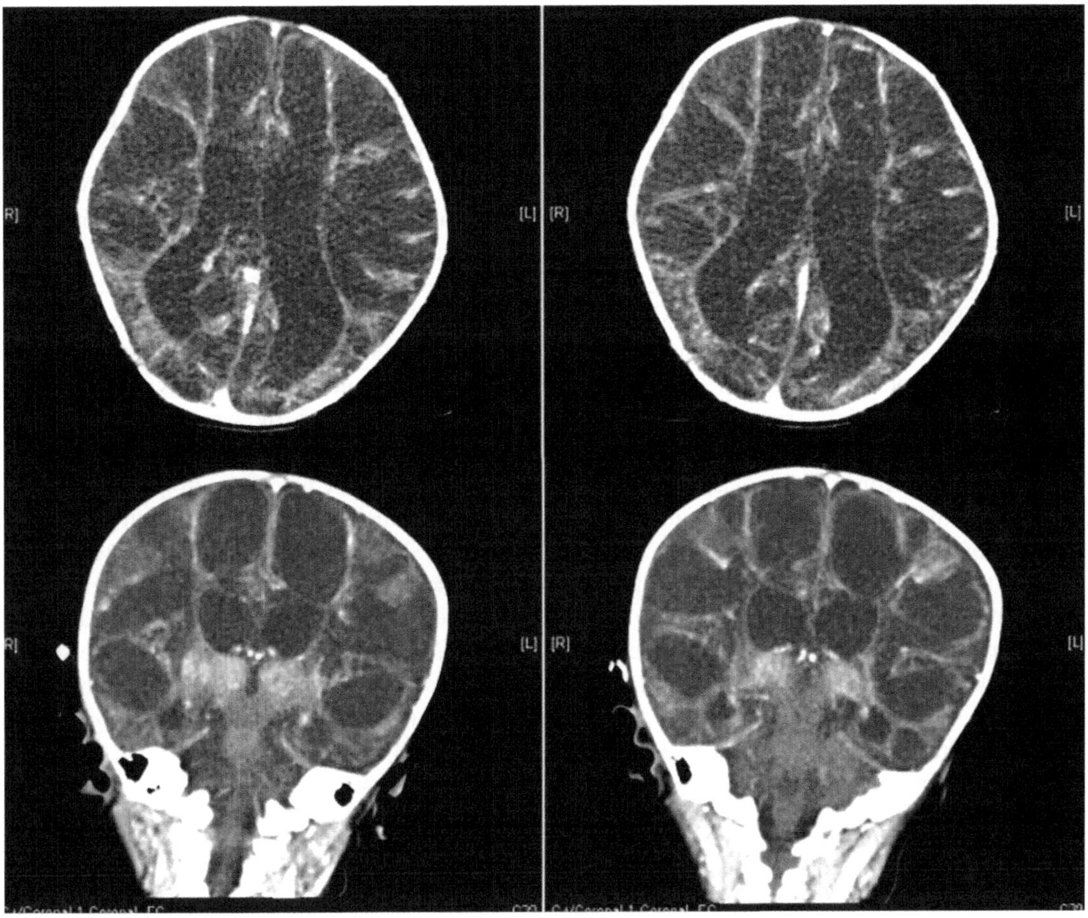

Fig. 2 Follow-up brain computed tomography 3 weeks after antiviral treatment showed diffuse encephalomalacia in axial plane (upper two films) and coronal plane (lower two films)

Discussion

Herpes simplex virus 1 and 2 (HSV-1 and HSV-2) are linear, enveloped, double stranded DNA viruses. It belongs to the family *Herpesviridae*, subfamily *Alphaherpesviridae*. Following primary infection, they become latent in the sensory neural ganglia with periodic reactivation to cause recurrent symptomatic disease or asymptomatic viral shedding. Both types of HSV cause common infections in healthy children and adults, and clinical manifestations vary, ranging from asymptomatic and mild common infections to life threatening in neonates and immune-compromised hosts.

HSV has a worldwide distribution, and humans are the only reservoir. Symptomatic or asymptomatic persons with primary or recurrent infections can transmit the virus. HSV-1 infection is more frequent and occurs earlier than HSV-2 infection. Most primary HSV-1 infections beyond the neonatal period are transmitted primarily through oral shedding. Primary HSV-2 infections are acquired after the onset of sexual activity, and genital herpes infections are among the most common sexually transmitted infections (STIs).

More than 90% of adults have antibodies to HSV-1 by their 40s. The prevalence of antibodies to HSV-1 increases with age and is inversely correlated with socioeconomic status. HSV-2 seroprevalence correlates with the onset of sexual activity and is higher in women. The global

HSV-2 prevalence is estimated at 11.3% among 15–49 years of age. In Taiwan, the HSV-1 seropositive rate was 19.2% for individuals less than 5 years old, increased to 46.4% for those 5–13 years old, 60.9% for those 14–29 years old, and 95.0% for those over 30 years old. In contrast, the HSV-2 seropositive rate was 1.6% for those less than 30 years old, 10.1% for those aged 30–39 years, and 31.2% for those aged over 60 years. The overall HSV-2 seropositive rate was twice as high in females than in males. Female gender and rural residence were independent factors for HSV-2 seropositivity. A recent meta-analysis of HSV-1 epidemiology in Asia showed that the seroprevalence was 50% for children and 76.5% for adults. HSV-1 contributes to one-fifth of genital herpes cases.

A cohort study of neonatal HSV infection from a multistate Medicaid population from 2009 to 2015 reported a corrected incidence rate of 4.5 per 10,000 births. The in-hospital mortality rate was stable at 6%. Population-based surveillance in Australia reported an incidence of 3.27 cases per 100,000 live births. HSV-1 infection was more common than HSV-2. Overall mortality rate 18.8%. The risk of transmission to a neonate born to a mother with primary genital HSV infection near the time of delivery is 25% to 60%. The risk to a neonate born to a mother with reactivation of infection during the first half of pregnancy or earlier is less than 2%.

Clinical manifestations of HSV infection depend on the site, type of virus, age, and immune status. Classic infections are small skin vesicles surrounded by an erythematous base, evolving in a few days into shallow ulcers. Most infections are asymptomatic. Gingivostomatitis is the most common primary infection of HSV-1 during childhood and is characterized by fever, irritability, oral ulcers in the anterior and posterior parts of the oral cavity, gum swelling/bleeding, and exudate-coated tonsils. HSV infection of the fingers or toes was occasionally seen in children with symptomatic or subclinical oral HSV who suck their thumbs or fingers. The most common manifestation of recurrent HSV-1 infection is herpes labialis.

Genital herpes infection is common in sexually experienced adolescents and young adults. Recurrences are more frequent with HSV-2. Primary genital herpes infections are most often asymptomatic, and they are usually not recognized or diagnosed. Primary genital HSV infection is rare in infants and children, and its presence should raise concern about sexual abuse.

Neonatal HSV infection can be caused by HSV-1 and HSV-2. Transmission can occur intrauterine, perinatal, and postnatal. Neonatal HSV disease presents in the first 4 weeks of life, and the majority is acquired by perinatal exposure to HSV. Signs and symptoms occur during the first 7 to 21 days of life. Clinical syndromes manifest as localized to the skin, eyes, and mouth (SEM disease); CNS disease with or without SEM disease; and disseminated disease. Forty-five percent of cases were SEM disease, 30% CNS disease, and 25% disseminated disease. Identifying the source of herpes simplex encephalitis (HSE) in neonatal disease can be difficult, as a history of known maternal HSV disease (mostly genital, occasionally oral) is not universal, and maternal disease may be asymptomatic. Skin lesions may be present and may appear later in the clinical course than the presenting fever, lethargy, or even seizures.

Herpes simplex encephalitis (HSE) is a devastating disease and is difficult to diagnose in its early stages. The mortality rate without antiviral treatment is 70%, with most survivors suffering from permanent neurologic sequelae. The incidence is 1 in 64,000 infants per year and 1 in 230,000 children per year. Childhood HSE clinical features are fever, altered mental state (encephalopathy), deteriorating level of consciousness, focal seizures, and focal neurologic abnormalities. Encephalopathy can be a change in behavior, sleepiness, or confusion. Children with normal behavior at presentation may become confused later as encephalitis progresses. Only 10% have a prior history of mucosal symptoms such as cold sores or conjunctivitis. The infective source is usually elusive. HSV infection of the eye may initially appear asymptomatic. Keratoconjunctivitis may progress to chorioretinitis, resulting in permanent vision impairment.

Neonatal HSV infection can be subtle on presentation, and physicians need to be vigilant to diagnose HSV promptly and initiate antiviral treatment. However, beyond the neonatal period, routine herpes testing and empiric acyclovir treatment may lead to increased medical costs and risks to patients.

Diagnosis of HSV infection is usually based on clinical findings. A definitive laboratory diagnosis is necessary for serious infections. Clinically, CSF analysis can show pleocytosis, and elevated protein levels are helpful but not diagnostic. Detection of intrathecal HSV-specific IgM by ELISA at 10 to 14 days after onset of symptoms suggestive of a neuroinvasive infection. PCR for HSV DNA from the CSF is the gold standard for the diagnosis of HSE. HSV is almost never grown from the CSF culture. MRI is the most sensitive imaging method to detect temporal lobe involvement. The typical EEG pattern is periodic lateralizing epileptiform discharges in the temporal lobe with slow wave complexes.

Polymerase chain reaction (PCR) is the preferred diagnostic method for CNS infection and disseminated disease. In cases in which repeated CSF PCR assays are negative, histologic examination and viral culture of brain biopsy is the most definitive diagnosis of HSV encephalitis. For evaluation of neonates with suspected HSV infection, specimens from the mouth, eye, anus, and skin vesicles should be obtained for HSV culture or PCR; CSF and whole blood specimens should be obtained for PCR and liver enzymes should be used for indirect evidence of HSV dissemination.

For genital herpes, virus culture and PCR are the preferred tests; however, failure to detect HSV in the genital lesion does not exclude HSV infection because viral shedding is intermittent. Serology is diagnostic of the type of infection. Western blot assay measuring HSV-1-specific and HSV-2-specific antibodies is the most accurate available serologic test and has a sensitivity and specificity of greater than 98% for distinguishing HSV-1-specific and HSV-2-specific antibodies.

Current antiviral agents available for medical treatment are acyclovir, valacyclovir, and famciclovir. Neonatal HSV infections, children with encephalitis, or infections in immune-compromised patients need parenteral acyclovir and aggressive intensive care for optimal outcomes. Treatment of increased intracranial pressure, seizures, and respiratory support may also be required for herpes encephalitis. Neonatal HSV disease should have an ophthalmologic examination and neuroimaging studies. After neonatal HSE, HSV can reactivate months to years after the initial infection, mostly presenting as dermal flares or as encephalitis as devastating as the initial illness. Early-life infection impairs the development of an effective adaptive immune response, but prolonged antiviral prophylaxis can prevent recurrence. Survivors of neonatal HSV infections given oral acyclovir suppression at 300 mg/m^2/dose three times daily for 6 months after the completion of parenteral therapy showed improved neurodevelopment of infants with CNS infection and prevented cutaneous recurrences.

Hypothetical management of patients with adjuvant corticosteroids in HSV encephalitis can reduce both viral load and the excessive inflammatory response and result in less damage to the brain. The level of biomarkers of inflammation in the CSF or serum should be determined. Empiric intravenous acyclovir should be initiated pending the results of CSF and MRI and continued for 14 to 21 days if the PCR is positive. Adjunctive corticosteroid therapy (dexamethasone 10 mg IV every 6 h for 4 days) should be started later during the rise of the inflammatory response and should be limited in time to prevent undesired effects.

Ocular involvement should receive topical ophthalmic drugs (1% trifluridine or 0.15% ganciclovir) and parenteral antiviral therapy. Primary or recurrent genital infections should receive antiviral therapy to shorten the duration of illness and viral shedding. Many children with severe HSV gingivostomatitis may require inpatient management due to dehydration. Oral acyclovir (15 mg/kg/dose 5 times a day PO for 7 days; max: 1 g/day) started within 72 h of onset has been shown to reduce the severity and duration of illness.

Further Reading

Bennett JE, Dolin R, Blaser MJ. Mandell, Douglas, and Bennett's principles and practice of infectious diseases. 9th edition. Philadelphia, PA: Elsevier/Saunders, 2020.

Shen JH, Huang KY, Chao-Yu C, Chen CJ, Lin TY, Huang YC. Seroprevalence of Herpes Simplex Virus Type 1 and 2 in Taiwan and Risk Factor Analysis, 2007. PLoS One 2015;10(8):e0134178. . Published 2015 Aug 7.

Khadr L, Harfouche M, Omori R, Schwarzer G, Chemaitelly H, Abu-Raddad LJ. The epidemiology of herpes simplex virus type 1 in Asia: systematic review, meta-analyses, and Meta-regressions. Clin Infect Dis 2019;68:757–772.

Patton ME, Bernstein K, Liu G, Zaidi A, Markowitz LE. Seroprevalence of herpes simplex virus types 1 and 2 among pregnant women and sexually active, Nonpregnant women in the United States, Clin Infect Dis 2018;67(10):1535–1542.

Mahant S, Hall M, Schondelmeyer AC, et al. Neonatal herpes simplex virus infection among medicaid enrolled children: 2009–2015. Pediatrics 2019;143(4): e20183233

Jones CA, Raynes-Greenow C, Isaacs D; Neonatal HSV Study Investigators and Contributors to the Australian Paediatric Surveillance Unit. Population-based surveillance of neonatal herpes simplex virus infection in Australia, 1997–2011. Clin Infect Dis 2014;59:525–31

American Academy of Pediatrics. Red Book: 2018-2021. Report of the Committee on Infectious Diseases, 31st ed, Kimberlin DW, Brady MT, Jackson MA, et al., American Academy of Pediatrics, Itasca, IL 2018.

Huang CW, Hsieh CH, Lin MR, Huang YC. Clinical features of gingivostomatitis due to primary infection of herpes simplex virus in children. BMC Infect Dis. 2020;20:782.

Le Doare K, Menson E, Patel D, Lim M, Lyall H, Herberg J. Fifteen minute consultation: managing neonatal and childhood herpes encephalitis. Arch Dis Child Educ Pract Ed 2015;100:58–63.

Gaensbauer JT, Birkholz M, Pfannenstein K, Todd JK. Herpes PCR testing and empiric acyclovir use beyond the neonatal period. Pediatrics 2014;134:e651–6.

Piret J, Boivin G. Immunomodulatory Strategies in Herpes Simplex Virus Encephalitis. Clin Microbiol Rev 2020;33:e00105–19.

Kimberlin DW, Baley J. Guidance on management of asymptomatic neonates born to women with active genital herpes lesions. Committee on infectious diseases, Committee on fetus and newborn. Pediatrics 2013;131:e635.

Case 3. A Premature Newborn with Respiratory Distress and Poor Activity: Bacterial Meningitis in Neonates

Chen-Yen Kuo

Keywords

Meningitis · Neonates

Key Points in Bacterial Meningitis in Neonates

- Neonatal meningitis can be categorized as early and late onset.
- The distribution of causative pathogens is related to birth gestational age, postnatal age, and geographic region.
- Clinical signs are often subtle and nonspecific.
- CSF culture is the gold standard for diagnosis of bacterial meningitis.
- Prompt treatment with appropriate antibiotics is essential to improve outcomes.
- For cases with relapse of bacterial meningitis in spite of adequate antibiotic therapy, it is mandatory to perform brain image studies to explore possible pus accumulations that may delay a complete sterilization of infection focus.

C.-Y. Kuo (✉)
Division of Pediatric Infectious Diseases, Chang Gung Memorial Hospital at Linkou, Taoyuan, Taiwan

Case Report

A female baby was born by vaginal delivery at 31st week of gestation with a birth weight of 1850 g after premature rupture of membrane. Apgar score was seven and eight points on one-minute and 5-min check, respectively. She was admitted to the neonatal unit due to respiratory distress after birth. On admission, the baby was poor in activity with a body temperature of 36 °C, pulse rate of 170/min, respiratory rate of 43/min, blood pressure of 56/38 mmHg and pulse oximetry of 80%. Physical examinations were essentially normal except for respiratory distress with chest wall retractions that needed endotracheal intubation. Initial laboratory data showed white blood cell (WBC) count of 7600/μL (immature neutrophils 23%, segmented neutrophil 18%, lymphocytes 27%, monocytes 16%, eosinophil 6%,), thrombocytopenia (platelet count 146,000/μL), and hemoglobin (Hb) 13.1 g/dL. Blood biochemistry data showed sugar of 110 mg/dL, and C-reactive protein (CRP) 97.8 mg/L (reference: <5 mg/L). Treatment with ampicillin and cefotaxime was initiated under the impression of early-onset sepsis. On the next day, *Escherichia coli* was isolated from blood culture. The strain had intermediate resistance to ceftriaxone. Meropenem (110 mg/kg/day) was substituted for ampicillin and cefotaxime on Day 2. Lumbar puncture was arranged, and cerebrospinal fluid (CSF) analysis showed decreased level of sugar (35 mg/dL), elevated level of protein (267.6 mg/dL) and pleocyto-

Y.-C. Huang et al. (eds.), *Paediatric Infectious Diseases*,
https://doi.org/10.1007/978-981-19-7276-8_3

sis (WBC 3150/μL), but there was no bacterial growth from CSF sample. She was extubated on Day 6. Blood culture on Day 7 and CSF culture on Day 15 were both negative. Brain magnetic resonance imaging (MRI) on Day14 revealed no evidence of ventriculitis. She was discharged after 21 days of meropenem therapy.

Two weeks later after discharge, the baby was admitted to the neonatal unit again due to poor appetite for 2 days and poor activity with upward gaze for one day. On admission, vital signs were body temperature 36.6 °C, pulse rate 181/min, respiratory rate 23/min, blood pressure 92/54 mmHg, and pulse oximetry 90%. Initial laboratory data showed leukopenia (WBC 2300/μL, immature neutrophils 9%, segmented 39%, lymphocytes 31%, monocytes 18%), platelet 274,000/μL, and hemoglobin 13.7 g/dL. Blood biochemistry data showed CRP of 39.2 mg/L. Lumbar puncture was arranged, and CSF analysis showed decreased level of sugar (5 mg/dL), elevated level of protein (393.4 mg/dL) and pleocytosis (WBC 1350/μL). Gram stain of CSF revealed gram-negative bacilli. We initiated empiric antibiotics with ampicillin and meropenem on Day 1. Due to unstable oxygen saturation, she received endotracheal intubation on Day 2. Besides, anticonvulsant with phenobarbital was used on Day 2 due to seizures. Electroencephalography revealed multifocal epileptiform activity over bilateral centroparieto-temporal areas. *E. coli* with intermediate resistance to ceftriaxone was isolated from blood and CSF again. Ampicillin was discontinued on Day 4. On Day 3 Brain MRI revealed subdural empyema on left lateral temporal fossa. Extubation was performed on Day 16 because the patient's respiratory condition improved gradually. On Day 45, follow-up brain MRI revealed subdural empyema of bilateral temporal areas. CSF analysis on Day 59 showed mild pleocytosis (WBC 11/μL), decreased level of sugar (45 mg/dL), and elevated level of protein (62.8 mg/dL). Blood culture on Day 16, 20 and CSF culture on Day 18, 30, 44, and 59 were all negative. The patient received meropenem 120 mg/kg/day for 60 days (Day 1–61) combined with 2 weeks of gentamicin.

However, she had fever, cough, and rhinorrhea 2 days after discontinuation of meropenem (on Day 63). Respiratory syncytial virus infection was diagnosed by positive respiratory syncytial virus antigen of sputum. Due to elevated CRP (136.7 mg/L) on Day 65, lumbar puncture was performed again, and CSF analysis showed pleocytosis (WBC 84 μL), decreased level of sugar (18 mg/dL), and elevated level of protein (126.8 mg/dL). Meropenem 120 mg/kg/day was administered on Day 65. *E. coli* with complete resistance to ceftriaxone was isolated from CSF sample again. No bacteria grew from blood specimen. Surgical debridement of subdural empyema was performed on Day 75. Finally, the patient received meropenem therapy for 73 days (Day 65–138) with resolution of subdural empyema in left frontal and right temporal regions shown by brain MRI on Day 122, normalization of CSF protein level (43.4 mg/dL) and normal CSF WBC count on Day135. No severe neurologic sequelae except for neurodevelopmental delay was noted during follow up.

All four *E. coli* clinical isolates from the case infant were characterized by pulsed field gel electrophoresis (PFGE) and shared a same PFGE pattern, indicating infection with a same strain throughout the clinical course.

Possible factors that may be associated with recurrence of meningitis were evaluated. No anatomic defects were detected by brain and spine MRI (on day 73). Screening tests for primary immunodeficiency (serum immunoglobulin and complement levels, lymphocyte surface markers and neutrophil function tests) were all normal for her age.

Discussion

Meningitis is the acute inflammation of the meninges, subarachnoid space, and brain vasculature, resulting from infection. Bacterial meningitis in the neonates is a devastating disease associated with high mortality and morbidity. Mortality from neonatal meningitis in developed countries and developing countries ranges from 10 to 15% and 40 to 58%, respectively. Neurological impairment was noted in up to 50% of infants with a history of bacterial meningitis, with 25% having severe disability. Prompt diagnosis and treatment are essential to improve outcomes.

Neonatal meningitis can be categorized as early and late onset, defined by the presence of signs of infection and organism isolation from CSF cultures at ≤72 h and > 72 h of life, respectively. Early onset of meningitis is primarily maternal in origin. Pathogens can be transmitted through the vagina to ruptured amniotic membranes, or due to contact of the neonate's skin during passage through the birth canal. Late onset of meningitis is largely nosocomial in nature. Hence, the distribution of causative pathogens in neonatal meningitis is related to birth gestational age, postnatal age and geographic region. Primary bloodstream infection with secondary hematogenous distribution to the central nervous system (CNS) is the most common mechanism in the development of neonatal meningitis. The distribution of organisms in neonatal meningitis is similar to those in neonatal sepsis. In all early-onset infections, group B Streptococcus (GBS) is the most common cause of neonatal sepsis and meningitis, followed by *Escherichia coli*. Listeria is also found in early-onset meningitis, which should be covered in empiric antibiotic. In all late-onset infections, *E. coli* (5%) and *Klebsiella* (4%) spp. are the most common Gram-negative pathogens, while GBS is also the most common cause. Empiric antibiotics for late-onset meningitis should cover pathogens in the nosocomial environment, including *Pseudomonas aeruginosa* and methicillin-resistant *Staphylococcus aureus*.

The clinical signs of neonatal meningitis can be subtle and nonspecific, including fever or hypothermia, irritability or lethargy, hypotonia, feeding intolerance, respiratory distress, apnea, bradycardia, hypotension, seizures, jaundice, bulging anterior fontanel, and hypo- or hyperglycemia. To confirm the diagnosis of neonatal meningitis, a lumbar puncture (LP) is needed and CSF analysis should include cell count, glucose, protein, gram stain, and culture. Growth on the CSF culture can provide identification of the pathogen and enables adjusting antibiotic therapy. Whenever possible, the LP should be performed prior to the administration of antibiotics. Because the normal values of CSF parameters (leukocyte count, protein, and glucose) in infants are poorly defined due to considerable overlap between infants with and without confirmed meningitis, CSF culture is still the gold standard for diagnosis of bacterial meningitis.

Prompt initiation of antibiotics is critical. Delays in treatment are associated with increased mortality and morbidity. Empiric antibiotics require adequate CSF penetration and sensitivity against the most probable pathogens, including ampicillin and cefotaxime. Antibiotics should be adjusted upon identification of the pathogen and its susceptibilities. For uncomplicated meningitis, the minimal recommended treatment durations are 14 days for GBS, *L. monocytogenes*, and 21 days for *Pseudomonas* and gram-negative enteric bacteria such as *E. coli*. Longer treatment courses are recommended for infants with meningitis and delayed clinical improvement after initiating therapy or with complications such as brain abscesses, ventriculitis, or brain infarctions. There has been debate about the need for a repeat LP during treatment in an infant with confirmed meningitis. Some experts recommend routinely repeating an LP in all patients at 48 hours, whereas others suggest repeating an LP only if clinical conditions are not improved by 24–72 h after beginning therapy.

Bacterial meningitis may be also complicated by reappearance of bacteria in the CSF during antibiotic therapy (recrudescence) or within three weeks after antibiotics have been stopped (relapse). Host immunity and inappropriate use of antibiotics including poor blood–brain barrier penetration, inadequate dosage or treatment duration can lead to recrudescence or relapse of bacterial meningitis. Recrudescence is usually caused by ineffective therapy, but relapse after adequate antibiotic therapy is usually ascribed to persistence of infection in meningeal or parameningeal foci.

This patient had two relapses of *E. coli* meningitis. The first and the second relapses manifested 2 weeks and 2 days after discontinuation of antibiotic, respectively. The first time of relapse might be ascribed to the presence of subdural empyema. With a diagnosis of *E. coli* meningitis complicated by subdural empyema, treatment for the first relapse was continued for 60 days, and sterilization was evidenced by a series of negative CSF cultures. Due to a rapid relapse of *E. coli* meningitis after 60 days of antibiotic treatment, treatment duration of the second relapse was determined by a complete resolution of subdural empyema and normalization of CSF parameters, including leukocyte count, protein level, and glucose level. The treatment was successful without relapse and with acceptable neurological sequelae. For cases with relapse of bacterial meningitis in spite of adequate antibiotic therapy, it is mandatory to perform brain image studies to explore possible pus accumulations that may delay a complete sterilization of infection focus.

Further Reading

Lin MC, Chiu NC, Chi H, Ho CS, Huang FY. Evolving trends of neonatal and childhood bacterial meningitis in northern Taiwan. J Microbiol Immunol Infect 2015;48: 296–301.

Heath PT, Okike IO, Oeser C. Neonatal meningitis: can we do better? Adv Exp Med Biol 2011; 719: 11–24.

Gaschignard J, Levy C, Romain O, Cohen R, Bingen E, Aujard Y, Boileau P. Neonatal Bacterial Meningitis: 444 Cases in 7 Years. Pediatr Infect Dis J 2011; 30:212–7.

Furyk JS, Swann O, Molyneux E. Systematic review: neonatal meningitis in the developing world. Trop Med Int Health 2011; 16: 672–9.

Ku LC, Boggess KA, Cohen-Wolkowiez M. Bacterial meningitis in infants. Clin Perinatol 2015; 42: 29–45.

Stoll BJ, Hansen NI, Sánchez PJ, Faix RG, Poindexter BB, Van Meurs KP et al; Eunice Kennedy Shriver National Institute of Child Health and Human Development Neonatal Research Network. Early onset neonatal sepsis: the burden of group B Streptococcal and *E. coli* disease continues. Pediatrics 2011;127:817–26.

Stockmann C, Spigarelli MG, Campbell SC, Constance JE, Courter JD, Thorell EA, et al. Considerations in the pharmacologic treatment and prevention of neonatal sepsis. Paediatric Drugs 2014;16:67–81.

Gordon SM, Srinivasan L, Harris MC. Neonatal Meningitis: Overcoming Challenges in Diagnosis, Prognosis, and Treatment with Omics. Front Pediatr 2017; 5:139

Greenberg RG, Benjamin DK Jr, Cohen-Wolkowiez M, Clark RH, Cotten CM, Laughon M, Smith PB. Repeat lumbar punctures in infants with meningitis in the neonatal intensive care unit. J Perinatol. 2011;31:425–9.

Korang SK, Safi S, Gluud C, Lausten-Thomsen U, Jakobsen JC. Antibiotic regimens for neonatal sepsis - a protocol for a systematic review with meta-analysis. Syst Rev 2019;8:306.

van der Flier M. Neonatal meningitis: small babies, big problem. Lancet Child Adolesc Health 2021;5:386–7

Part II

Central Nervous System Infection

Case 4. A 6-Year-Old Boy with Fever for 10 Days and Lethargy: Tuberculous Meningitis

Ming-Han Tsai and Yhu-Chering Huang

Keywords

Tuberculosis · Children · Meningitis · Tuberculoma

Key Points in Tuberculous Meningitis

- TB meningitis may present with subacute and nonspecific symptoms, but have a seriously unfavorable outcome if not treated early and adequately.
- TB meningitis should be highly suspected in a patient who has symptoms/signs of meningitis and has a cerebrospinal fluid analysis similar to those of bacterial meningitis, but negative for traditional bacterial culture, particularly in a tuberculosis- prevalent region.
- Communication hydrocephalus is frequently seen in patients with TB meningitis. A brain image can be arranged two weeks after symptoms onset.
- Once TB meningitis is suspected, anti-tuberculosis medication should be prompted and should not be delayed until proved otherwise.
- The adjuvant treatment with corticosteroids may reduce mortality, but does not significantly alter the long-term sequelae.
- Paradoxical development of tuberculoma during therapy does not represent a failure of anti-tuberculosis drugs, and continuation of therapy may achieve a complete resolution.

M.-H. Tsai (✉)
Department of Pediatrics, Chang Gung Memorial Hospital at Keelung, Keelung, Taiwan

Chang Gung University College of Medicine, Taoyuan, Taiwan
e-mail: a12270@cloud.cgmh.org.tw

Y.-C. Huang
Department of Pediatrics, Chang Gung Memorial Hospital, Chang Gung University, Taoyuan, Taiwan

Case Report

A 6-year-old, previously healthy boy was admitted to the hospital because of fever for 10 days. There was no cough nor night sweats. Both his father and grandfather in the same household had pulmonary tuberculosis (TB) but completed anti-TB therapy several years ago. On admission, the patient was lethargic and had a body temperature of 37.6 °C, a respiratory rate of 26 breaths per minute, and a heart rate of 98 beats per minute. Neither cervical lymphadenopathy nor organomegaly was found. The lung was clear, and no focal neurologic sign was observed.

Laboratory data showed the following: leukocyte count, 23,400/mm^3 with 77% segmented

Y.-C. Huang et al. (eds.), *Paediatric Infectious Diseases*,
https://doi.org/10.1007/978-981-19-7276-8_4

neutrophils, 15% lymphocytes, 6% monocytes, 1% eosinophils, and 1% basophils; hemoglobin, 13.3 g/dL; and platelet count, 512,000/mm^3. Due to his lethargic appearance and prolonged fever, a lumbar puncture was performed and cerebrospinal fluid (CSF) showed 475 leukocytes/mm^3 with 76% lymphocytes, 6% neutrophils, and 13% monocytes; a glucose level of 39 mg/dL; and a protein concentration of 124.7 mg/dL. CSF study was negative for bacteria and virus. Polymerase chain reaction for herpesvirus was also negative (Tsai et al. 2004).

The chest radiograph showed mildly diffuse infiltrates. Electroencephalogram revealed cortical dysfunction over the right occipital area, and computed tomographic scan of brain showed mild ventriculomegaly (Fig. 1). Meningoencephalitis was impressed, and penicillin G (400,000 U/kg/day) and acyclovir (10 mg/kg dose every 8 h) were empirically administered. On the second day, anti-TB therapy with isoniazid (10 mg/kg/day), rifampin (15 mg/kg/day), pyrazinamide (25 mg/kg/day), and streptomycin (20 mg/kg/day) were added because TB meningitis was also considered. On the third day, consciousness declined, and the patient was transferred to the pediatric intensive care unit. Repeated CSF examination on the sixth day yielded 700 leukocytes/mm^3 with 59% lymphocytes, 28% neutrophils, and 11% monocytes, a glucose level of 43 mg/dL, and a protein level of 124 mg/dL. Penicillin and acyclovir were discontinued on the fifteenth day of hospitalization, and dexamethasone was added at that time. Fever subsided, and he was discharged on day 19. Streptomycin was discontinued after treatment for 16 days; isoniazid, rifampin, and pyrazinamide were continuously used. Steroid therapy was withdrawn gradually and discontinued after treatment for 48 days (Tsai et al. 2004).

CSF culture yielded *Mycobacterium tuberculosis* subsequently, and the result showed susceptible to all tested anti-TB drugs. However, 7 weeks after discharge, the patient complained of blurred vision. Eye examination documented impaired visual acuity (left eye 1/10, right eye 8/10), and visual field examination revealed bilateral temporal hemianopsia. Magnetic resonance imaging of brain (Fig. 2) at this point showed multiple tuberculomas in the basal ganglia, cerebellopontine angle, prepontine cisterns, brainstem, and right temporal lobe. The optic chiasm was involved and hydrocephalus was present.

The patient was admitted again 10 weeks after the onset of illness. Follow-up CSF examination revealed 4 leukocytes/mm^3, a glucose level of 62 mg/dL, and a protein concentration of 32.5 mg/dL. No organism was observed by Gram

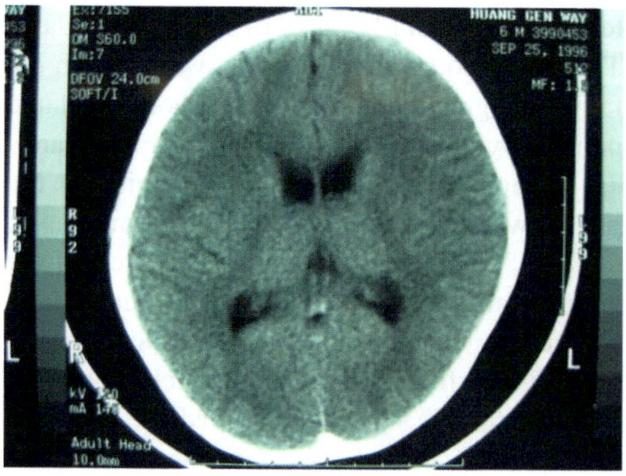

Fig. 1 Computerized tomography scan of brain performed on admission showed mild ventriculomegaly. (Reproduced with permission from (Tsai et al. 2004))

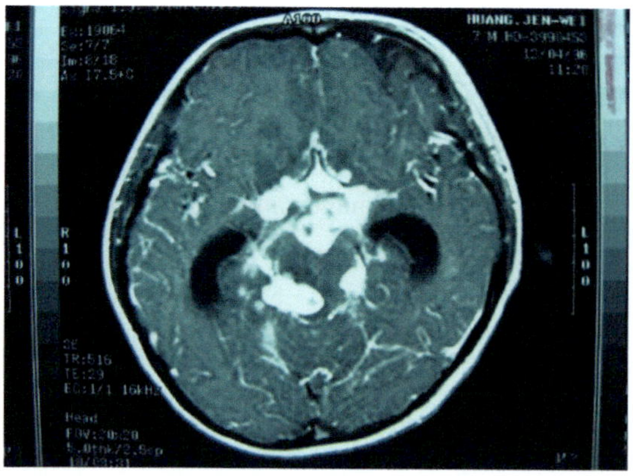

Fig. 2 Magnetic resonance imaging of brain performed at the time when impaired visual acuity developed revealed multiple tuberculomas in basal, cerebellopontine angle, prepontine cisterns, brain stem and right temporal lobe, involving optic chiasma with hydrocephalus (transverse T1-weighted image after intravenous contrast enhancement; TR516/TE29) (Reproduced with permission from (Tsai et al. 2004))

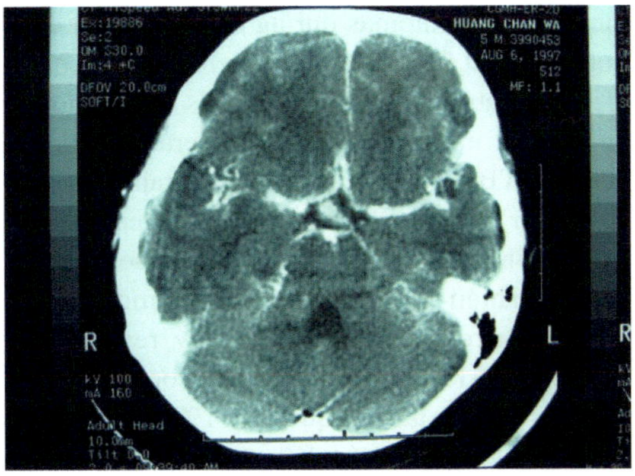

Fig. 3 Computerized tomography scan of brain performed one year later revealed increased leptomeningeal enhancement and suprasellar enhancement and mild dilated ventricles, but complete resolution of tuberculomas (Reproduced with permission from (Tsai et al. 2004))

stain, acid-fast stain, or culture for *M. tuberculosis*. A ventriculoperitoneal shunt was placed on the second day of this hospitalization. Streptomycin and steroid were added again. He was then discharged on day 9 of the second hospitalization and anti-TB therapy and steroids were continuously prescribed. Steroid therapy was gradually withdrawn and discontinued 7 weeks after reinstitution. Visual acuity improved 9 weeks after the onset of visual acuity impairment and returned to normal 24 weeks later. The recovery of visual field was also observed at the same time. Follow-up computed tomographic scan of brain (Fig. 3) 1 year later revealed relatively increased leptomeningeal and suprasellar enhancement with mildly dilated ventricles, but complete resolution of tuberculomas. All anti-TB drugs were discontinued after an 18-month treatment course. No neurologic sequela except excessive body weight gain was observed (Tsai et al. 2004).

Discussion

Tuberculosis (TB) is a communicable disease, which is one of the most common ten causes of death worldwide, and the leading cause of death from a single infectious agent. It is caused by the bacillus *Mycobacterium tuberculosis*, which is spread when people being sick with TB expel the agent into the air (e.g., by coughing). Thus, the disease primarily affects the lungs (pulmonary TB), but may also affect other sites (extrapulmonary TB). Close contacts of patients with infectious TB are at increased risk of developing *M. tuberculosis* infection, mostly latent (LTBI), and disease (mostly pulmonary TB). The risk of developing tuberculosis disease in individuals with LTBI is estimated to be 5%–10% over the course of a lifetime, mostly occurring within the first two years after exposure, and the risk is higher in children less than 3 years of age.

Although most people who develop tuberculosis disease are adults, children can be affected worldwide. According to the latest report issued by the WHO in 2020, children aged less than 15 years accounted for 12% of the people who developed TB. However, most children with active TB have not been reported, due to the low detection rate. Thus, the prevention of childhood TB is still a challenging task.

Children are often evaluated for TB after presenting with symptoms suggestive of disease (passive case finding) or as a result of contact evaluation (active case finding). The most common TB presentation in children are pulmonary disease and associated intrathoracic adenopathy. Besides, TB of the superficial lymph nodes and of the central nervous system are the most common forms of extrapulmonary disease in children. Infants may have the highest risk of progression to tuberculosis disease with dissemination and meningeal involvement. In a 20-year retrospective cohort study reported by van Well GT et al., TB meningitis mainly affects young children aged less than 5 years, with the mean age of 37 months.

TB meningitis is the most severe form of tuberculosis, which causes substantial morbidity and mortality in children. The clinical manifestations of TB meningitis include development of tuberculoma, cranial nerve palsies, hydrocephalus, and brain infarctions. The diagnosis of definite TB meningitis is made when AFB are seen, *M. tuberculosis* is cultured, or *M. tuberculosis* is detected by a reliable molecular method from the CSF in someone with symptoms or signs suggestive of meningitis. Symptoms and signs of meningitis may include headache, irritability, vomiting, fever, neck stiffness, convulsions, focal neurological deficits, altered consciousness, or lethargy. A retrospective cohort study in South Africa showed that most children with TB meningitis had nonspecific symptoms existing for longer than 1 week, including decreased level of consciousness, poor weight gain, and any type of motor deficit. Thirty-nine percent of patients had ≥1 sign of brainstem dysfunction. Cranial nerve palsies occurred in 27% of children.

The CSF findings of TB meningitis is characterized by a predominantly lymphocytic pleocytosis (>50%), an elevated protein level (>100 mg/dL), and a low glucose concentration (less than 40 mg/dL). However, rare cases of culture-proven TB meningitis without other CSF abnormalities have been reported. In a patient who has CSF findings similar to those of bacterial meningitis, but negative traditional bacterial culture, TB meningitis may also be considered.

The performance of cerebral imaging is not essential to, but can help, establish a diagnosis of definite or probable TB meningitis. On CT of brain, about 80% of pediatric patients have hydrocephalus and 75% have basal meningeal enhancement; if negative findings initially but TB meningitis is still highly suspected, CT of brain can be repeated 2 weeks later. Infarcts (8–44%) and tuberculoma (8–31%) are also seen in certain cases. MRI has higher sensitivity than CT for the detection of abnormalities, including meningeal enhancement, infarcts, and tuberculoma, especially of lesions involving the brainstem. Of the reported case, tuberculoma developed after anti-tuberculosis therapy was initiated. Thwaites et al. reported that tuberculoma may occur in 74% of patients during treatment, most of which were asymptomatic. The cause of the paradoxical development of tuberculomas during anti-tuberculosis therapy remains unclear. Most investigators presume that the occurrence of new tuberculomas is an interplay between the host's immune responses and the direct effects of mycobacterial products. Hence, paradoxical development of tuberculomas during therapy often does not represent failure of anti-tuberculosis therapy.

The treatment of TB meningitis should not be delayed in immunologically vulnerable children because TB in young children can rapidly progress with serious sequelae. Delayed treatment of TB meningitis may result in the disease progression with high rates of morbidity and mortality. A 20-year retrospective cohort study reported by van Well GT et al. showed that only 16% of patients did not have sequelae, 71% had any type of sequelae, and 13% of the children died as a consequence of TB meningitis. Anti-TB drug resistance should be considered in children from areas with a high prevalence of drug-resistant tuberculosis and in those who have had documented contact with a person with drug-resistant disease.

Corticosteroids may reduce mortality, but do not significantly alter the long-term sequelae of TB meningitis. The benefit of corticosteroids in TB meningitis is proven by several studies, but the mechanism is unknown. Corticosteroids do reduce brain edema, and might reduce cytokine production and subsequent brainstem encephalopathy. Additionally, the adjuvant treatment with corticosteroids in these studies led to improved survival, but not to a decrease in motor deficits. The optimal duration of TB meningitis therapy has not been established. WHO recommends that children with TB meningitis should receive a standard regimen for four-drug treatment comprising isoniazid, rifampicin, pyrazinamide, and ethambutol for 2 months (the intensive phase). Aminoglycoside (parenteral streptomycin, kanamycin, amikacin, or capreomycin) should be initiated, if possible. When susceptibility to first-line drugs is established, the ethambutol or aminoglycoside can be discontinued. Pyrazinamide is given for a total of 2 months, and isoniazid and rifampicin are given for a total of 9 to 12 months.

In summary, TB meningitis affects mainly children less than 5 years of age. The presentation is often subacute, and early symptoms are nonspecific. The diagnosis of TB meningitis is made when AFB are seen, *M. tuberculosis* is cultured, or *M. tuberculosis* is detected by a reliable molecular method from the CSF. The treatment of TB meningitis should not be delayed because tuberculosis in young children may rapidly disseminate with serious sequelae. Once a child with TB meningitis, even on anti-TB therapy, presents with neurologic deterioration or new symptoms, the development of intracranial tuberculomas should also be considered. Because paradoxical development of tuberculoma during therapy does not represent a failure of anti-TB drugs, continuation of therapy can usually achieve a complete resolution of the tuberculomas.

Further Reading

World Health Organization. Global tuberculosis report 2020. Geneva: World Health Organization; 2020.

Yang R, Liu M, Jiang H, Zhang Y, Yin J, Li Q, et al. The epidemiology of pulmonary tuberculosis in children in Mainland China, 2009-2015. Arch Dis Child 2020; 105:319–25.

Jenkins HE. Global burden of childhood tuberculosis Pneumonia 2016; 8:24.

Perez-Velez CM, Marais BJ. Tuberculosis in children. N Engl J Med 2012; 367:348–61.

van Well GTJ, Paes BF, Terwee CB, Springer P, Roord JJ, Donald PR, et al. Twenty years of pediatric tuberculous meningitis: a retrospective cohort study in the western Cape of South Africa. Pediatrics 2009; 123:e1–8.

Marais S, Thwaites G, Schoeman JF, Torok ME, Misra UK, Prasad K, et al. Tuberculous meningitis: a uniform case definition for use in clinical research. Lancet Infect Dis 2010; 10:803–12.

Donald PR, Schoeman JF. Tuberculous meningitis. N Engl J Med 2004; 351:1719–20.

Thwaites GE, Macmullen-Price J, Tran TH, Pham PM, Nguyen TD, Simmons CP, et al. Serial MRI to determine the effect of dexamethasone on the cerebral pathology of tuberculous meningitis: an observational study. Lancet Neurol 2007; 6:230–6.

Tsai MH, Huang YC, Lin TY. Development of tuberculoma during therapy presenting as hemianopsia. Pediatr Neurol 2004; 31:360–3.

World Health Organization. Rapid advice: Treatment of tuberculosis in children. Geneva: WHO; 2010.

Case 5. A 2-Year-Old Girl with Fever, Lethargy, and Bilious Vomiting and Petechiae and Purpura: Meningococcal Meningitis and Sepsis

Chien-Yu Lin and Yhu-Chering Huang

Keywords

Meningococcus · *Neisseria meningitidis*
Meningococcemia · Purpura fulminans

Key Points in Meningococcal Infection

- The incidence of invasive meningococcal infection is low, but the disease is fulminant and life-threatening with high mortality and morbidity.
- Clinical manifestations are initially nonspecific and skin lesions as purpura fulminans are pathognomonic.
- High index of suspicion is required to initiate appropriate antimicrobial treatment.
- Currently, serogroup B is prevalent in most countries worldwide.
- Meningococcal vaccination is effective against meningococcus, but not yet included in the national immunization programs in most Asian countries.

Case Report

Case 1

A 6-month-old male infant presented with fever and cough for 1 week. Influenza vaccination was administered 1 week ago and no obvious travel or contact history was reported. No vomiting, diarrhea, or skin lesions were noted. The initial laboratory data revealed leukocytosis (white blood cell 18,600/μL, immature neutrophils 4%, segmented 59%, lymphocytes 27%, monocytes 7%, eosinophil 0%, metamyelocyte 3%) without anemia (hemoglobin 11.1 g/dL) or thrombocytopenia (platelet count 395,000/μL). Blood biochemistry testing showed elevated C-reactive protein level (106.6 mg/L, normal <5 mg/L)) and elevated liver enzymes (aspartate aminotransferase 58 IU/L, alanine transaminase 228 IU/L). Spinal tap revealed pleocytosis with low cerebrospinal fluid (CSF) glucose level (Pandy's test: positive, white blood cell count: 78/mm^3, lymphocyte: neutrophil = 68:9, CSF glucose 34 mg/dL, blood glucose 149 mg/dL). Empirical antibiotics with cefotaxime was given. Both CSF and blood cultures obtained on admission subsequently yielded a non-resistant *Neisseria menin-*

C.-Y. Lin (✉)
Division of Pediatric Infectious Diseases, Department of Pediatrics, Hsinchu MacKay Memorial Hospital and Hsinchu Municipal MacKay Children's Hospital, Hsinchu City, Taiwan

Department of Medicine, MacKay Medical College, New Taipei City, Taiwan

Y.-C. Huang
Pediatrics, Chang Gung Memorial Hospital, Chang Gung University, Taoyuan, Taiwan

Y.-C. Huang et al. (eds.), *Paediatric Infectious Diseases*,
https://doi.org/10.1007/978-981-19-7276-8_5

gitidis. Antibiotics was administered for 21 days. He recovered smoothly but visual evoked potential (VEP) test showed bilateral prolonged p100 latency. The brain sonography demonstrated left ventricular dilatation and he continued to be followed up at our hospital. The strain was characterized as serogroup B by the central laboratory of Taiwan Centers for Disease Control.

Case 2

A 2-year-old girl was transferred for fever, lethargy, and bilious vomiting for 2 days. Multiple petechiae and purpura over trunk and legs developed on the next day (Fig. 1). Blood tests showed normal white blood cell count 4880/μL (segment 73.9%, monocyte 6.8%, lymphocyte 19.1%), high C-reactive protein (300 mg/L) and coagulopathy (prothrombin time 14.8 s, international normalized ratio 1.4, activated partial thromboplastin time 44.9 s). She was treated at pediatric intensive care unit and received fresh frozen plasma transfusion and empiric antibiotics with vancomycin plus cefotaxime treatment. A Spinal tap revealed pleocytosis (white blood cell count: 1322/mm^3, lymphocyte: neutrophil = 5:85), protein 58.5 mg/dL. The blood culture yielded a non-susceptible *Neisseria meningitidis* (minimal inhibitory concentration of penicillin: 0.25 μg/mL, intermediate; susceptible for ceftriaxone and meropenem) on hospital day 3 and vancomycin was discontinued. Intravenous cefotaxime dosage was kept within 300–400 mg/kg/day. Fever still fluctuated. A computed tomography of brain was arranged on hospital day 8 for possible intracranial complications of meningitis and revealed no significant abnormal findings. Auditory evoked potential (AEP) test showed within normal limit on hospital day 11. Fever persisted and limping gait was noted on day 13. A magnetic resonance imaging of lower extremities revealed right thigh myositis, over quadriceps of right distal thigh, anterior and lateral aspect, and minimal joint effusion of right knee (Fig. 2). Antibiotics was continued and the condition of right lower extremity improved gradually. Intravenous antibiotics was used for a total of 21 days and fever subsided since hospital day 22. She was discharged on day 28 with an uneventful recovery. The final diagnosis was meningococcal sepsis with meningitis and myositis over right distal thigh.

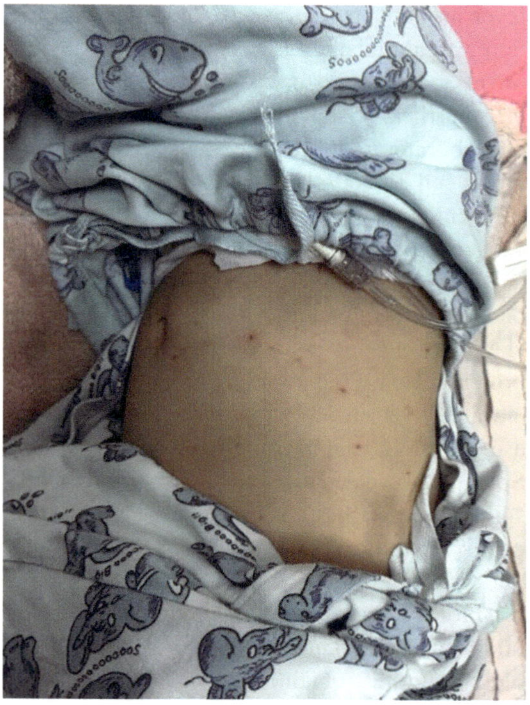

Fig. 1 Multiple petechiae and purpura over trunk and legs developed in a 2-year-old girl with invasive meningococcal disease

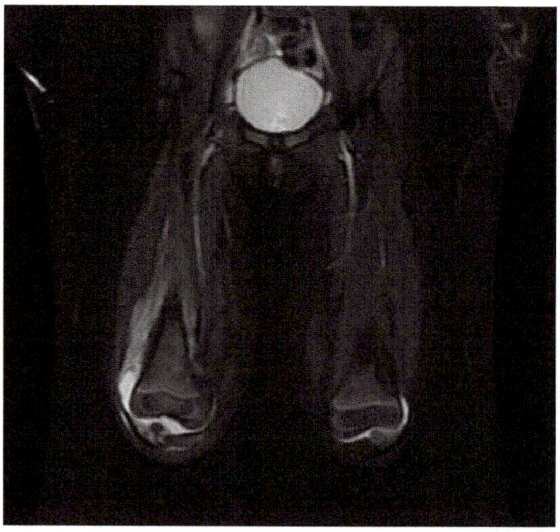

Fig. 2 A magnetic resonance imaging of lower extremities revealed right thigh myositis, over quadriceps of right distal thigh, anterior and lateral aspect, and minimal joint effusion of right knee in coronal view

Discussion

Invasive meningococcal disease (IMD) refers to severe infection caused by Gram-negative diplococci, *Neisseria meningitidis*, and usually manifests as sepsis and meningitis. The incidences of IMD vary in different countries and the annual attack rates ranges from 0.02 to 0.2 cases per 100,000 persons per year in Asia-Pacific area. The incubation period ranges from 1 to 10 days and is typically 3 to 4 days. The initial symptoms are protean and include fever, nausea or vomiting, headache, ill appearance, muscle ache, and skin rashes. The pathognomonic purpura fulminans denotes to non-blanching erythematous macules that evolve to purple-black hemorrhagic necrotic lesions within hours (Fig. 3). IMD may progress to fatal emergency rapidly and a high case fatality with 10% to 15% has been reported. Accurate and early diagnosis ensures initiation of timely and appropriate antimicrobial treatment and better outcome. The presence and early recognition of purpura fulminans may provide a clue for early diagnosis of IMD and contributes to starting timely treatment. A broad range of physical, neurological, and psychological sequelae have been identified in 10% to 20% survivors and impairment of quality of life is common. Although IMD is uncommon, it's an important health threat for its fulminant clinical course, high case fatality rate, and high complication rate.

Invasive infection is usually preceded by prior carriage and nasal carriage is observed in approximately one-tenth of population. People with complement deficiency, functional or anatomical asplenia, HIV infection, or other immunocompromised status are at increased risk of invasive meningococcal disease. Young infants are most susceptible to IMD and followed by adolescents and young adults with group settings, such as college students and military recruits. Increased risks of transmission and disease have been reported in outbreaks and post-exposure chemoprophylaxis is recommended for close contacts and in outbreak settings. Several antibiotics have been used for post-exposure prophylaxis, including rifampin, ceftriaxone, ciprofloxacin, and azithromycin. For managing patients with IMD, treatment of shock and increased intracranial pressure is crucial. Empirical antimicrobial agents with cefotaxime or ceftriaxone are recommended. Penicillin and meropenem are alternative choices and the concern of increasing resistance is rising.

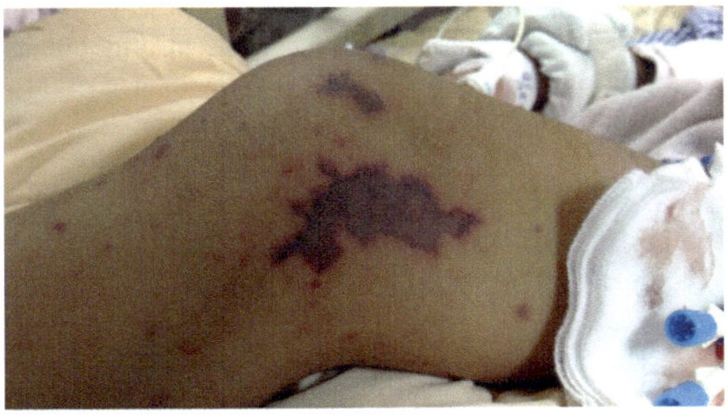

Fig. 3 Purpura fulminans in a child with invasive meningococcal disease

Based on capsular serogroups, at least 13 serogroups of *Neisseria meningitidis* have been identified and almost all human diseases are caused by serogroups A, B, C, W, X, and Y. The distribution of prevalent serogroup varies in different countries and is affected by meningococcal vaccination. For example, serogroup A is the mainstream serogroup in "meningococcal belt" in Africa before the introduction of vaccines and has drastically declined after vaccination. Currently, serogroup B is the most prevalent serogroup in the USA and most European countries. In Asia-Pacific regions, circulating serogroups are different in different countries, but serogroup B is prevalent across various countries. Serogroup B accounts for more than the half cases of IMD in Taiwan and Australia, one third in China, and 20% cases of IMD in Japan. Serogroup W is rising in some countries, such as the Philippines, Australia, and New Zealand. Continuous surveillance is crucial for prevention and management of IMD.

There are several available vaccines against meningococcus with different coverage of serogroups, including vaccines against serogroup A (MenA), serogroup B (MenB), serogroup C (MenC), serogroups A, C, W, and Y (MenACWY). Meningococcal vaccines are effective against

IMD with tolerable adverse effects. For people with risk factors, such as immunocompromised patients, complement deficiency or asplenia, meningococcal vaccination is recommended in most countries. Meningococcal vaccination is also recommended for people travelling to endemic areas. For the general population, the vaccine strategies of meningococcal vaccines vary across countries for their own epidemiological characteristics, availability and feasibility of vaccines, coverage of vaccination program, risk-benefit balance, and cost-effectiveness considerations. Vaccine strategies also evolve by time. In the UK, MenC has been replaced with MenACWY for the rise in serogroup W. MenB vaccination for young infants and MenACWY for adolescents are included in the UK national immunization program (NIP) since 2015. On the contrary, the Centers for Disease Control recommends MenACWY for young infants in the United States and MenB is approved for people aged 10 years or older. In Asia-Pacific region, MenA and MenC are incorporated in the NIP in China, and MenB and MenACWY are included in NIP in Australia. Meningococcal vaccination is not included in NIP in other countries.

In summary, IMD is fulminant and life-threatening. The incidences are rare in most countries, but the disease course is rapid and unpredictable. High case fatality rate is associated and timely diagnosis and management are crucial for successful treatment. Recognition of purpura fulminans may provide a clue for early diagnosis and empirical antimicrobial agent with cefotaxime or ceftriaxone is recommended. Currently, serogroup B meningococcus is prevalent in most areas and there are available vaccines against meningococcus. Vaccine strategies vary across countries and continuous surveillance is warranted.

Further Reading

Aye AMM, Bai X, Borrow R, Bory S, Carlos J, Caugant DA, et al. Meningococcal disease surveillance in the Asia-Pacific region: The global meningococcal initiative. J Infection. 2020;81:698–711.

MacNeil JR, Blain AE, Wang X, Cohn AC. Current Epidemiology and Trends in Meningococcal Disease-United States, 1996–2015. Clin Infect Dis 2018;66:1276–81.

Olbrich KJ, Müller D, Schumacher S, Beck E, Meszaros K, Koerber F. Systematic review of invasive meningococcal disease: sequelae and quality of life impact on patients and their caregivers. Infect Dis Ther 2018;7:421–38.

Christensen H, May M, Bowen L, Hickman M, Trotter CL. Meningococcal carriage by age: a systematic review and meta-analysis. Lancet Infect Dis 2010;10:853–61.

Taha MK, Weil-Olivier C, Bouée S, Emery C, Nachbaur G, Pribil C, et al. Risk factors for invasive meningococcal disease: a retrospective analysis of the French national public health insurance database. Hum Vaccin Immunother 2021;17:1858–66.

Mbaeyi S, Pondo T, Blain A, Yankey D, Potts C, Cohn A, et al. Incidence of meningococcal disease before and after implementation of quadrivalent meningococcal conjugate vaccine in the United States. JAMA Pediatr 2020;174:843–51.

Parikh SR, Campbell H, Bettinger JA, Harrison LH, Marshall HS, Martinon-Torres F, et al. The ever-changing epidemiology of meningococcal disease worldwide and the potential for prevention through vaccination. J Infect 2020;81:483–98.

Martinón-Torres F, Taha MK, Knuf M, Abbing-Karahagopian V, Pellegrini M, Bekkat-Berkani R, et al. Evolving strategies for meningococcal vaccination in Europe: Overview and key determinants for current and future considerations Pathog Glob Health 2021:1–14.

Pizza M, Bekkat-Berkani R, Rappuoli R. Vaccines against meningococcal diseases Microorganisms 2020;8: 1521.

Chiu NC, Huang LM, Willemsen A, Bhusal C, Arora AK, Reynoso Mojares Z, et al. Safety and immunogenicity of a meningococcal B recombinant vaccine when administered with routine vaccines to healthy infants in Taiwan: A phase 3, open-label, randomized study. Hum Vaccin Immunother 2018;14:1075–83.

Case 6. A 2-Year-Old Boy with Fever, Hand-Foot-Mouth Disease, and Myoclonic Jerk: Enterovirus A71 Infection

Kuan-Ying A. Huang

Keywords

Enterovirus A71 · Children · Neurological complications · Stage-based treatment · Vaccine

Key Points in Enterovirus A71 Infection

- Enterovirus A71 (EV-A71) is one of the major causative pathogens of hand, foot, and mouth disease in children.
- EV-A71 infection could cause neurological diseases, include meningitis, polio-like syndrome, myelitis, and brainstem encephalitis.
- Frequent myoclonic jerks, consciousness change, and autonomic dysregulation are warning signs of brainstem encephalitis.
- The stage-based management reduces morbidity and mortality associated with severe EV-A71 infections.
- EV-A71 vaccine is effective against hand, foot, and mouth disease and neurological diseases.

K.-Y. A. Huang (✉)
Graduate Institute of Immunology and Department of Pediatrics, National Taiwan University Hospital, College of Medicine, National Taiwan University, Taipei, Taiwan
e-mail: arthurhuang1726@ntu.edu.tw

Case Report

Case 1

A 2-year-old boy was admitted due to fever and the occurrence of myoclonic jerk for one day. Rashes on the soles, palms, and buttocks and oral ulcers had developed since three days ago. The vital signs on admission were body temperature 36.8 °C, heart rate 140/min, respiratory rate 28/min, and blood pressure 128/88 mmHg. The initial laboratory data showed white blood count 11,900/μL, lymphocytes 21.0%, monocytes 8.2%, neutrophils 70.2%, platelet 346,000/μL, hemoglobin 14.4 g/dL, C-reactive protein 10.0 mg/L, and glucose 101 mg/dL. The pulse oximetric saturation was 97% under room air and his capillary refilling time was less than 2 s. The initial diagnosis is hand, foot, and mouth disease and supportive care was administered.

On day 1 of admission, he had two episodes of vomiting and increased frequency of myoclonic jerk. On the second day of admission, he still had intermittent fever and episodes of vomiting. On the same day, frontal headache developed at midnight and hypertension (blood pressure of 171/89 mmHg) was noted with normal body temperature and pulse rate. Within half an hour, cold sweating and irritability occurred, accompanied by increased heart rate of 140/min and hyperglycemia (glucose 231 mg/dL). One hour later, his consciousness deteriorated to a Glasgow Coma Score of 12 (E3, V3, M6) and was transferred to a tertiary hospital for further intensive care.

Y.-C. Huang et al. (eds.), *Paediatric Infectious Diseases*,
https://doi.org/10.1007/978-981-19-7276-8_6

While arriving at the tertiary hospital (two hours after the episode of headache and hypertension), he had decompensated shock with hypotension (blood pressure 69/34 mmHg), tachycardia (pulse rate 161/min), and poor distal perfusion. He also had tachypnea and cough with pink and foamy secretions. Hypoxia with severe respiratory acidosis was noted and he was intubated. Meanwhile, the laboratory data showed leukocytosis with thrombocytosis (white blood count 28,900/μL, lymphocytes 20.5%, monocytes 5.0%, neutrophils 71.0%, platelet 535,000/μL, hemoglobin 14.1 g/dL), elevated Troponin-I level (1.97 mg/dL), and hyperglycemia (glucose 281 mg/dL). The chest radiograph showed bilateral lung congestions. He died three hours after arrival to the transferred hospital. Enterovirus A71 (EV-A71) was isolated from both his throat and rectal swabs.

Case 2

A 2-year-old girl was admitted due to fever and oral ulcers for 2 days. Occasional myoclonic jerk occurred during sleep. On admission her vital signs were body temperature 37.9 °C, heart rate 145/min, respiratory rate 32/min, and blood pressure 98/72 mmHg. Laboratory data showed normal leukocyte count (white blood count 8600/μL, lymphocytes 28.9%, monocytes 6.9%, neutrophils 64.1%), hemoglobin 11.6 g/dL, platelet 382,000/μL, C-reactive protein 5.0 mg/L and glucose 114 mg/dL. The initial diagnosis is herpangina and supportive care was given. In addition, her elder brother had herpangina one week ago.

On day 2 of admission, she became lethargic and had unsteady gait. Hypertension (blood pressure 125/97 mmHg), tachycardia (>150/min) and hyperglycemia (capillary glucose 327 mg/dL) were reported. At the same time, she has elevated Troponin-I level (3.39 mg/dL) and N-terminal pro-B-type natriuretic peptide (NT-proBNP, 9536 pg/mL). She was transferred to the intensive care unit and received intravenous immunoglobulin and milrinone immediately. Her fever subsided after day 3 of admission. Her blood pressure and heart rates returned to within normal level after day 4 of admission. On day 6 of admission, she was transferred from the intensive care unit to the general ward. Real-time reverse transcription polymerase chain reaction tests revealed that both throat and rectal samples were positive with EV-A71. Besides, EV-A71 was isolated from her throat swab and the sequence analysis showed that this strain belongs to the B5 genotype.

On day 7 of admission, she began to complain of left calf pain and could not stand on her own. Decreased strength (3 out 5) of her left lower leg was also noted. Deep-tendon reflexes and the Babinski sign were normal. Nerve conduction studies revealed decreased amplitudes of left peroneal compound muscle action potential and absent H-reflex of left lower leg. Left peroneal neuropathy was impressed. She had a regular neurology follow-up and the neuropathy recovered spontaneously.

Discussion

EV-A71 is a non-enveloped RNA virus and was first identified in 1969 from a child with encephalitis in California, United States. This virus can be divided into seven different genogroups, of which genogroups B and C are predominantly circulating in endemic regions. The seroprevalence study revealed the age-specific seropositive rate rises from infancy (8%, 0.5–0.9 years) to childhood (42%, 3–5.9 years) and reaches a plateau of around 60% among individuals aged 6–11 years old and above, which suggests that young children are at greatest risk of new EV-A71 infection.

The EV-A71 transmission mainly occurs through the oral–fecal or oral–oral route, but it could possibly occur through contact with virus-contaminated vesicular fluid, surfaces, or fomites. The respiratory and intestinal tract are probably initial infection sites where the virus replicates. Viremia occurs with the onset of illness and may play a role in spreading the virus to target organs, including the central nervous system. Animal studies also imply that EV-A71 may invade the central nervous system via retrograde axonal transport.

Clinical stages of symptomatic EV-A71 infection are as follows, hand, foot, and mouth disease or herpangina (Stage 1), central nervous system involvement (Stage 2), autonomic dysregulation and/or cardiopulmonary failure (Stage 3), and convalescence (Stage 4). Previous household EV-A71 study showed an over 50% transmission rate among household contacts, among infected children 6% were asymptomatic, 73% of them had uncomplicated illness (hand, foot, and mouth disease, herpangina, and febrile illness), and other 21% developed neurological illness. Supportive treatment is the mainstay of uncomplicated illness (Stage 1) and full recovery with sequelae is typically seen in uncomplicated cases.

Some symptomatic patients could develop central nervous system involvement (Stage 2), such as meningitis, myelitis, polio-like syndrome, or encephalitis, and clinical presentations include meningism, ataxia, limb weakness, myoclonic jerk, lethargy, or seizure; importantly, a few patients would progress to much more severe neurological conditions, followed by cardiopulmonary failure and mortality, which is usually associated with brainstem encephalitis (Stage 3). Sudden onset of autonomic dysregulation, i.e., tachycardia, transient hypertension, profuse sweating, paralytic ileus, neurogenic bladder, or increased startle reflex, is the warning sign of brainstem encephalitis. Hyperglycemia and leukocytosis could be found at this stage. Identification of central nervous system involvement and progression and close monitoring of cardiopulmonary status are suggested for patients with Stages 2 and 3 illnesses. Intravenous immunoglobulin therapy is recommended for those patients with central nervous system involvement. Milrinone treatment could reduce the mortality in patients with brainstem encephalitis. Respiratory and cardiovascular supports should be promptly administered for critically ill patients. Patients without progression to Stage 3 usually recover without sequelae. By contrast, a high mortality is seen in patients that progress to Stage 3 and develop hypotension or shock.

The autopsy of mortality case reveals extensive inflammation in the meninges and central nervous system, with brainstem and spinal cord being severely involved. EV-A71 is isolated from brain tissues, whereas there is no evidence of inflammation in the lung and heart. The cardiopulmonary failure associated with brainstem encephalitis has been proposed to be neurogenic, caused by the EV-A71 invasion of the vasomotor and respiratory centers in the lower brainstem. Besides, the immunopathological study reveals that viral destruction is predominantly located in the medial and caudal areas of the medulla oblongata where are considered to be central depressor areas of autonomic control, which supports the association of brainstem lesions and autonomic dysregulation in the advanced stage of EV-A71 infection.

Long-term neurological or recognitive sequelae are often observed in survivors from brainstem encephalitis with cardiopulmonary failure. The long-term sequelae include limb weakness and atrophy, tube feeding dependency, ventilator dependence, and delayed neurodevelopment.

There are no approved antiviral drugs available for the prevention and treatment of EV-A71 infection in the clinical setting. Several EV-A71 vaccines are successfully developed. Three inactivated, adjuvanted genotype C4 vaccines show promising safety and efficacy in the phase III clinical trial and are approved by China's Food and Drug Administration.

In summary, EV-A71 mostly causes hand, foot, and mouth disease and herpangina in children that are usually self-limiting illnesses; however, severe infections that are associated neurological diseases could occur in the outbreaks. Following the eradication of polio in the developed countries, EV-A71 has become one of major enteroviruses that are prone to cause severe neurological complications. A prompt recognition of signs of disease progression and administration of stage-based management would reduce mortality and morbidity associated with severe EV-A71 infections.

Further Reading

Chang LY, Lin HY, Gau SS, Lu CY, Hsia SH, Huang YC, Huang LM, Lin TY. Enterovirus A71 neurologic complications and long-term sequelae. J Biomed Sci 2019;26:57.

Chea S, Cheng YB, Chokephaibulkit K, Chotpitayasunondh T, Rogier van Doorn H, Hafy Z, et al. Workshop on use of intravenous immunoglobulin in hand, foot and mouth disease in Southeast Asia. Emerg Infect Dis 2015;21:e140992.

Chi CY, Khanh TH, Thoa le PK, Tseng FC, Wang SM, Thinh le Q, et al. Milrinone therapy for enterovirus 71-induced pulmonary edema and/or neurogenic shock in children: a randomized controlled trial. Crit Care Med 2013;41:1754–1760.

Hsia SH, Lin JJ, Chan OW, Lin TY. Cardiopulmonary failure in children infected with Enterovirus A71. J Biomed Sci 2020;27:53.

Huang KA, Huang PN, Huang YC, Yang SL, Tsao KC, Chiu CH, et al. Emergence of genotype C1 Enterovirus A71 and its link with antigenic variation of virus in Taiwan. PLoS Pathog 2020;16:e1008857.

Liang Z, Wang J. EV71 vaccine, an invaluable gift for children. Clin Transl Immunol 2014;3:e28.

McMinn PC. Recent advances in the molecular epidemiology and control of human enterovirus 71 infection. Curr Opin Virol 2012;2:199–205.

Ooi MH, Wong SC, Lewthwaite P, Cardosa MJ, Solomon T. Clinical features, diagnosis, and management of enterovirus 71. Lancet Neurol 2010;9:1097–1105.

Teoh HL, Mohammad SS, Britton PN, Kandula T, Lorentzos MS, Booy R, et al. Clinical characteristics and functional motor outcomes of enterovirus 71 neurological disease in children. JAMA Neurol 2016;73:300–307.

Zhu W, Jin P, Li JX, Zhu FC, Liu P. Correlates of protection for inactivated enterovirus 71 vaccine: the analysis of immunological surrogate endpoints. Expert Rev Vaccines 2017;16:945–949.

Case 7. A 15-Year-Old Adolescent with Right Upper Limb Weakness Following Upper Respiratory Infection: Acute Flaccid Myelitis Caused by Enterovirus D68

Jainn-Jim Lin and Wing-Lung Cheng

Keywords

Acute flaccid paralysis · Myelitis · Enterovirus D68

Key Points in Acute Flaccid Myelitis Caused by Enterovirus D68

- Acute flaccid myelitis (AFM) is characterized by rapid progressive asymmetric weakness, together with a spinal gray matter lesion on magnetic resonance imaging.
- It is preceded by a short prodromal respiratory illness followed by acute flaccid paralysis with or without respiratory failure.
- A high index of suspicion with neuroimaging findings is key to an early diagnosis.
- Treatment options for EV-D68-associated AFM are limited to supportive care.
- The outcome is usually poor, with a high a rate of neurologic sequelae.

J.-J. Lin (✉)
Division of Pediatric Critical Care Medicine and Pediatric Neurocritical Care Center, Chang Gung Children's Hospital and Chang Gung Memorial Hospital, Chang Gung University College of Medicine, Taoyuan, Taiwan
e-mail: lin0227@cgmh.org.tw

W.-L. Cheng
Department of Pediatrics, Mennonite Christian Hospital, Hualien, Taiwan

Case Report

A 15-year-old previously healthy boy presented to the pediatric emergency department with the acute onset of right upper limb weakness for 2 days. He had a 7-day history of high-grade fever, productive cough, and rhinorrhea. On examination, his GCS (Glasgow coma scale) was 15/15 and he was afebrile (36 °C); pulse rate, 112/min; respiratory rate, 28/min; blood pressure, 102/76 mm Hg; and SpO_2, 100%. Chest and abdominal findings were normal. A neurological examination revealed mild neck stiffness and muscle weakness of the right upper limbs with grade 1/5 at proximal portions and grade 4/5 at distal portions. Notably, he also had right pathological extensor plantar responses. There were no other focal neurological findings. Initial laboratory findings revealed no leukocytosis (9940/μL) with normal C-reactive protein (0.09 mg/L). Liver and renal function tests were within normal range (AST 33 U/L, ALT 13 U/L, BUN 7 U/L, Cr 0.73 U/L). He was admitted to a regional hospital, and initial brain computed tomography (CT) and magnetic resonance imaging (MRI) showed no specific findings. Routine cerebrospinal fluid (CSF) analysis revealed leukocytosis (WBC 73/μL) with lymphocyte predominance (51.3%), mildly increased total protein (49 mg/L) and normal glucose level (69 mg/L). He was initially treated for presumed encephalitis with intravenous ceftriaxone, acyclovir, and oral doxycycline therapy.

Y.-C. Huang et al. (eds.), *Paediatric Infectious Diseases*,
https://doi.org/10.1007/978-981-19-7276-8_7

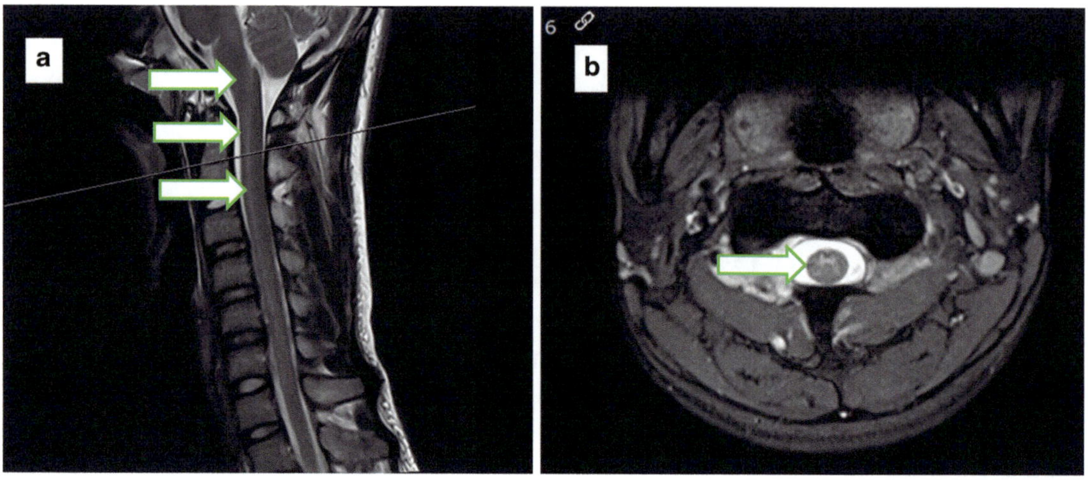

Fig. 1 Magnetic resonance imaging (MRI) of the cervical spinal on day 2 after admission showed T2-flare hyperintensity involving the pons, lower medulla, and anterior horn at levels C1–C6 of the spinal cord (**a**, **b**), indicating the presence of inflammation

However, 12 h after admission, his condition rapidly deteriorated. Central facial palsy with difficulty in swallowing and mild respiratory distress were noted. In addition, low muscle weakness was noted in both upper limbs with grade 1/5 at the left upper limb, grade 0/5 at the right upper limb, and normal muscle power of both lower limbs. Notably, pathological extensor plantar responses progressed bilaterally. Spinal MRI was arranged, which showed abnormal signals in the brainstem and cervical and thoracic spinal cord, possibly indicating inflammatory lesions (Fig. 1a, b). He also received a combination of intravenous solu medrol (methylprednisolone sodium succinate) 40 mg Q8H and plasmapheresis every 2 days for five courses. Polymerase chain reaction (PCR) for influenza from a throat swab and serological tests for *Mycoplasma pneumoniae* were all negative. Other relevant investigations included negative blood and CSF cultures. CSF viral isolation was also negative. Only a nasopharyngeal swab tested positive for Enterovirus-D68 by reverse-transcriptase PCR (RT-PCR).

Ten days after admission, his muscle weakness mildly improved, and he received rehabilitation at the hospital. He was stable upon discharge at day 14 of illness and had good motor and cognitive ability after three months of follow-up. Five years later, he had no seizures or obvious neurologic signs and normal school performance.

Discussion

Human enterovirus D68 (EV-D68) is a member of the species enterovirus D of the Picornaviridae family. It is usually asymptomatic or mildly symptomatic with respiratory illness, but occasionally causes severe respiratory illnesses. In 2014, an outbreak of EV-D68 occurred in children in the US, and it was reported to be linked to acute flaccid paralysis in a subset of patients. The term acute flaccid myelitis (AFM) was introduced after an upsurge of pediatric cases. Since then, an increasing number of cases have been reported worldwide. In terms of molecular epidemiology, Clades A, B, and C of EV-D68 were distributed worldwide. After 2014, the main strains in the world were clade B. In Taiwan, the popular EV-D68 clades from 2007 to 2013 were A1, A2, and B1, and moves to clade B3 after 2014. Meanwhile, clade A was dominant during 2006 and 2011 in China, but clade B strains emerged after 2011.

Different clades of EV-D68 may have different virulence and lead to different disease severity, which requires further research in the future.

The clinical picture of acute flaccid myelitis is usually preceded by a short prodromal respiratory illness, followed by acute asymmetric flaccid limb weakness (proximal muscle weakness worse than distal) with or without bulbar palsy and respiratory failure. CSF analysis may show mild to moderate pleocytosis, and neurophysiological testing may show reduced compound motor action potentials with normal conduction velocities and the absence of conduction blocks compatible with anterior horn cell disease. Neuroimaging may show typical hyperintensity in spinal grey matter on T2-flare MRI, and the dorsal brainstem is involved in some cases. Clinically, the presentation of EV-D68-associated AFM may be similar to Guillain-Barré syndrome and acute transverse myelitis. However, MRI findings of spinal grey matter are supportive of AFM.

There are three different stages in the pathogenesis of EV-D68 infections in humans: respiratory infection, systemic dissemination, and CNS invasion. However, the causal relationship between EV-D68 infections and AFM and the exact pathogenesis of AFM remain unclear. In general, viruses can enter the CNS via peripheral nerves or a hematogenous route. Therefore, the following mechanisms have been suggested: (1) EV-D68 enters the CNS via cranial nerves; (2) EV-D68 hematogenously disseminates to invade the CNS through the blood-brain-barrier or blood-CSF barrier; (3) EV-D68 enters the CNS via the infection of lymphocytes or other immune cells that enter the CNS. Even though the exact mechanism of CNS invasion is not known, it is possible that different invasion strategies used by the virus can explain the different disease manifestations.

The confirmed diagnosis of EV-D68-associated AFM is based on clinically acute asymmetric weakness, together with specific findings on MRI during periods of EV-D68 circulation and the detection of enteroviruses in a respiratory specimen obtained from the lower respiratory tract (Table 1). One of the challenges of the diagnosis is that EV-D68 is not always detected in clinical samples from AFM patients. Indeed, detection of EV-D68 in CSF is uncommon and has only been reported in a handful of cases. In addition, EV-D68 is not readily detected in fecal samples, and it has a rhinovirus-like replication cycle in the nasal cavity. The recently published PAHO/WHO report recommends including a respiratory sample if acute flaccid paralysis (AFP) is suspected.

Treatment options for EV-D68-associated AFM are limited to supportive care. There are

Table 1 Case definition of acute flaccid myelitis caused by human enterovirus-D68

1.	**Possible case** A possible case is defined as a person presenting with symptoms of either acute myelitis/paralysis or Guillain-Barré Syndrome, particularly during periods of EV-D68 circulation indicated by epidemiological alerts or systematic surveillance
2.	**Probable case** A probable case is defined as a person presenting with symptoms of either acute myelitis/paralysis or Guillain-Barré syndrome and at least one of the following criteria: – **MRI:** Abnormality presenting with T2 hyperintensity in spinal cord grey matter with or without hyperintensity at the dorsal brain stem – **Neurophysiologic investigations:** Showing an axonal neuropathy, including reduced compound motor action potentials with normal conduction velocities, and the absence of conduction blocks compatible with anterior horn cell disease – **Laboratory findings:** Detection of enteroviruses in a respiratory specimen obtained from the lower respiratory tract during periods of EV-D68 circulation
3.	**Confirmed case** A confirmed case is defined as a person presenting with the following criteria: – **Symptoms:** Acute flaccid myelitis/paralysis – **MRI:** Abnormality presenting with T2 hyperintensity in spinal cord grey matter with or without hyperintensity at the dorsal brain stem – **Laboratory findings:** Detection of enterovirus-D68-specific nucleic acids in a respiratory specimen using a validated PCR assay targeting the VP1 gene with subsequent sequencing and typing

Modified from references (CDC and NCIRD 2015) and (Kramer 2019) with reproduce permission currently no approved specific antiviral drugs. Immunomodulatory drugs have been proposed, including intravenous immunoglobulin (IVIG), steroids, plasmapheresis, or a combination of these treatments. IVIG has been recommended according to evidence in human EV-A71-associated encephalomyelitis and a mouse model of EV-D68-associated AFM. Steroids were not recommended in a mouse model study of EV-D68-associated AFM, as steroid treatment led to an increased viral load and deterioration of motor symptoms. However, steroids have an anti-inflammatory effect and may be beneficial in AFM cases with spinal cord edema or white matter involvement. While scientific proof is still lacking, Helfferich et al. recommend IVIG in the acute phase, combined with maximal supportive care with ventilatory support and intensive rehabilitation.

The outcome is usually poor, with a high rate of neurologic sequelae. Only 5–39% of patients with EV-D68-associated AFM recover partially or completely. On follow-up, most patients retain significant residual motor deficits, and residual proximal weakness tends to be more severe than distal weakness. Cranial nerve deficits usually recover well over time; however, some cases still need long-term ventilatory support. While not much is known about the prognostic factors, more severe disability and weakness at the nadir and the persistence of denervation seem to be associated with worse outcomes.

In conclusion, EV-D68-associated AFM is a polio-like condition characterized by the combination of acute flaccid paralysis and a spinal gray matter lesion on MRI. There are currently no effective treatment options for EV-D68-associated AFM. IVIG has been recommended, but with only minimal improvement over time in most cases. Insights from basic research are needed to make progress in the diagnosis, treatment, and prevention of this new polio-like disease.

Further Reading

Hu YL, Chang LY. Current status of enterovirus D68 worldwide and in Taiwan. Pediatr Neonatol 2020; 61: 9–15.

Messacar K, Schreiner TL, Maloney JA, Wallace A, Ludke J, Oberste MS, et al. A cluster of acute flaccid paralysis and cranial nerve dysfunction temporally associated with an outbreak of enterovirus D68 in children in Colorado, USA, Lancet. 2015;385: 1662–71.

Maloney JA, Mirsky DM, Messacar K, Dominguez SR, Schreiner T, Stence NV. MRI findings in children with acute flaccid paralysis and cranial nerve dysfunction occurring during the 2014 enterovirus D68 outbreak. AJNR Am J Neuroradiol 2015;36:245–50.

Knoester M, Helfferich J, Poelman R, Van Leer-Buter C, Brouwer OF, Niesters HGM; 2016 EV-D68 AFM Working Group. Twenty-nine Cases of Enterovirus-D68-associated Acute Flaccid Myelitis in Europe 2016: A Case Series and Epidemiologic Overview. Pediatr Infect Dis J 2019;38:16–21.

Yea C, Bitnun A, Robinson J, Mineyko A, Barton M, Mah JK, et al. Longitudinal outcomes in the 2014 acute flaccid paralysis cluster in Canada. J Child Neurol 2017;32:301–7.

Chong PF, Kira R, Mori H, Okumura A, Torisu H, Yasumoto S, et al; Acute Flaccid Myelitis Collaborative Study Investigators. Clinical Features of Acute Flaccid Myelitis Temporally Associated With an Enterovirus D68 Outbreak: Results of a Nationwide Survey of Acute Flaccid Paralysis in Japan, August-December 2015. Clin Infect Dis. 2018;66:653–64.

CDC and NCIRD (2015). For Clinicians: Diagnosing Acute Flaccid Myelitis (AFM) in the United States. Available at: https://www.cdc.gov/acute-flaccid-myelitis/downloads/AFM-Diagnosis-Classification-508.pdf. Accessed Dec 29 2020

Helfferich J, Knoester M, Van Leer-Buter CC, Neuteboom RF, Meiners LC, Niesters HG, et al. Acute flaccid myelitis and enterovirus D68: lessons from the past and present. Eur J Pediatr. 2019;178:1305–15.

Sooksawasdi Na Ayudhya S, Laksono BM, van Riel D. The pathogenesis and virulence of enterovirus-D68 infection. Virulence 2021;12:2060–72.

Cassidy H, Poelman R, Knoester M, Van Leer-Buter CC, Niesters HGM. Enterovirus D68—The New Polio? Front Microbiol 2018;9:2677.

Kramer R, Lina B, Shetty J. Acute flaccid myelitis caused by enterovirus D68: Case definitions for use in clinical practice. Eur J Paediatr Neurol 2019;23:235–9.

Case 8. A 7-Year-Old Girl with Acute Onset of Hallucinations and Unsteady Gait: Acute Necrotizing Encephalopathy of Childhood

Jainn-Jim Lin

Keywords

Acute encephalopathy · Viral febrile infection · MRI · Thalamus · Methylprednisolone · Childhood

Key Points in Acute Necrotizing Encephalopathy of Childhood

- Acute necrotizing encephalopathy (ANE) is a rare but fulminant type of acute encephalopathy.
- It is characterized by acute encephalopathy in previously healthy children following viral infections.
- Macrophage activation and hypercytokinemia (cytokine storm) may play a major role in the development of ANE.
- The hallmark neuroimaging findings are multifocal symmetric brain lesions that mainly affect the bilateral thalamus.
- A high index of suspicion with neuroimaging findings are the keys to an early diagnosis.
- Early methylprednisolone pulse therapy may help in selected cases.
- The outcome is still poor with high mortality and morbidity.

J.-J. Lin (✉)
Division of Pediatric Critical Care Medicine and Pediatric Neurocritical Care Center, Chang Gung Children's Hospital and Chang Gung Memorial Hospital, Chang Gung University College of Medicine, Taoyuan, Taiwan
e-mail: lin0227@cgmh.org.tw

Case Report

A 7-year-1-month-old previously healthy girl presented to the pediatric emergency department with acute onset of hallucinations and unsteady gait. She had a two-day history of high-grade fever, headache, and multiple bouts of diarrhea and vomiting. On examination, her Glasgow Coma Scale (GCS) was 12/15 and she was afebrile (36 °C); pulse rate, 108/min; respiratory rate, 28/min; blood pressure, 92/56 mm Hg; and SpO_2, 100%. Chest and abdominal findings were normal except for a mildly distended abdomen. A neurological examination revealed normal cranial nerve function; however, she had hypertonia and hyperreflexia of all limbs. There were no other focal neurological findings. Initial laboratory findings revealed no leukocytosis (7600/L) with mildly elevated serum C-reactive protein (11.7 mg/L). Liver enzyme tests were normal (AST 33 U/L, ALT 13 U/L), and the ferritin level was 219.9 ng/mL (normal range: 10–291 ng/mL). Initial brain computed tomography (CT) showed no specific findings (Fig. 1a). She was then admitted to our hospital.

Y.-C. Huang et al. (eds.), *Paediatric Infectious Diseases*,
https://doi.org/10.1007/978-981-19-7276-8_8

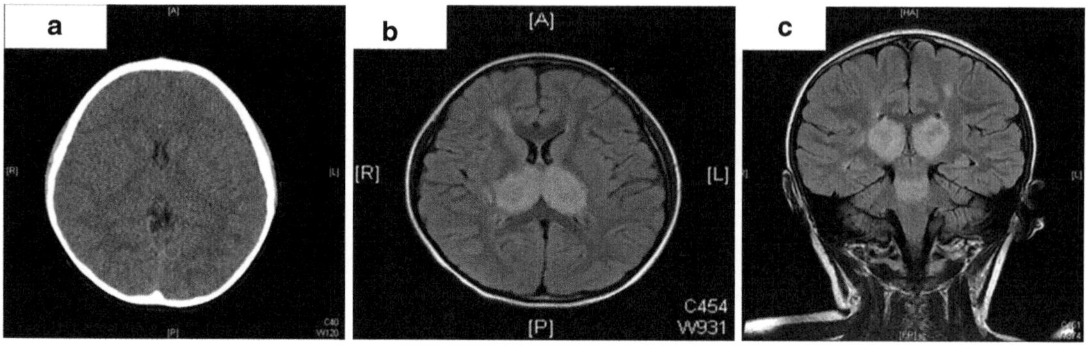

Fig. 1 Brain computerized tomography (CT) on admission showed no specific findings (**a**). Brain magnetic resonance imaging (MRI) on day 3 after admission showed T2-flare hyper-intensity involving the bilateral medial thalamus (**b**, **c**) and midbrain (**c**)

At admission, she developed generalized tonic-clonic seizures, and her mental status deteriorated to coma (GCS 8/15). She was intubated and received ventilator support. She was started on antibiotics (vancomycin 15 mg/kg/dose four times a day, ceftriaxone 50 mg/kg/dose twice a day intravenously, and azithromycin 10 mg/kg/dose once a day enterally), and antivirals (acyclovir 10 mg/kg/dose three times a day intravenously, and oseltamivir 45 mg twice a day enterally). She also received combined intravenous methylprednisolone 30 mg/kg/day for 3 days and intravenous immunoglobulin (IVIG) 400 mg/kg/day for 5 days as well as the anticonvulsive drug phenobarbital.

Cerebrospinal fluid (CSF) analysis showed a leukocyte count of 1 cell/mm^3 (all lymphocytes), normal sugar and proteins, and negative gram stain. Polymerase chain reaction (PCR) for influenza and herpes simplex viruses were negative. Other relevant investigations included negative blood and CSF cultures, and CSF viral isolation was also negative. Only a nasopharyngeal swab tested positive for influenza B by reverse transcriptase-PCR. Brain magnetic resonance imaging (MRI) on day 3 after admission showed involvement of the bilateral thalamus and pons (Fig. 1b, c). Diffusion weighted imaging (DWI)/apparent diffusion coefficient (ADC) sequence showed restricted diffusion at all of the affected sites. Mild enhancement was seen on post-gadolinium images.

Her GCS improved on day 5 after admission, and she received rehabilitation at hospital. She was stable upon discharge on day 35 of illness. After 3 months, she had good motor and cognitive ability. After 5 years of follow-up, she had no seizures, no obvious neurological signs and normal school performance.

Discussion

Acute necrotizing encephalopathy (ANE) is a rare but fulminant type of acute encephalopathy. It is characterized by acute encephalopathy in previously healthy children following viral infections. It was first proposed by Mizuguchi et al. in 1995, and predominantly affects infants and young children. It is most prevalent in East Asia, especially Taiwan and Japan, but it has also been reported in other areas of the world. A nationwide survey on the epidemiology of acute encephalopathy in children in Japan using a questionnaire showed that ANE ranked third of acute encephalopathy associated with viral infections, with an incidence of 4.1% between 2007 and 2010 and 2.8% between 2014 and 2017. In 2016, the Japanese Society of Child Neurology published "Guidelines for the Diagnosis and Treatment of Acute Encephalopathy in Childhood," which made recommendations and comments on the general aspects of acute encephalopathy, and on individual syndromes.

ANE is usually preceded by a virus-associated febrile illness followed by rapid deterioration. The most common pathogens of the preceding infection are influenza virus (41.0%) and HHV-6 (20.5%). No cases of bacterial infection have been reported. However, the causal relationship between viral infections and ANE and the exact pathogenesis of ANE remain unclear. Hypercytokinemia (cytokine storm) may play a major role in the development of ANE. The levels of inflammatory cytokines are usually higher in serum than in CSF, and in severe cases, patients also often have signs of systemic inflammatory response syndrome. An association between hemophagocytic syndrome and ANE has also been reported. These clinical findings indicate that macrophage activation and hypercytokinemia participate in the pathogenesis of ANE.

The pathologic findings of ANE are diffuse brain edema with evidence of local breakdown of the blood-brain barrier. Increased biomarkers of vascular endothelial injury, such as serum E-selectin, thrombomodulin and VCAM-1 also suggests that vascular edema plays a pathologic role in encephalopathy in ANE. Vascular injury has been ascribed to endothelial damage by inflammatory cytokines, although the precise mechanism remains unknown. In addition to diffuse brain edema, necrotic lesions with petechial hemorrhage in the bilateral thalamus as well as other brain regions such as the putamina, cerebral, and cerebellar deep white matter, and brainstem tegmentum have been reported.

Interestingly, most cases of ANE are sporadic, although a few cases are recurrent and with familial episodes. Missense mutations in the gene encoding the nuclear pore protein Ran Binding Protein 2 (RANBP2) have been identified in the recurrent and familial forms of ANE.

ANE often affects infants and children younger than 5 years of age. It has been reported in previously healthy children with presenting symptoms of acute encephalopathy following 2–4 days of a viral febrile disease, and it runs a fulminant course with rapid deterioration in the level of consciousness, and even coma. Almost all patients also develop seizures accompanied with decerebrate or decorticate posture. In reported fatal cases, ANE diagnoses were made between 4.5 h and 4 days after the initial neurological symptoms. Importantly, severe cases often also showed signs of systemic inflammatory response syndrome, with higher levels of liver enzymes and creatinine at initial examination, and then gradual increases in sodium. All patients met the criteria of shock, disseminated intravascular coagulation (DIC) and multiple organ failure within 14 h of symptom detection. Despite aggressive therapies, the patients were diagnosed with brain death from 16 h to 4 days after the initial neurological symptoms.

Although the clinical course of ANE is diverse, the hallmark neuroimaging findings are multifocal symmetric brain lesions that mainly affect the bilateral thalamus, plus the involvement of other regions in the brain including upper brainstem tegmentum, cerebral periventricular white matter, internal capsule, putamen, and cerebellar medulla, which can be demonstrated by CT and MRI. In particular, DWI is both sensitive and also capable of distinguishing vascular and cellular edema based on the ADC.

The diagnosis of ANE is based on a combination of clinical symptoms, laboratory findings, and neuroimaging findings. Suggested diagnostic criteria for ANE are listed in Table 1. In summary, the clinical picture of ANE is dominated by disturbance of consciousness of acute onset with GCS < 11 for duration of 24 h or longer during the course of an infectious disease. The cardinal symptoms are also often accompanied by convulsions or seizures and signs of increased intracranial pressure. Other clinical and laboratory findings in the acute stage are nonspecific, although increased CSF protein, elevation of serum aminotransferases of varying degrees, and no increase in blood ammonia are also characteristic of ANE. Although bilateral sympathetic thalamic lesions are characteristic, making the diagnosis of ANE also requires differentiation from clinically similar conditions, such as Reye syndrome and encephalitis/meningitis, and from radiological viewpoints such as acute disseminated encephalomyelitis and Leigh and Wernicke encephalopathies.

There is still no general consensus on the treatment of ANE. In general, intensive support-

Table 1 Diagnostic criteria for acute necrotizing encephalopathy of childhood

1	**Clinical symptoms** Acute encephalopathy following a viral febrile disease. Rapid deterioration in the level of consciousness. Convulsions
2.	**Cerebrospinal fluid (CSF) findings** No CSF pleocytosis. Increase in CSF protein commonly observed
3.	**Neuroimaging findings** CT or MRI evidence of symmetric, multifocal brain lesions. Involvement of the bilateral thalamus. Lesions also common in the cerebral periventricular white matter, internal capsule, putamen, upper brain stem tegmentum, and cerebellar medulla. No involvement of other CNS regions
4.	**Other laboratory findings** Elevation of serum aminotransferases of varying degrees. No increase in Blood ammonia
5	**Exclusion of resembling diseases**
	A. Differential diagnosis from a clinical viewpoint Overwhelming bacterial and viral infections, and fulminant hepatitis Toxic shock, hemolytic uremic syndrome and other toxin-induced diseases Reye syndrome, hemorrhagic shock and encephalopathy syndrome, and heat stroke
	B. Differential diagnosis from a radiological viewpoint Acute disseminated encephalomyelitis, acute hemorrhagic leucoencephalitis, other types of encephalitis and vasculitis Leigh encephalopathy and related mitochondrial cytopathies Glutaric acidemia, methylmalonic acidemia, and infantile bilateral striatal necrosis Wernicke encephalopathy, and carbon monoxide poisoning Arterial or venous infection, and the effects of severe hypoxia or head trauma

Reproduced with permission from references (Hoshino 2012) and (Mizuguchi 2021)

ive therapies, including respiration, circulation, central nervous system, blood sugar/electrolytes, and nutrition should be maintained. In terms of CNS, serial observations of the level of consciousness (GCS) and brainstem reflexes are suggested. Continuous monitoring of electroencephalography (EEG) may also be useful. Management of convulsive status epilepticus and electrographic seizures and increased intracranial pressure (ICP) are important parts of neurocritical care. However, intensive supportive therapy alone is not as effective.

Since 2000, Japanese pediatricians have treated their patients with more aggressive therapies, many of them designed either to combat a cytokine storm or to protect the brain. Anti-inflammatory therapies such as IVIG and steroids and neuroprotective strategies such as brain-targeted temperature management (hypothermia or normothermia) have also been proposed. Okumura et al. conducted a retrospective study to examine the efficacy of anti-inflammatory treatment, including steroids and IVIG in children with ANE, and they found that early methylprednisolone pulse therapy within 24 h after the onset was related to better outcomes in the children without brainstem lesions. Outcomes were not correlated with IVIG treatment. Brain hypothermia have multiple neuroprotective effects, including decreased excitotoxicity, apoptosis, inflammation, and free radical production, as well as improved blood-brain barrier integrity. However, at present, little information is available for the efficacy of brain hypothermia in children with ANE. Given the possibility of secondary neuronal damage in the early stage of ANE, brain hypothermia should be attempted according to the severity in select patients.

The outcome is usually poor, with high mortality (26.8 to 28.2%). However, the overall full recovery rate has improved from about 12.8% (between 2007 and 2010) to about 22.6% (between 2014 and 2017). Nevertheless, many of the survivors have severe neurologic sequelae, and moderate to severe motor disabilities with focal neurologic signs are usually more severe than mental deficits.

In conclusion, ANE is a rare but fulminant type of acute encephalopathy. It is characterized by acute encephalopathy in previously healthy children following viral infections. The hallmark neuroimaging findings are multifocal symmetric brain lesions that mainly affect the bilateral thalamus, as demonstrated by MRI. The exact pathogenesis of ANE remains unclear. Macrophage activation and hypercytokinemia (cytokine storm) may play a major role in the development of ANE. The diagnosis of ANE is based on a combination of clinical symptoms, laboratory findings, and neuroimaging findings. There is still no general consensus on the treatment of ANE. The earlier methylprednisolone pulse therapy is started, the better the outcome. However, the outcome is still poor with high mortality and moderate to severe neurologic sequelae.

Further Reading

Mizuguchi M. Acute necrotizing encephalopathy of childhood: a novel form of acute encephalopathy prevalent in Japan and Taiwan. Brain Dev 1997;19:81–92.

Hoshino A, Saitoh M, Oka A, Okumura A, Kubota M, Saito Y, Takanashi J, Hirose S, Yamagata T, Yamanouchi H, Mizuguchi M. Epidemiology of acute encephalopathy in Japan, with emphasis on the association of viruses and syndromes. Brain Dev 2012;34:337–43.

Kasai M, Shibata A, Hoshino A, Maegaki Y, Yamanouchi H, Takanashi JI, Yamagata T, Sakuma H, Okumura A, Nagase H, Ishii A, Goto T, Oka A, Mizuguchi M. Epidemiological changes of acute encephalopathy in Japan based on national surveillance for 2014–2017. Brain Dev 2020;42:508–14.

Mizuguchi M, Ichiyama T, Imataka G, Okumura A, Goto T, Sakuma H, Takanashi JI, Murayama K, Yamagata T, Yamanouchi H, Fukuda T, Maegaki Y. Guidelines for the diagnosis and treatment of acute encephalopathy in childhood. Brain Dev 2021;43:2–31.

Kansagra SM, Gallentine WB. Cytokine storm of acute necrotizing encephalopathy. Pediatr Neurol 2011;45:400–2.

Lin YY, Lee KY, Ro LS, Lo YS, Huang CC, Chang KH. Clinical and cytokine profile of adult acute necrotizing encephalopathy. Biomed J. 2019;42:178–86.

Mizuguchi M, Yamanouchi H, Ichiyama T, Shiomi M. Acute encephalopathy associated with influenza and other viral infections. Acta Neurol Scand 2007;115:45–56.

Neilson DE, Adams MD, Orr CMD, Schelling DK, Eiben RM, Kerr DS, et al. Infection-triggered familial or recurrent cases of acute necrotizing encephalopathy caused by mutations in a component of the nuclear pore, RANBP2. Am J Hum Genet 2009;84:44–51.

Tomioka K, Nishiyama M, Nagase H, Ishida Y, Tanaka T, Tokumoto S, et al. Detailed clinical course of fatal acute encephalopathy in children. Brain Dev. 2019;41:691–8.

Okumura A, Mizuguchi M, Kidokoro H, Tanaka M, Abe S, Hosoya M, Aiba H, Maegaki Y, Yamamoto H, Tanabe T, Noda E, Imataka G, Kurahashi H. Outcome of acute necrotizing encephalopathy in relation to treatment with corticosteroids and gammaglobulin. Brain Dev 2009;31:221–7.

Case 9. A 5-Year-Old Girl with Acute Onset of Generalized Tonic-Clonic Seizures for Ten Minutes: *Mycoplasma Pneumoniae*-Associated Encephalitis

Jainn-Jim Lin

Keywords

Mycoplasma Pneumoniae · Encephalitis
Childhood

Key Points

- Neurological manifestations are one of the most severe common extrapulmonary complications of M. pneumoniae infection.
- The pathogenesis of M. pneumoniae-associated encephalitis remains undefined.
- Three distinct disease patterns were observed: Ddirect invasion, immune-mediated, and vascular.
- The combined use of acute-phase serology and molecular biology tests may be able to identify M. pneumoniae DNA.
- Antibiotic therapy should be considered for all children suspected of having the direct type of M. pneumoniae encephalitis.
- Immune modulating therapies should be considered in those suspected of having the immune-mediated type of M. pneumoniae-associated encephalitis.

J.-J. Lin (✉)
Division of Pediatric Critical Care Medicine and Pediatric Neurocritical Care Center, Chang Gung Children's Hospital and Chang Gung Memorial Hospital, Chang Gung University College of Medicine, Taoyuan, Taiwan
e-mail: lin0227@cgmh.org.tw

Case 1

A 5-year-3-month-old previously healthy girl presented to our pediatric emergency department with the acute onset of generalized tonic-clonic seizures for ten minutes. She had a 7-day history of productive cough and rhinorrhea with intermittent headache over bilateral parietal-occipital areas, but without fever. She also had a 1-day history of intermittent abdominal pain without vomiting or diarrhea. She visited a local medical doctor, and an upper respiratory tract infection was impressed for which symptomatic medication was prescribed. Due to acute onset of seizures, she was sent to our emergency department.

On examination, her Glasgow coma scale (GCS) was E1V2M4 (7/15) and she was afebrile (37.1 °C); pulse rate, 120/min; respiratory rate, 40/min; blood pressure, 105/41 mm Hg; and SpO_2, 100%. Chest and abdominal findings were normal. A neurological examination revealed mild neck stiffness and bilateral muscle weakness grade 4/5. Notably, she also had bilateral pathological extensor plantar responses. There

Y.-C. Huang et al. (eds.), *Paediatric Infectious Diseases*,
https://doi.org/10.1007/978-981-19-7276-8_9

were no other focal neurological findings. Initial laboratory findings revealed no leukocytosis (11,800/μL) with normal C-reactive protein (4.21 mg/L). Liver and renal function tests were within normal range (AST 26 U/L, ALT 10 U/L, BUN 9.2 mg/dL, Creatinine (Cr) 0.24 mg/dL). She was admitted to our hospital, and initial brain computed tomography (CT) and magnetic resonance imaging (MRI) showed no specific findings. Routine cerebrospinal fluid (CSF) analysis revealed no leukocytosis (WBC 5/μL) with lymphocyte predominance (83.8%), mildly increased total protein (15 mg/L) and normal glucose level (48 mg/L). She was initially treated for presumed encephalitis with intravenous acyclovir and oral azithromycin therapy. In addition, the anti-epileptic drug phenytoin was also prescribed.

Twenty-four hours after admission, her consciousness gradually improved; however, her parents reported a personality change. Brain MRI on day 3 was arranged, which showed no specific findings. Electroencephalography (EEG) on day 4 showed a mild slow background over the right temporal-occipital area, indicating possible postictal findings. Polymerase chain reaction (PCR) for influenza from a throat swab and for herpes simplex virus from CSF were both negative. Other relevant investigations included negative blood and CSF bacterial cultures. CSF viral isolation was also negative, and only a serological test for *M. pneumoniae* immunoglobulin M (IgM) was positive.

Seven days after admission, she had clear consciousness without seizures or personality change. She was discharged on day 10 of illness and had good motor and cognitive abilities after 12 months of follow-up. Five years later, she had no seizures or obvious neurologic signs and normal school performance.

Case 2

A 6-year-11-month-old previously healthy girl presented to our pediatric emergency department with the acute onset of upward gaze, lips cyanosis, and generalized tonic-clonic movement for 2–3 min. She had a 4-day history of high-grade fever, but no history of productive cough, rhinorrhea, vomiting, or diarrhea. On examination, her GCS was 3/15 and she was febrile (39 °C); pulse rate, 128/min; respiratory rate, 28/min; blood pressure, 92/56 mm Hg; and SpO_2, 100%. Chest and abdominal findings were normal. A neurological examination revealed no other focal neurological findings or neck stiffness, but she had bilateral pathological extensor plantar responses. Initial laboratory findings revealed no leukocytosis (4600/μL) with normal C-reactive protein (<0.2 mg/L). Liver and renal function tests were within normal range (AST 33 U/L, ALT 13 U/L, BUN 4.1 mg/dL, Cr 0.31 mg/dL). She was admitted to our hospital. She was intubated due to apnea 2 h after admission; however, initial brain CT and MRI showed no specific findings. Routine CSF analysis revealed no leukocytosis (WBC 1/μL) with lymphocyte predominance (100%), normal total protein (17.6 mg/L) and normal glucose level (91 mg/L).

She was initially treated for presumed encephalitis with intravenous vancomycin, ceftriaxone and acyclovir, and oral oseltamivir and azithromycin therapy. In addition, the antiepileptic drug luminal was also prescribed. Due to suspected immune-mediated encephalitis, she also received a combination of intravenous methylprednisolone pulse therapy 30 mg/kg/day for 3 days and intravenous immunoglobulin (IVIG) 400 mg/kg/day for 5 days. PCR for influenza and *Mycoplasma pneumoniae* from a throat swab were both negative. Other relevant investigations included negative blood and CSF bacteria cultures. CSF viral isolation was also negative, and only a CSF sample tested positive for *M. pneumoniae* by real time PCR.

Her respiratory condition and consciousness gradually improved, and she was extubated on day 3 after admission and transferred to a general ward on day 7. She was stable upon discharge on day 14 of illness and had good motor and cognitive abilities after 3 months of follow-up. Four years later, she had no seizures or obvious neurologic signs and normal school performance.

Discussion

Mycoplasma pneumoniae is mainly considered to be a respiratory pathogen and is a common cause of community-acquired pneumonia in children. Neurological manifestations are one of the most severe common extrapulmonary complications of *M. pneumoniae* infection and occur without respiratory symptoms in a great number of cases. Previous studies have reported that 5–10% of acute, febrile patients presenting with central nervous system manifestations are associated with *M. pneumoniae* infection, and the most common clinical syndrome of *M. pneumoniae*-associated neurologic manifestations is encephalitis. Patients with *M pneumoniae*-associated encephalitis are predominantly children, and they frequently require intensive care with prolonged hospitalization.

The pathogenesis of *M. pneumoniae*-associated encephalitis remains undefined. Three distinct disease patterns have been demonstrated. The first pattern is the direct type, which occurs in the early phase (<7 days) of the infection with no prodrome, less frequent respiratory manifestations, and detection of *M. pneumoniae* in the CSF but not in the respiratory tract. This type could be related to direct invasion of the central nervous system. The second pattern is the indirect type, which occurs in the late phase (≥7 days) of disease with respiratory manifestations, an IgM response in peripheral blood, and detection of *M. pneumoniae* in the respiratory tract, but not the CSF. This type has been proposed to be immune mediated. Encephalitis has been described to be both a direct and indirect mechanism. The third pattern is the vascular type, in which local vasculitis or thrombotic vascular occlusion occurs through a direct or indirect mechanism. The mechanisms are not mutually exclusive, which explains why lesions related to different pathogeneses can be detected in some patients.

The diagnosis of *M. pneumoniae* encephalitis remains challenging due to the lack of knowledge with regards to the true pathogenesis. The diagnosis should be based on the clinical case definition for acute encephalitis (Table 1) and strong evidence of *M. pneumoniae* infection in nervous tissue or CSF, including detection of the organism in a culture or using molecular detection techniques in addition to serology and exclusion of other potential etiologies. Because the culture of *M. pneumoniae* is complicated and slow, the combined use of acute-phase serology and molecular biology tests to identify *M. pneumoniae* DNA has been suggested. *M. pneumoniae*-associated encephalitis is classified into three categories: (1) confirmed: defined as detection of *M. pneumoniae* by PCR in CSF or of intrathecal synthesis of specific antibodies; (2) probable: defined as ≥four-fold rise in specific serum antibody titer; and (3) possible: defined as detection of *M. pneumoniae* by PCR in respiratory specimens and/or single raised specific serum antibody titer (Table 1).

Table 1 Case definition of *Mycoplasma pneumoniae*-associated encephalitis in children

1.	Children ≤16 years of age
2.	The clinical case definition for acute encephalitis **Major criterion (required):** Altered mental status lasting ≥24 h with no alternative cause identified **Minor criteria** (two required for possible encephalitis; ≥3 required for probable or confirmed encephalitis) Fever ≥38 °C (100.4 °F) within the 72 h before or after presentation Seizures New onset of focal neurologic findings CSF WBC count ≥5/cubic mm Abnormality of brain parenchyma on neuroimaging Abnormality on electroencephalography
3.	The case definition for acute encephalitis caused by *M. pneumoniae*
	Confirmed possible case A confirmed case is defined as detection of *M. pneumoniae* by PCR in CSF or of intrathecal synthesis of specific antibodies
	Probable case A probable case is defined as ≥four-fold rise in specific serum antibody titer
	Possible case A possible case is defined as detection of *M. pneumoniae* by PCR in respiratory specimens and/or single raised specific serum antibody titer

Modified from references (Britton 2017).
CSF cerebrospinal fluid, *PCR* polymerase chain reaction

The latency between a previous respiratory episode and the development of neurological manifestations can be useful to distinguish cases due to direct invasion of *M. pneumoniae* from those associated with an immune-mediated mechanism. However, when *M. pneumoniae* infection is suspected, the identification of a recent episode of *M. pneumoniae* infection is often impossible because the signs and symptoms of the disease are not specific, and laboratory tests do not always offer adequate support.

The lack of knowledge of the true pathogenesis of *M. pneumoniae*-associated encephalitis explains why treatment is not precisely defined. Antibiotic therapy should be considered for all children suspected of having the direct type of *M. pneumoniae* encephalitis. Antibiotics with good blood-brain barrier penetration, such as ciprofloxacin, doxycycline, and azithromycin, are recommended, even though the best drug, dosage, and duration of therapy have not been established. The benefits of immune modulating therapies such as methylprednisolone, IVIG, and plasmapheresis are still unclear, but should be considered in those suspected of having immune-mediated *M. pneumoniae*-associated encephalitis in order to limit autoimmune-related neurologic damage. In cases with progressively worsening *M. pneumoniae*-associated encephalitis, steroids, IVIG, and plasma exchange have been reported to be valid therapeutic options. However, there is no conclusive evidence for the use of immunomodulating therapy. Further studies are needed to find the best therapy for those with suspected immune-mediated encephalitis.

In conclusion, *M pneumoniae*-associated encephalitis is one of the most severe common extrapulmonary complications of *M. pneumoniae* infection, and it occurs without respiratory symptoms in a great number of cases. The pathogenesis of *M pneumoniae*-associated encephalitis is not always known, and it can depend on direct invasion of *M. pneumoniae* or a pathological immune-mediated response to *M. pneumoniae*. The mainstay of treatment is antibiotics with good blood-brain barrier penetration, such as ciprofloxacin, doxycycline, or azithromycin; however, the role of immunomodulation therapy is unclear. Knowledge of the pathogenesis of the different manifestations should guide strategies for diagnosis and treatment.

Further Reading

Narita M. Classification of Extrapulmonary Manifestations Due to *Mycoplasma pneumoniae* Infection on the Basis of Possible Pathogenesis. Front Microbiol 2016;7:23.

Pönkä A. Central nervous system manifestations associated with serologically verified *Mycoplasma pneumoniae* infection. Scand J Infect Dis 1980;12:175–84.

Al-Zaidy SA, MacGregor D, Mahant S, Richardson SE, Bitnun A. Neurological Complications of PCR-Proven *M. pneumoniae* Infections in Children: Prodromal Illness Duration May Reflect Pathogenetic Mechanism. Clin Infect Dis 2015;61:1092–8.

Christie LJ, Honarmand S, Talkington DF, Gavali SS, Preas C, Pan CY, et al. Pediatric encephalitis: what is the role of *Mycoplasma pneumoniae*? Pediatrics 2007;120:305–13.

D'Alonzo R, Mencaroni E, Di Genova L, Laino D, Principi N, Esposito S. Pathogenesis and Treatment of Neurologic Diseases Associated With *Mycoplasma pneumoniae* Infection. Front Microbiol 2018;9:2751.

de Groot RCA, Meyer Sauteur PM, Unger WWJ, van Rossum AMC. Things that could be *Mycoplasma pneumoniae*. J Infect 2017;Suppl 1:S95–S100.

Venkatesan A, Tunkel AR, Bloch KC, Lauring AS, Sejvar J, Bitnun A et al. Case Definitions, Diagnostic Algorithms, and Priorities in Encephalitis: Consensus Statement of the International Encephalitis Consortium. Clin Infect Dis 2013; 57:1114–28.

Waites KB, Xiao L, Liu Y, Balish MF, Atkinson TP. *Mycoplasma pneumoniae* from the Respiratory Tract and Beyond. Clin Microbiol Rev 2017;30:747–809.

Qu J, Gu L, Wu J, Dong J, Pu Z, Gao Y, et al.; Beijing Network for Adult Community-Acquired Pneumonia (BNACAP). Accuracy of IgM antibody testing, FQ-PCR and culture in laboratory diagnosis of acute infection by *Mycoplasma pneumoniae* in adults and adolescents with community-acquired pneumonia. BMC Infect Dis 2013;13:172.

Meyer Sauteur PM, Moeller A, Relly C, Berger C, Plecko B, Nadal D; Swiss Pediatric Surveillance Unit (SPSU). Swiss national prospective surveillance of paediatric *Mycoplasma pneumoniae*-associated encephalitis. Swiss Med Wkly 2016;146:w14222.

Britton PN, Bag SK, Booy R, Sharpe C, Owen KB, Zhao J, et al. Probable epidemic *Mycoplasma pneu-*

moniae disease activity in metropolitan Sydney, 2015: combining surveillance data to cross-validate signal detection. Commun Dis Intell Q Rep 2017;41:E295–E307.

Cunha BA, Cunha CB. Pharmacokinetic considerations in selecting optimal antibiotic therapy for *Mycoplasma pneumoniae* encephalitis. Eur J Clin Microbiol Infect Dis 2019;38:631–5.

Daba M, Kang PB, Sladky J, Bidari SS, Lawrence RM, Ghosh S. Intravenous Immunoglobulin as a Therapeutic Option for *Mycoplasma pneumoniae* Encephalitis. J Child Neurol 2019;34:687–91.

Case 10. A 1-Year-Old Boy with Fever, Progressive Consciousness Change, and Seizure: Eosinophilic Meningoencephalitis

Hao-Ting Hsu and Po-Yen Chen

Keywords

Child · Seizure · Eosinophil · Meningoencephalitis

Key Points

- Eosinophilic meningoencephalitis may occur in endemic area with consumption of raw or undercooked freshwater snails, slugs, raw vegetable juice (can be cluster), or in children crawling on the ground (sporadic).
- Eosinophilic meningoencephalitis can attack any age of patients.
- Diagnosis is based on clinical manifestations and microscopic identification of eosinophils in cerebrospinal fluid.
- Optional treatment may include steroid and anti-parasitic drugs.
- Prognosis is generally good.

Case Report

A 1-year-old boy had low-grade fever (38°–38.5 °C), cough, and running nose since 1 month prior to this admission. He ever received some symptomatic medications at local medical clinics. He was ever admitted to a regional hospital due to persistent symptoms. Physical examination on his admission revealed a 9 kg boy with only congested throat and fine rhonchi of his lung field. The initial laboratory data showed WBC 24,900/μL, Neutrophil 38%, Lymphocyte 38%, Myelocyte 3%, Eosinophil count 19%, band form 1%, Hgb = 12.8 g/dL (Table 1). The blood culture, stool analysis and culture, urine analysis and culture were all negative finding. He received empirical ampicillin. He was found to have drowsy consciousness and stiff neck on the sixth hospital day. He received lumbar puncture on the sixth day, and was found to have abnormal CSF (Cerebrospinal fluid) analysis (Table 2). The CSF antigen screen for bacteria, Gram stain, and acid-fast stain and culture were all negative. He received high dose ampicillin and cefotaxime initially, and later chloramphenicol, metronidazole, amikacin, and acyclovir due to persistent fever. Other investigation studies included serologic tests for HSV, VZV, rubella, toxoplasma, VDRL, stool for parasite, IHA (Indirect hemagglutination assay for amoeba), and CT scan of brain, and were all negative. The follow-up CBC analysis 2 weeks later still showed leukocytosis, high eosinophil count (11%) and CRP 2.87 mg/dL.

H.-T. Hsu
Department of Pediatrics, Taichung Veterans General Hospital, Taichung, Taiwan

P.-Y. Chen (✉)
Pediatrics, Taichung Veterans General Hospital, National Chung Hsing University, Taichung City, Taiwan

Y.-C. Huang et al. (eds.), *Paediatric Infectious Diseases*, https://doi.org/10.1007/978-981-19-7276-8_10

Table 1 Serial follow-up of peripheral complete blood count during the clinical course

Hospital day	WBC (/μL)	Hb (g/dL)	Hct (%)	Plt (×1000/μL)	Neut (%)	Lym (%)	Mon (%)	Eos (%)
Hospital 1								
Day 1	24,900	12.8			38	38		19
Day 9	20,800				49	28		15
Day 14	23,300	9.7			53	28		11
Hospital 2								
Day 16	10,720	8.5	26.0	643 K	42	18	14	6
Day 17	13,510	13.6	40.7	668 K	40	25	6	9
Day 20	13,980	12.3	38.8	710 K	44	35	5	6
Day 27	10,000	12.3	39.5	–	10	52	8	30

WBC white blood cell count, *Hb* hemoglobin, *Hct* hematocrit, *Plt* platelet count, *Neut* segmented neutrophils, *Lym* lymphocytes, *Mon* monocytes, *Eos* eosinophils

Table 2 Series analysis of cerebrospinal fluid specimens

Hospital day	WBC	Neu/Lym	Eosinophil (%)	RBC	Protein (mg/dL)	Glucose (mg/dL)	Pressure (mmHg)
Hospital 1							
Day 6	410	25/75		45	42	42/146[a]	
Day 9	180	5/15		10	75	39	
Hospital 2							
Day 15	152	19/81	0	2	83	27/103[a]	200
Day 16	180	11/15	15	270	87	24/132[a]	280/180
Day 19	298	42/58	0	67	79	33	200
Day 21	1008	37/32	31	45	90	37	335/250
Day 22	1000	8/17	73	54	93	36	350/300
Day 27	323	13/50	34	2	84	35	335/300
Day 28	318	3/37	58	837	91	47	–

Neu neutrophils, *Lym* lymphocytes, *WBC* white blood cell, *RBC* red blood cell
[a]CSF/Serum

Whole body gallium scan showed increased uptake in spleen only. On hospital day 15, sudden onset of generalized tonic-clonic convulsion, loss of consciousness, trismus, and upward gazing developed and totally for three episodes, with a duration of 3–6 min in each episode. He was then referred to a medical center for further evaluation and management.

On arrival at the medical center, the boy was in drowsy state with hypotonic posture. He had tachypnea (70–80/min.), tachycardia (180/min), congested throat, stiff neck, and coarse breathing sound. He had no fever, normal eardrum, no lymphadenopathy, no hepatosplenomegaly, no skin rash. He still had leukocytosis, thrombocytosis, anemia, and elevated eosinophil count (Table 1), BUN/Cr. = 2/0.3, Alb = 2.7 g/dL, no electrolyte imbalance, normal liver enzymes (GOT/GPT = 21/36 U/L), blood glucose 103 mg/dL, ammonia 30 mg/dL. He received repeated lumbar puncture and had abnormal data (Table 2). Gram stain, KOH stain and India ink stain of CSF specimens were all negative. He received ampicillin, ceftriaxone, and acyclovir again. Follow-up peripheral blood WBC revealed increasing eosinophilia (6–30%) and thrombocytosis. The follow-up CSF examination revealed elevated WBC count, high eosinophil count, elevated protein level, low glucose level and high intracranial pressure.

Microbiologic and immunological evaluations included Chlamydia (IgG, Ig A, IgM), HSV (IgG, IgM), EBV (EBVCA IgM, IgG), Mycoplasma pneumoniae (IF), CSF *M. tuberculosis* PCR, and culture of CSF and blood were all negative. The sonogram of brain revealed hydrocephalus, while the abdominal and heart sonogram were normal.

MRI of brain revealed moderate dilated ventricle and a small lesion over paraventricular region. EEG revealed a generalized slow background with abnormal sleep pattern. The fresh CSF fluid under low power microscopic examination was found to have many filamentous larvae. The fundal examination revealed 2 subretinal microlarvae standstill at right posterior pole (0.6 mm). He received mebendazole 100 mg twice a day for 3 days under the impression of eosinophilic meningoencephalitis, caused by *Angiostrongylus cantonensis*. He got better with less drowsiness, and was discharged in stable condition. He was followed up regularly at OPD for years and no major neurologic sequelae (including hearing and visual response) was found.

Discussion

Eosinophilic meningoencephalitis was not a rare disease two decades ago in Taiwan, particularly in children. The diagnosis of eosinophilic meningoencephalitis is based on clinical manifestations and microscopic identification of eosinophils and the larvae identity present in cerebrospinal fluid (CSF). The presence of eosinophils in the CSF should always be considered an abnormal finding. Helminthic infections are the most common cause of eosinophilic meningoencephalitis. Though less common, CSF-specific eosinophilia may also be associated with other types of infections, neoplastic diseases, drug use, prosthesis reactions, and miscellaneous idiopathic conditions.

Angiostrongylus cantonensis is the most important etiological agent of eosinophilic meningitis. The filiform worms are 20–40 mm in size. The infection is acquired by consumption of raw or undercooked freshwater snails, slugs, raw vegetable juice, prawns, or crabs containing third-stage larvae. Infection may also be acquired by ingestion of vegetables or other fomites contaminated with infectious larvae. It may be caused by ingesting larvae contained in the slime during the time that child (toddler) crawled on the ground in rural area, and mainly sporadic. The epidemiology of eosinophilic meningitis has changed during the past two decades in Taiwan and occurs mainly in adults in the setting of outbreaks. Outbreaks of central nervous system infection with *A. cantonensis* had occurred many times in southern Taiwan, including recruited Thai workers and family clusters, who usually ate raw or under-cooked snails. Human and some other domestic animals are incidental hosts that could subsequently cause disease.

Fever and neurological symptoms are the main symptoms. In infants and young children, fever and change of consciousness are predominant. Diagnosis can be made by peripheral and CSF eosinophilic pleocytosis, tortuous tracts of various sizes in brain tissue, visible larvae in CSF or fundus and Ag detected by ELISA. MRI scans can find high signal intensities over the globus pallidus and brain tissue on TI-weighted imaging, leptomeningeal enhancement, ventriculomegaly, and punctate areas of abnormal enhancement within the cerebral and cerebellar hemispheres on gadolinium-enhancing T1 imaging, and a hyperintense signal on T2-weighted images. There is a significant correlation between severity of headache, CSF pleocytosis, and CSF and blood eosinophilia with MRI signal intensity in T1-weighted imaging.

Management is mainly symptomatic and conservative. Repeated spinal taps provide some therapeutic benefit, as they serve to decrease intracranial pressure. Oral prednisolone therapy may be useful to reduce increased intracranial pressure significantly. Anti-parasitic drugs do not influence the outcome of infection, though mebendazole or thiabendazole is sometimes suggested. One of the controversies about the use of anti-helminths is that the larvae of *A. cantonensis* usually die soon after their arrival in the brain tissue, and the dead larvae may be more dangerous than the live ones.

The prognosis is generally good. Only a few cases reported neurologic sequelae, including visual loss, hydrocephalus, or mortality.

Further Reading

Graeff-Teixeira C, da Silva AC, Yoshimura K. Update on eosinophilic meningoencephalitis and its clinical relevance. Clin Microbiol Rev. 2009;22:322-48.

Tseng YT, Tsai HC, Sy CL, Lee SS, Wann SR, Wang YH, Chen JK, Wu KS, Chen YS. Clinical manifestations of eosinophilic meningitis caused by Angiostrongylus cantonensis: 18 years' experience in a medical center in southern Taiwan. J Microbiol Immunol Infect. 2011;44:382-9.

Tsai HC, Liu YC, Kunin CM, Lai PH, Lee SS, Chen YS, Wann SR, Lin WR, Huang CK, Ger LP, Lin HH, Yen MY. Eosinophilic meningitis caused by Angiostrongylus cantonensis associated with eating raw snails: correlation of brain magnetic resonance imaging scans with clinical findings. Am J Trop Med Hyg 2003;68: 281-5.

Tsai HC, Lee SS, Huang CK, Yen CM, Chen ER, Liu YC. Outbreak of eosinophilic meningitis associated with drinking raw vegetable juice in southern Taiwan. Am J Trop Med Hyg 2004;71: 222-6.

Tsai TH, Liu YC, Wann SR, Lin WR, Lee SJ, Lin HH, Chen YS, Yen MY, Yen CM. An outbreak of meningitis caused by Angiostrongylus cantonensis in Kaohsiung. J Microbiol Immunol Infect 2001;34: 50-6.

Part III

Respiratory Tract Infection

Case 11. A 14-Year-Old Boy with Nasal Congestion and Cough for Days Followed by a Tender Bulging Mass on the Forehead: Acute Bacterial Sinusitis and Associated Complications

Yi-Ching Chen and Yhu-Chering Huang

Keywords

Acute sinusitis · Orbital cellulitis · Pott puffy tumor

Key Points

- To distinguish bacterial sinusitis from common cold is important and may prevent unnecessary excessive antibiotic use.
- Three clinical patterns are favorable for the diagnosis of bacterial sinusitis and include persistence of nasal symptoms ≥10 days, severe symptoms with high fever, purulent nasal discharge for days, and worsening symptoms of fever and nasal discharge.
- Common orbital complications of acute sinusitis include periorbital and orbital cellulitis.
- Intracranial complications of acute sinusitis include epidural abscess, meningitis, cavernous sinus thrombosis, subdural empyema, and brain abscess.
- Pott puffy tumor is a rare complication of acute sinusitis which has a typical triad of frontal sinusitis, subperiosteal (extradural) abscess, and frontal bone osteomyelitis.

Case 1

A 14-year-9-month previously healthy boy visited the emergency department (ED) because of a tender bulging mass on his forehead for 10 days. Two weeks prior to admission, he had nasal congestion and cough and the symptoms persisted despite the over-the-counter (OTC) medications use. Ten days before admission, a progressively enlarging, tender mass was noted accompanied by new-onset fever, headache, and severe nasal congestion. He was taken to a local hospital for help, where an oral antibiotic was prescribed. However, fever persisted in the following days, and the forehead mass enlarged day by day despite the oral antibiotic use. He was then transferred to the ED of a tertiary medical center, and admission was arranged.

Y.-C. Chen (✉)
Division of Pediatric Infectious Diseases, Department of Pediatrics, Chang Gung Memorial Hospital, Taoyuan, Taiwan

Y.-C. Huang
Division of Pediatric Infectious Diseases, Department of Pediatrics, Chang Gung Memorial Hospital, Chang Gung University, Taoyuan, Taiwan
e-mail: ychuang@cgmh.org.tw

Y.-C. Huang et al. (eds.), *Paediatric Infectious Diseases*,
https://doi.org/10.1007/978-981-19-7276-8_11

Upon admission, physical examination revealed a large forehead mass around 7 centimeters in diameter with local tenderness and swelling (Fig. 1). No erythema, local heat, or open wound was observed over the mass. Furthermore, severe headache and nasal congestion were complained. Laboratory tests revealed normal white blood cell (WBC) count (9800/μL, neutrophil 74.2%, lymphocyte 18.4%), normocytic anemia (hemoglobin 9.2 g/dL), thrombocytosis (platelet count 721,000/μL), and elevated C-reactive protein level (45.96 mg/L). Computed tomography of the brain was also performed, which revealed opacification of the right frontal, ethmoid and maxillary sinus, suggestive of right paranasal sinusitis; a small amount of fluid accumulation (6 × 36 mm in size) with marginal enhancement was also noted at the anterior paramedial frontal subgaleal region, and abscess formation was highly suspected (Fig. 2a, b). Intravenous (IV) amoxicillin/clavulanic acid was administered empirically. Echo-guided aspiration of the frontal abscess was also performed, and the pus culture subsequently yielded *Fusobacterium nucleatum*. Antibiotic was then shifted to aqua-penicillin according to the results of antibiotic susceptibility testing.

During the following hospital days, he received a functional endoscopic sinus surgery for severe maxillary sinusitis. However, headache and nausea sensation progressed gradually despite the IV antibiotic use. Bilateral eye protruding was also observed. Magnetic Resonance Imaging (MRI) of the brain was arranged and showed a 47 × 34 × 20 mm septate mass with enhanced thick wall and water restriction in the right anterior frontal lobe, which was compatible with brain abscess (Fig. 2c, d). He then received right frontal craniotomy with surgical drainage of the brain abscess and frontal sinus fistula. Antibiotics were also adjusted to vancomycin, gentamicin, and metronidazole. After 51 days of hospitalization, he was discharged from the hospital without neurologic sequelae. The final diagnosis was bacterial sinusitis complicated with Pott puffy tumor, post status of brain abscess drainage.

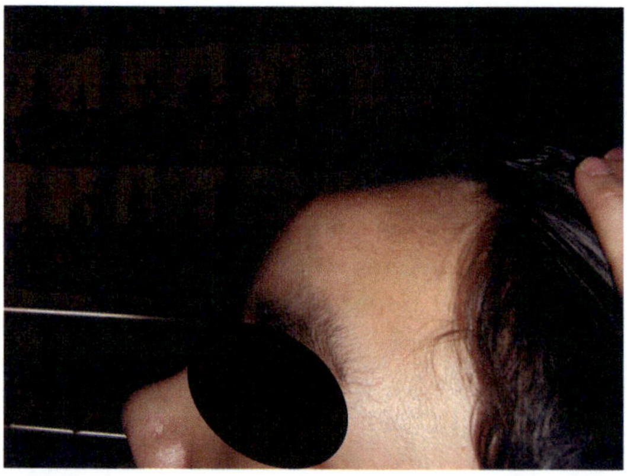

Fig. 1 Picture recorded at admission. A large forehead mass around 7 centimeters in diameter with local tenderness and swelling

Case Report: 2

A 10-year-5-month-old previously healthy boy visited the hospital due to fever for 10 days with progressive right eye swelling. He had no cough, rhinorrhea, sore throat, diarrhea, or vomiting. Two days prior to admission, he had progressive right eye swelling accompanied by orbital pain, blurred vision, and ptosis. Neither foreign body sensation nor photophobia was complained. Productive cough with yellowish, sticky sputum was also developed in the recent 2 days. Due to the new- onset ophthalmologic discomfort and prolonged fever, he was taken to our outpatient department and was admitted for further evaluation.

Upon admission, he looked mildly lethargic with moderate pain distress. Local swelling of the upper eyelid, ptosis, proptosis and injected conjunctiva of right eye was observed on examination. In addition, extraocular motility (EOM) limitation was noted in which the right eyeball could not turn upward and toward the medial side. Laboratory tests revealed leukocytosis (13,500/μL, neutrophil segment 84%, lymphocyte 9%), normal hemoglobin count (11.6 g/dL), thrombocytosis (platelet count 489,000/μL) and significant elevated C-reactive protein level (147.2 mg/L). Due to the limitation of EOM, CT of the brain was also arranged right upon admission under the impression of right orbital cellulitis, which revealed air–fluid levels in bilateral

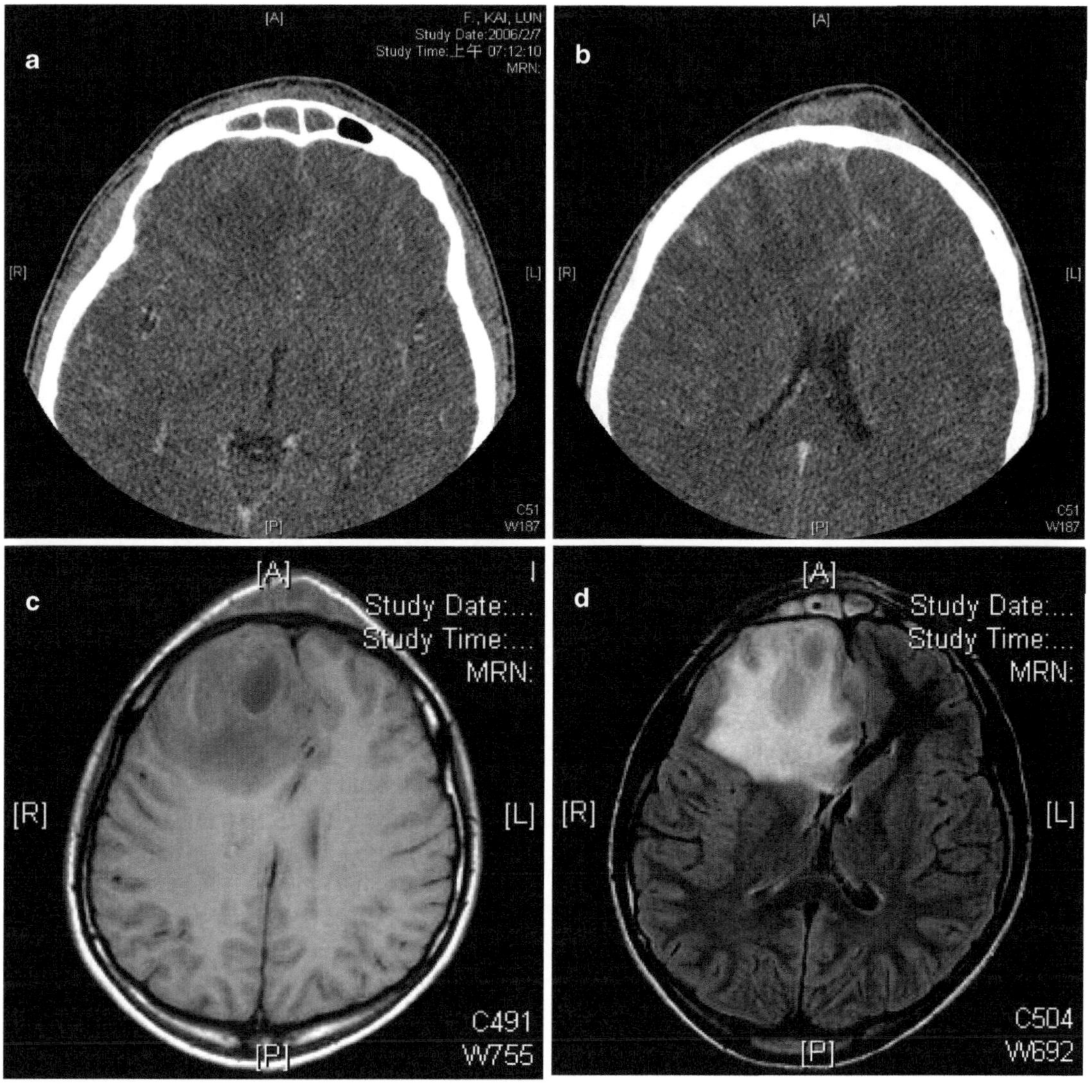

Fig. 2 (**a**, **b**) CT scan of head revealed frontal sinusitis with subperiosteal abscess formation. (**c**, **d**) MRI of brain showed a brain abscess at right frontal region with perifocal brain edema

maxillary and ethmoid sinuses with mucosal thickening; the inflammation at medial subperiosteal space of right orbit with swelling of the medial rectus muscle and eyelid was also noted, compatible with orbital cellulitis (Fig. 3). Empiric antibiotic with intravenous amoxicillin/clavulanic acid was given. Otolaryngologist and ophthalmologist consultations were arranged to evaluate the disease severity, and conservative treatment was recommended with meticulous monitoring of clinical progression. His clinical symptoms improved gradually after antibiotic use and range of motion (ROM) limitation also improved day by day. Fever subsided on the fourth day of antibiotic treatment. After 7 days of intravenous antibiotic treatment, he was discharged from the hospital with oral amoxicillin/clavulanic acid for additional 7 days. He recovered well during the follow-up at the outpatient clinic, and no associated ophthalmologic complication was observed. The final diagnosis was sinusitis complicated with right orbital cellulitis.

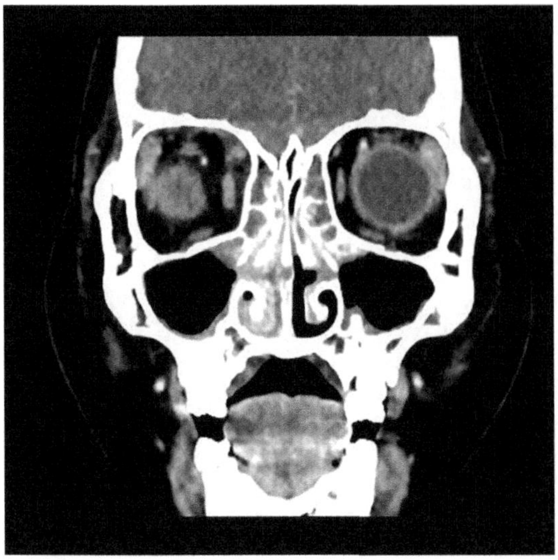

Fig. 3 CT scan of head reveal bilateral ethmoid sinus with right orbital involvement (medial site)

Discussion

Among respiratory tract infections, sinusitis is one of the common illnesses in childhood and adolescence. There are four paranasal sinuses in humans and include ethmoidal, maxillary, sphenoidal, and frontal sinus. The ethmoidal sinuses are present and pneumatized at birth, while the other sinuses are pneumatized later (maxillary sinuses: 4 years of age; sphenoidal sinuses: 5 years of age; frontal sinuses 7–8 years of age). Anatomically, they are located close to important anatomical structures, especially the orbital cavity and skull base, and are normally sterile because of the mucociliary clearance system.

Both viruses and bacteria can cause sinusitis. However, the viral rhinosinusitis is usually self-limited, while approximately 0.5–2% of viral upper respiratory tract infections are complicated by acute symptomatic bacterial sinusitis. The bacterial pathogens responsible for sinusitis include *Streptococcus pneumoniae*, nontypeable *Haemophilus influenzae*, and *Moraxella catarrhalis*. Clinical symptoms in children and adolescents with sinusitis are nasal congestion, purulent nasal discharge, and cough due to post-nasal drip. Other less common symptoms include headache, hyposmia, halitosis (bad smells) and pain, tenderness and swelling around eyes, cheeks, nose, or forehead.

To distinguish bacterial sinusitis from common cold is important and may prevent unnecessary excessive antibiotic use. The American Academy of Pediatrics published a guideline for sinusitis and suggested that the following three clinical patterns are favorable for the diagnosis of bacterial sinusitis: persistence (nasal symptoms and daytime cough persist ≥10 days without improvement); severe symptoms (temperature ≥39 °C with purulent nasal discharge for 3 days or longer); and worsening symptoms (recurrence of symptoms after an initial improvement or new symptoms of fever and nasal discharge). When interviewing children with non-specific respiratory symptoms, the clinician should trace the patient's history in a detailed manner to better differentiate a sinusitis from a common old and treat the patient in a timely way or avoid unnecessary antibiotic use. Initial empiric antibiotic therapy with amoxicillin (90 mg/kg/day divided bid) or amoxicillin-clavulanate (80–90 mg/kg/day of amoxicillin) is adequate for the majority of children with acute bacterial sinusitis of mild to moderate severity.

Due to the anatomical proximity of the paranasal sinuses to the skull base and orbital cavity, the complications of bacterial sinusitis could be dangerous and rapid-progressing, even life-threatening. Periorbital and orbital cellulitis are the most common orbital complications caused by bacterial sinusitis, mainly ethmoiditis. Infection can invade directly through the lateral wall of the ethmoidal sinus because of the thin bony structure. Periorbital cellulitis usually presents with swelling of the tissue surrounding the globe. Orbital cellulitis further involves the intraorbital cavity and may cause proptosis, chemosis, decreased visual acuity, double vision, impaired extraocular movements, and eye pain. Image studies, such as CT scan of orbit, should be performed accompanied by otolaryngology and ophthalmology consultations to define the disease severity and the potential indication of surgical drainage. As for the intracranial complications, epidural abscess, meningitis, cavernous sinus thrombosis, subdural empyema, and brain abscess have been reported secondary to bacterial sinusitis. Therefore, image studies should be arranged promptly once the abnormal neurological examination was found in patients with sinusitis, such as altered mental status, nuchal rigidity, severe headache, focal neurological signs, or signs suggestive of increased intracranial pressure.

Osteomyelitis of frontal bone with associated subperiosteal abscess, so-called Pott puffy tumor, was another uncommon complication. It was first described by an English surgeon Sir Percival Pott, who observed that this severe complication could be secondary to underlying infection in sinuses (most often frontal or mastoid) or after injury. The typical triad of Pott puffy tumor composes frontal sinusitis, subperiosteal (extradural) abscess, and frontal bone osteomyelitis. Compared to preschool-age children, adolescents aged 10–20 years had the highest probability of developing this condition. Clinical symptoms of Pott puffy tumor included headache, local swelling, fever, nuchal rigidity, altered mental status, focal neurological sign, and seizure. On examination, patients usually present with a tender, doughy soft tissue swelling that causes pitting edema over the frontal bone. Treatment usually needs prolonged antimicrobial agent treatment, accompanied by prompt surgical drainage for the optimal source control. Without prompt surgical drainage and parenteral antibiotic treatment, infection would further cause intracranial infection, causing epidural abscess, subdural empyema, meningitis, cerebral abscess, and dura-vein thrombophlebitis.

Further Reading

DeMuri G, Wald ER. Acute bacterial sinusitis in children. Pediatr Rev. 2013;34:429-437.

Jankowski R, Nguyen DT, Poussel M, Chenuel B, Gallet P, Rumeau C. Sinusology. Eur Ann Otorhinolaryngol Head Neck Dis. 2016;133:263-268.

Leung AK, Hon KL, Chu WC. Acute bacterial sinusitis in children: an updated review. Drugs Context. 2020;9:2020-9-3.

van Cauwenberge PB, Vander Mijnsbrugge AM, Ingels KJ. The microbiology of acute and chronic sinusitis and otitis media:a review. Eur Arch Otorhinolaryngol. 1993;250 Suppl 1:S3-S6.

Wald ER, Applegate KE, Bordley C, et al. Clinical practice guideline for the diagnosis and management of acute bacterial sinusitis in children aged 1 to 18 years. Pediatrics 2013;132:e262-e280.

Chang YS, Chen PL, Hung JH, et al. Orbital complications of paranasal sinusitis in Taiwan, 1988 through 2015: Acute ophthalmological manifestations, diagnosis, and management. PLoS One. 2017;12:e0184477. P

Sijuwola O, Adeyemo A, Adeosun A. Orbital complications of rhinosinusitis. Ann Ib Postgrad Med. 2007;5:6-8.

Bambakidis NC, Cohen AR. Intracranial complications of frontal sinusitis in children: Pott's puffy tumor revisited. Pediatr Neurosurg. 2001;35:82-89.

Tsai BY, Lin KL, Lin TY, et al. Pott's puffy tumor in children. Childs Nerv Syst. 2010;26:53-60.

Case 12. A 1-Year-3-Month-Old Boy with Cough, Rhinorrhea, Bilateral Eye Discharge, Fever, and Ear Discharge: Mastoiditis and Conjunctivitis-Otitis Media Syndrome

Ping-Ing Lee

Keywords

Haemophilus influenzae · Otitis media · Bacterial conjunctivitis · Mastoiditis

Key Points

- Mastoiditis, prevalent in young children, can lead to a variety of intracranial and extracranial complications, including meningitis; epidural, subdural, and brain abscesses; vascular thrombosis; osteomyelitis; and deep neck abscess.
- Persistent clinical manifestations, such as persistent ear discharge, after appropriate antibiotic treatment of otitis media are important diagnostic clue for silent mastoiditis.
- Masked/latent mastoiditis, usually chronic or recurrent, is an indolent, smoldering temporal bone infection with few clinical clues. In classic masked/latent mastoiditis, the tympanic membrane is intact and the middle ear shows no abnormalities at otoscopy,
- Most common bacterial pathogens for mastoiditis include *Streptococcus pneumoniae*, Group A streptococcus, *Staphylococcus aureus*, *Haemophilus influenzae*, *Moraxella catarrhalis*, and *Pseudomonas aeruginosa.*
- The link between *H. influenzae* conjunctivitis and otitis media is known as conjunctivitis–otitis media syndrome that may also be linked to paranasal sinusitis. Empiric antibiotic treatment should be active against β-lactamase-producing *H. influenzae* for such cases.

Case Report

A healthy 1-year-3-month-old boy had cough and rhinorrhea with bilateral eye discharge for 7 days. He was brought to a clinic because of fever for 2 days with some discharges from right ear. He had received two doses of 13-valent pneumococcal conjugate vaccine at 2 months and 4 months of age. The throat appeared injected, and the conjunctivae were injected bilaterally on his first visit. The left ear drum was injected, and the right ear canal was filled with pus discharge. With a diagnosis of bilateral otitis media, amoxicillin/clavulanic acid with a dose of 90 mg amoxicillin/kg/day 3 times per day was given. The fever sub-

P.-I. Lee (✉)
Department of Pediatrics, National Taiwan University Children's Hospital, National Taiwan University, Taipei, Taiwan
e-mail: pinging@ntu.edu.tw

Y.-C. Huang et al. (eds.), *Paediatric Infectious Diseases*,
https://doi.org/10.1007/978-981-19-7276-8_12

sided immediately after the treatment. However, right ear discharge persisted for 1 week, and bilateral ear drum appeared opaque during the follow-up visit. Bacteria cultures of right ear discharge and eye discharge grew *Haemophilus influenzae* that was β-lactamase-producing and was susceptible to amoxicillin-clavulanic acid. The mastoid X-ray examination showed haziness of bilateral mastoid air cells (Figs. 1, 2 and 3). Antibiotic treatment was continued for 4 weeks with complete recovery.

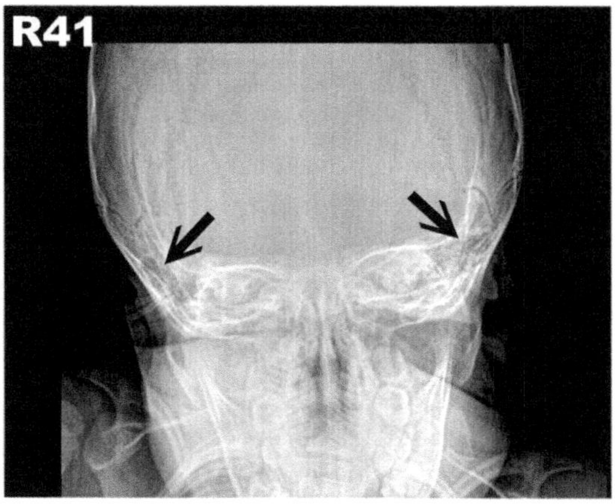

Fig. 1 Transorbital view of the skull. The arrows indicate haziness of bilateral mastoid air cells

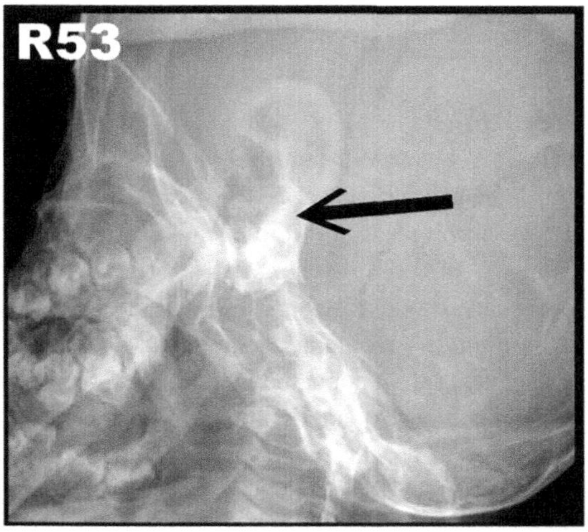

Fig. 2 Schuller view of right mastoid area. The arrow indicates haziness of right mastoid air cells

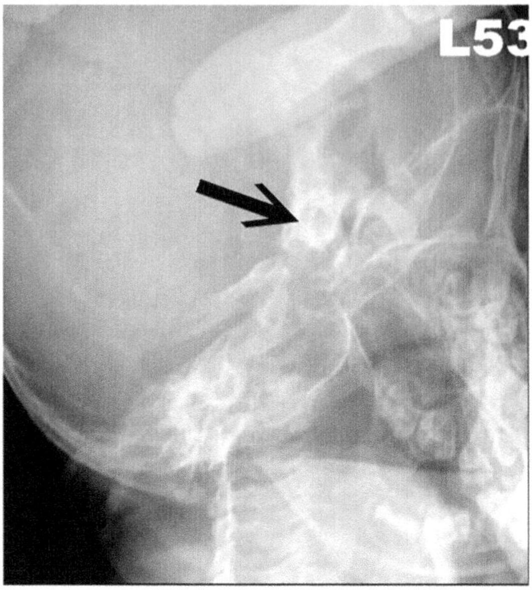

Fig. 3 Schuller view of left mastoid area. The arrow indicates haziness of left mastoid air cells

Discussion

Acute mastoiditis is the infection of the mastoid process of the temporal bone and is a frequently overlooked complication of acute otitis media. Prior to the antibiotic era, mastoiditis may be found in up to 20% of cases of acute otitis media. Extension of the infectious process beyond the mastoid system can lead to a variety of intracranial and extracranial complications, including meningitis; epidural, subdural, and brain abscesses; vascular thrombosis; osteomyelitis; and deep neck abscess. With the advent of antibiotics, cases of acute mastoiditis can still be seen in pediatric patients. Contemporary reports describe an increasing predisposition for younger children to become afflicted by acute mastoiditis, and a rise in hospital admission for pediatric acute mastoiditis cases. The emergence of antimicrobial resistance and the masking of clinical signs by prior antibiotic therapy are possible underlying reasons.

Patients with mastoiditis classically present with the triad of otalgia, auricular proptosis, and a bulging, erythematous tympanic membrane. A meta-analysis of acute mastoiditis showed that the most commonly observed physical findings included (1) postauricular reddish swelling with tenderness; (2) abnormal tympanic membrane findings, including erythema, dullness, and bulging; and (3) external auditory canal edema or sagging. However, most symptoms are nonspecific, including fever, lethargy, irritability, and poor feeding. No consensus exists on the exact diagnostic criteria of acute mastoiditis. The most commonly used diagnostic criteria are a recent episode of otitis media with at least two of the following symptoms: protrusion of the pinna, retroauricular swelling, retroauricular erythema, retroauricular tenderness, or abscess of the external auditory canal; or an intraoperative finding of acute mastoiditis (purulent secretion or acute infection in the mastoid process).

Obvious signs such as a postauricular reddish tender swelling may prompt a tentative diagnosis of mastoiditis (Fig. 4). In the absence of such obvious findings, a diagnosis of mastoiditis may be missed. As illustrated by the present case, the diagnosis of mastoiditis was suspected due to a partial treatment response with persistent ear discharge, while the antibiotic used was effective against the *H. influenzae* isolated from ear discharge.

"Silent mastoiditis" and "masked mastoiditis/latent mastoiditis" are used to describe mastoiditis that lacks typical manifestations of mastoiditis. Silent mastoiditis occurs when antibiotic therapy affords transient relief of clinical mastoid symptoms, while middle ear inflammation continues in a silent manner. Masked/latent mastoiditis, usually chronic or recurrent, is an indolent, smoldering temporal bone infection with few clinical clues, owing to the previous use of broad-spectrum antibiotics. In classic masked/latent mastoiditis, the tympanic membrane is intact and the middle ear shows no abnormalities at otoscopy, probably related to attic blockade and anaerobic infection. An important point is that a normal tympanic membrane usually, but not always, excludes acute mastoiditis. The most important diagnostic clue for mastoiditis in the present case was persistent ear discharge after appropriate antibiotic therapy. The clinical picture is consistent with silent mastoiditis.

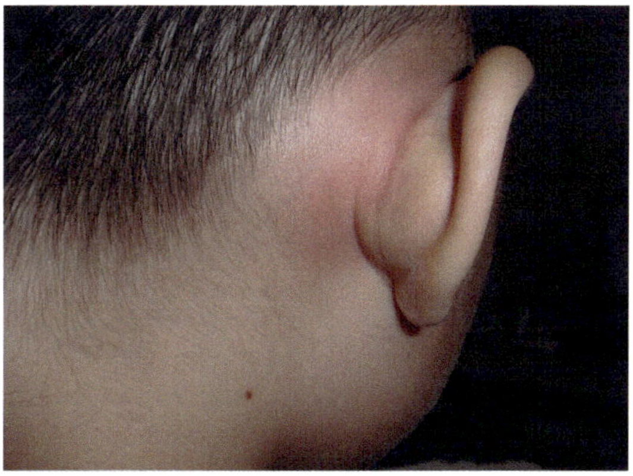

Fig. 4 Postauricular reddish tender swelling in an 8-year-old body with mastoiditis

The presence of mastoiditis has to be confirmed by image studies. Plain mastoid radiographs (Schuller view) are only marginally helpful in confirming the clinical diagnosis in most cases. However, nearly totally opacified mastoid air cells in present case can still support the diagnosis of bilateral mastoiditis. Computed tomography has traditionally been the initial imaging technique for mastoiditis and is efficient in evaluating bony structures. Magnetic resonance imaging is superior in evaluating soft tissues and intracranial structures that may be important in cases with suspected intracranial complication of mastoiditis.

Bacterial isolates from myringotomy or mastoidectomy specimens in patients with mastoiditis most frequently grow *Streptococcus pneumoniae*, Group A streptococcus, *Staphylococcus aureus*, *H. influenzae*, *Moraxella catarrhalis*, and *Pseudomonas aeruginosa*. An important diagnostic clue for the offending pathogen in the present case is the presence of bilateral eye discharge for 7 days. The link between *H. influenzae* conjunctivitis and otitis media has been known as conjunctivitis–otitis media syndrome that may also be linked to paranasal sinusitis. The pathogenic role of *H. influenzae* in present case is evidenced by the growth of *H. influenzae* in culture from both ear discharge and eye discharge.

Increasing prevalence of β-lactamase-producing *H. influenzae* strains are noted worldwide. Studies have reported percentages of β-lactamase-positive *H. influenzae* between 10% and 25% in most regions, including South Africa, Europe, the USA, Canada, Central America, and South America. In some regions, including Taiwan, Vietnam, Japan, and South Korea, β-lactamase-positive strains account for up to 55% of *H. influenzae* with a high prevalence of β-lactamase-negative ampicillin-resistant strains and β–lactamase–positive–amoxicillin–clavulanate resistant strains. Because of the possible etiological role of *H. influenzae* in present case, empiric antibiotics stable against β–lactamase should be used instead of amoxicillin.

Further Reading

Loh R, Phua M, Shaw CKL. Management of paediatric acute mastoiditis: systematic review. J Laryngol Otol 2018;132:96-104.

Laulajainen-Hongisto A, Aarnisalo AA, Jero J. Differentiating acute otitis media and acute mastoiditis in hospitalized children. Curr Allergy Asthma Rep 2016;16:72.

Lin HW, Shargorodsky J, Gopen Q. Clinical strategies for the management of acute mastoiditis in the pediatric population. Clin Pediatr (Phila) 2010;49:110-5.

Eugene Leibovitz. Complicated otitis media and its implications. Vaccine 2008; 23(Suppl 7):G16-9.

van den Aardweg MTA, Rovers MM, de Ru JA, Albers FWJ, Schilder AGM. A systematic review of diagnostic criteria for acute mastoiditis in children. Otol Neurotol 2008;29:751-7.

Mather M, Powell S, Yates PD, Powell J. Acute mastoiditis in children: contemporary opportunities and challenges. J Laryngol Otol 2020;134:434-9.

Tsai TC, Yu PM, Tang RB, Wang HK, Chang KC. Otorrhea as a sign of medical treatment failure in acute otitis media: two cases with silent mastoiditis complicated with facial palsy. Pediatr Neonatol 2013;54:335-8.

Spratley J, Silveira H, Alvarez I, Pais-Clemente M. Acute mastoiditis in children: review of the current status. Int J Pediatr Otorhinolaryngol 2000;56:33-40.

Vazquez E, Castellote A, Piqueras J, et al. Imaging of complications of acute mastoiditis in children. Radiographics 2003;23:359-72.

Goycoolea MV, Castro M, Galvez M, Montoya C, Fuentes J, Silva-Pinto V. Otitis media and mastoiditis in temporal bones of prehistoric Chilean populations. A paleopathological and paleoepidemiological study. Acta Otolaryngol 2019;139:340-4.

Hu YL, Lee PI, Hsueh PR, et al. Predominant role of *Haemophilus influenzae* in the association of conjunctivitis, acute otitis media and acute bacterial paranasal sinusitis in children. Sci Rep 2021;11:11.

Bingen E, Cohen R, Jourenkova N, Gehanno P. Epidemiologic study of conjunctivitis-otitis syndrome. Pediatr Infect Dis J 2005; 24: 731-2.

Cho YC, Chiu NC, Huang FY. et al. Epidemiology and antimicrobial susceptibility of non-typeable *Haemophilus influenzae* in otitis media in Taiwanese children. J Microbiol Immunol Infect 2019;52:75-80.

Case 13. A 3-Year-9-Month-Old Girl with Painful Swelling Over Left Face for 1 Week: Acute Parotitis

Chih-Ho Chen

Keywords

Parotitis · Children · Suppurative parotitis · Abscess · Mumps · Viral parotitis

Key Points

- Predisposed by some conditions and caused by a variety of infectious and noninfectious causes.
- Suppurative parotitis is characterized by acute- or subacute-onset, tender, and warm erythematous swelling with fluctuation.
- Suppurative parotitis, caused by aerobes and anaerobes, occurs mostly in neonates, immunocompromised, and debilitated children.
- Mumps, the most common cause, is confirmed by mumps IgM and RT-PCR under clinical suspicion.
- Juvenile recurrent parotitis, the second most common cause, is diagnosed based on presentation and exclusion of other causes.

Case Report

A previously healthy 3-year-9-month-old girl presented with a one-week history of pain and swelling on the left side of her face. She did not have fever, cough, or rhinorrhea. She was brought to a local clinic. Oral amoxicillin-clavulanate and prednisolone were administered there, but the response was poor. She was referred to our pediatric emergency department for management.

At the emergency department, she was acutely ill, with a temperature of 36.7 °C, a pulse of 108 per minute, respiratory rate of 20 per minute, and a blood pressure of 120/64 mmHg. On physical examination, 4 × 5 cm firm tender erythematous swelling with central fluctuation over left preauricular area was noted. No contact history was found. Laboratory studies were remarkable for white blood cell count of 14,300/mm^3 (segmented neutrophils 76.8%) and a C-reactive protein level of 23.7 mg/L (normal, <5 mg/L). Chest radiography showed no active lung lesion. Under the impression of presumed acute parotitis, she was admitted for further management.

After admission, intravenous amoxicillin-clavulanate was initiated. On hospital day 3, sonography of neck revealed that a 2.2 × 1.7 × 2.0 cm hypoechoic lesion over left parotid gland without flow signal compared with unremarkable right parotid gland. On the same day, incision and aspirational drainage was performed extraorally. Aspirated pus was sent for aerobe, anaerobe, and fungal culture. After aspi-

C.-H. Chen (✉)
Division of Pediatric Infectious Diseases, Department of Pediatrics, Kaohsiung Chang Gung Memorial Hospital, and Chang Gung University College of Medicine, Kaohsiung, Taiwan

Y.-C. Huang et al. (eds.), *Paediatric Infectious Diseases*,
https://doi.org/10.1007/978-981-19-7276-8_13

rational drainage, her left preauricular swelling declined in size and became softer. Culture of the parotid gland aspirate yielded Viridans streptococcus, *Prevotella melaninogenica*, and *Prevotella nanceiensis*. The susceptibility test showed that both *P. melaninogenica* and *P. nanceiensis* isolates were susceptible to ampicillin/sulbactam, clindamycin, and metronidazole, but nonsusceptible to penicillin and piperacillin. On hospital day 7, a second aspirational drainage was performed. On the same day, laboratory tests were remarkable for an amylase level of 453 U/L (normal range 28–100), a white blood cell count of 8300/mm^3, and a C-reactive protein level of 1.3 mg/L. No fungus was identified on fungal culture. After a 10-day course of intravenous amoxicillin-clavulanate, her the lesion declined in size to 3 × 3 cm. She was discharged with oral antibiotics on hospital day 12.

At follow-up outpatient clinics, oral amoxicillin-clavulanate was administered continuously. Her left preauricular swelling improved gradually. Laboratory studies showed an amylase level of 163 U/L (normal range 28–100), and a white blood cell count of 6600/mm^3 (normal range 6700–11,800). After a 21-day course of oral amoxicillin-clavulanate, her left preauricular swelling declined to 1.5 × 1.5 cm. There was no more erythema or tenderness over her left face.

Discussion

Parotid glands are located anteroinferior to ears and consist of superficial and deep lobes, which the facial nerve passes through. Saliva is secreted through parotid duct (Stensen duct) into the mouth. The opening of the Stensen duct is located opposite the maxillary second molar. Parotitis, inflammation of parotid glands, is characterized by swelling of parotid glands that obscure the mandibular angle. Dehydration, medication or disease-related xerostomia (dry mouth), and Stensen duct obstruction could predispose to parotitis. Salivary stasis, caused by ductal ectasia, inflammation, stone, and stricture, facilitates retrograde migration of oral bacteria and increases the risk of infection. Acute parotitis can be caused by a variety of causes, which are generally categorized into infectious and noninfectious causes. Infectious causes include aerobes, anaerobes, viruses, and mycobacteria. Noninfectious causes include Sjögren syndrome, salivary stones, radiation, iodine, tumor, trauma, juvenile recurrent parotitis, and bulimia nervosa.

Acute parotitis is often diagnosed clinically. Detailed history taking and physical examination could help identify the possible causes. History includes systemic diseases, medications use, radiation or iodine exposure, dental procedures, and vaccination history should be inquired into. Parotid glands could be examined by gentle massage intraorally and extraorally. Suppurative discharge from the Stensen duct and surrounding erythema may be checked. Gram stain and culture of discharge from the Stensen duct could provide microbiological evidence. Leukocytosis and neutrophil predominance could differentiate bacterial suppurative parotitis from viral parotitis and noninfectious parotitis. A serum amylase level may be elevated. Sonography could be arranged to screen ductal stones and abscess formation. Computed tomography is used to identify the anatomical abnormalities, radiolucent stones, or abscess formation. X-ray sialography is the gold-standard method to identify the abnormalities of the Stensen duct. However, X-ray sialography is contraindicated in acute infection. By contrast, magnetic resonance sialography is not contraindicated in acute infection and does not need manipulation of the Stensen duct.

Suppurative parotitis occurs mostly in neonates, immunocompromised, and debilitated children. Dehydration, xerostomia, trauma, and salivary stasis predispose subjects to suppurative bacterial infection. Suppurative parotitis is usually unilateral, but bilateral suppurative parotitis has been reported in 17% of cases. It usually presents with acute- or subacute-onset, tender, and warm erythematous swelling of parotid glands with fluctuation. Accompanied manifestations include fever, trismus, dysphagia, malaise, and purulent discharge from the Stensen duct. Generally, the pathogens responsible for bacterial parotitis are the flora in the oral cavity. The common bacteria identified include *Staphylococcus aureus*,

Streptococcus pneumoniae, *Streptococcus pyogenes*, Viridans streptococci, and gram-negative bacilli. Anaerobic bacteria, including *Peptostreptococcus*, *Prevotella*, *Fusobacterium*, and *Actinomyces*, were rarely identified pathogens in suppurative parotitis. Most suppurative parotitis could be treated with antibiotics and/or surgical drainage successfully. Without prompt treatment, suppurative parotitis can lead to parapharyngeal abscess, airway compression, osteomyelitis, facial palsy, and fistula formation.

Even in the vaccine era, mumps is still the most common cause of acute parotitis. In Taiwan, children aged 5–6 years have the highest incidence of mumps, while adults aged ≥20 years have the lowest incidence. Mumps is characterized by a low-grade fever, myalgia, and headache, followed by bilateral parotid glands swelling. Laboratory testing may reveal leukopenia, relative lymphocytosis, and an elevated serum amylase level. The diagnosis may be made by the detection of mumps immunoglobulin M and reverse-transcription polymerase chain reaction. Mumps is usually self-limited. Most patients' parotitis resolve within 1 week without complications. Some patients may develop orchitis or oophoritis a few days later. Those without full vaccination have a higher risk of complications and hospitalization. Other causative viruses, including coxsackievirus, Epstein-Barr virus, parainfluenza virus, human herpes virus 6, and human immunodeficiency virus may also cause parotitis.

Juvenile recurrent parotitis (JRP) is the second most common cause of parotitis in children. JRP usually occurs in children aged 3–6 years. The etiology of JRP remains unclear. It is thought to be caused by inflammation of the parotid gland and duct, leading to impaired salivary flow. It is characterized by recurrent episodes of acute parotitis without abscess formation. Clinical manifestations include unilateral or alternatively bilateral parotid gland swelling, pain, and fever. Flares usually resolve within 1 week. The diagnosis is usually established based on clinical presentation and exclusion of other causes. The treatment for JRP is mainly conservative. Conservative approaches include pain control, the use of sialagogic agents such as lemon juice and chewing gum, massage, and mouth rinses. Antibiotics are sometimes used during acute flares to prevent secondary bacterial infection and scar formation of parotid gland. Although some studies suggested that sialography and sialendoscopic dilatation may reduce recurrent episodes (Papadopoulou-Alataki et al. 2019). However, sialendoscopy is often performed under general anesthesia in children. No randomized controlled studies have demonstrated the effectiveness of these treatment options yet. Most cases of JRP resolve by puberty.

Further Reading

Wilson M, Pandey S. Parotitis. In: StatPearls. Treasure Island (FL): StatPearls Publishing; August 11, 2021.

Al-Dajani N, Wootton SH. Cervical lymphadenitis, suppurative parotitis, thyroiditis, and infected cysts. Infect Dis Clin North Am. 2007;21:523-viii.

Abu-Taleb NSM, Abdel-Wahed N, Amer ME. The Role of Magnetic Resonance Imaging and Magnetic Resonance Sialography in the Diagnosis of Various Salivary Gland Disorders: An Interobserver Agreement. J Med Imaging Radiat Sci. 2014;45:299-306.

Mori T, Shimomura R, Ito T, et al. Neonatal suppurative parotitis: Case reports and literature review. Pediatr Int. 2022; 64:e14762

Ismail EA, Seoudi TM, Al-Amir M, Al-Esnawy AA. Neonatal suppurative parotitis over the last 4 decades: report of three new cases and review. Pediatr Int. 2013;55:60-64.

Srivanitchapoom C, Yata K. Clinical characteristics that predict parotid abscess: An observational cohort study. Ann Med Surg (Lond). 2021;64:102230.

Chen CC, Lu CC, Su BH, Chen KT. Epidemiologic features of mumps in Taiwan from 2006 to 2011: a new challenge for public health policy. World J Pediatr. 2015;11:141-147.

Davidkin I, Jokinen S, Paananen A, Leinikki P, Peltola H. Etiology of mumps-like illnesses in children and adolescents vaccinated for measles, mumps, and rubella. J Infect Dis. 2005;191:719-723.

Wood J, Toll EC, Hall F, Mahadevan M. Juvenile recurrent parotitis: Review and proposed management algorithm. Int J Pediatr Otorhinolaryngol. 2021;142:110617.

Papadopoulou-Alataki E, Dogantzis P, Chatziavramidis A, et al. Juvenile Recurrent Parotitis: The Role of Sialendoscopy. Int J Inflam. 2019;2019:7278907.

Case 14. A 5-Year-Old Boy with Fever, Sore Throat, Odynophagia, and Torticollis: Deep Neck Infection

Ming-Ru Lin and Yhu-Chering Huang

Keywords

Group A streptococcus · Deep neck infection

Key Points

- Deep neck infection can lead to life-threatening complications, including airway compromise, jugular vein thrombosis, and mediastinal extension.
- Fever, local swelling, or mass and limited rotation of the neck are the most common presentations of pediatric deep neck infection.
- Most cases of deep neck infection are caused by polymicrobials.
- Head and neck computed tomography image study can be considered in children with a suspicion of deep neck infection.
- Surgical drainage may be indicated in patients with unresponsiveness to antibiotic therapy or complications.

M.-R. Lin (✉)
Division of General and Emergency Medicine, Department of Pediatrics, Linkou Chang Gung Memorial Hospital, Taoyuan, Taiwan

Y.-C. Huang
Pediatrics, Chang Gung Memorial Hospital, Chang Gung University, Taoyuan, Taiwan
e-mail: ychuang@cgmh.org.tw

Case Report

A 5-year-11-month-old boy was generally healthy without underlying chronic disease and received vaccination as scheduled. He experienced fever off and on for 3 days and visited the pediatric emergency department of a medical center. He suffered from sore throat, odynophagia, and torticollis (unable to rotate his neck to the left side due to pain) these days. On physical examination, his head tilted to the right with mild local tenderness on the left side of his neck. Injected throat without enlargement or exudates of both tonsils was found. Other physical examinations were essentially negative. A throat swab for rapid antigen test for group A Streptococcus was done and revealed a positive result. Initial laboratory data showed WBC 22900/μL (segmented 91.5%, lymphocytes 4%, monocytes 4.5%), platelet count 326,000/μL, hemoglobin (Hb) 11.6 g/dL, and C-reactive protein (CRP) 178.3 mg/L (normal, <5 mg/L). A plain film of lateral view of C-spine was taken and showed widening of pre-vertebral space (near 1.5 times to the length of the vertebral body) from C2 to C5 (Fig. 1a). Due to suspected deep neck infection, a computed tomography (CT) scan with contrast enhancement of head and neck was done and disclosed bilateral multiple cervical lymphadenitis with abscess formation at left side retropharyngeal region over naso-to-oro-pharynx level (Fig. 2). Intravenous amoxicillin-clavulanic acid was administered empirically for

Y.-C. Huang et al. (eds.), *Paediatric Infectious Diseases*,
https://doi.org/10.1007/978-981-19-7276-8_14

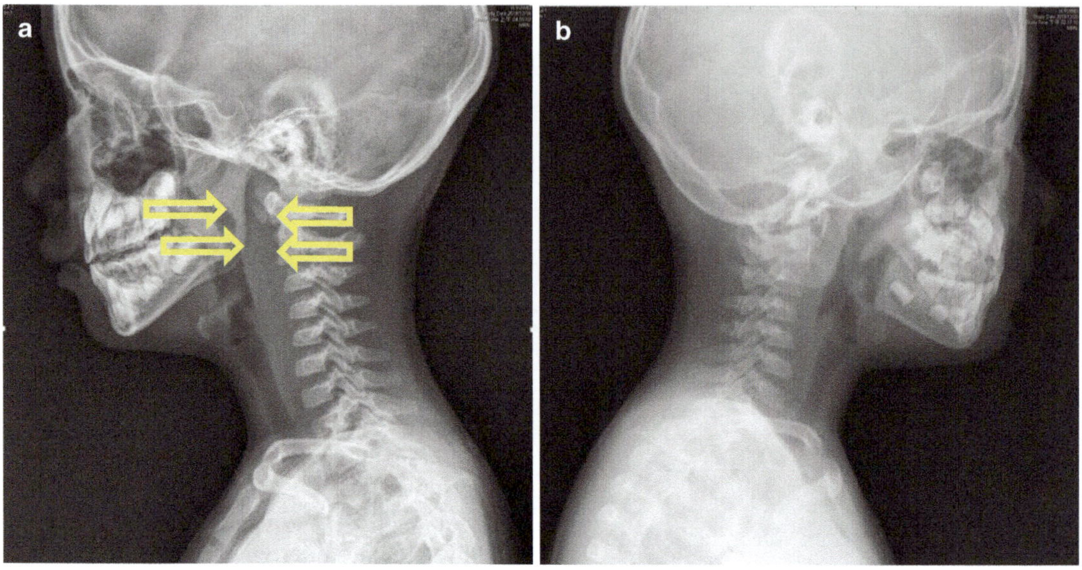

Fig. 1 C-spine plain films showed widening of pre-vertebral space (approximately 1.5 times to the length of the vertebral body, arrows) from C2 to C5 on admission (**a**) and no more widening of prevertebral space after treatment (**b**)

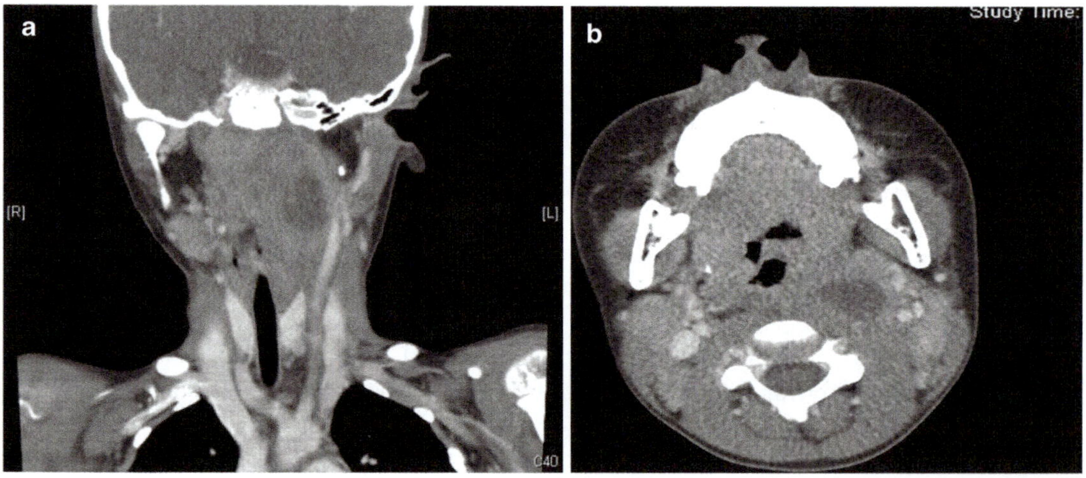

Fig. 2 Head and neck CT scan showed cervical lymphadenitis, bilateral with abscess formation at left side retropharyngeal region of naso- and oropharynx level in coronal plane (**a**) and axial plane (**b**)

covering anaerobes of oral cavity in addition to group A Streptococcus. Intravenous teicoplanin was added on hospital day 3 for coverage of possible methicillin-resistant *S. aureus* infection due to persistent pain and fever. His fever gradually subsided accompanied with improvement on range of motion of his neck. No more widening of prevertebral space was noted by plain film on hospital day 5 (Fig. 1b). Blood culture obtained on admission showed negative result. He was discharged on hospital day 8. Oral amoxicillin-clavulanic acid was given for additional 6 days to complete the treatment. He recovered uneventfully.

Discussion

Despite an uncommon disease in children, deep neck space infection (DNI) can lead to life-threatening complications, including airway obstruction, jugular vein thrombosis, and mediastinal involvement in a rapid progress. Timely diagnosis of DNI is important to improve clinical outcome. However, early diagnosis of DNI in children remains a challenge for physicians due to its subtle initial clinical presentations. Moreover, children usually poorly cooperate during physical examination, and they often describe their symptoms ineffectively, which may lead physicians to make other diagnoses such as tonsillitis, viral pharyngitis, and lymphadenitis. Fever, local swelling or mass, and limited rotation of the neck are the most common presentations of pediatric DNI and clinical physicians should always take DNI into consideration, regardless of the age of patients. Like in adults, preceding upper respiratory tract infection (tonsillitis, sinusitis), odontogenic infection, and congenital anomalies (such as bronchogenic cyst) are the leading causes of DNI in children. Nevertheless, a congenital cyst with secondary infection more frequently occurs in children and tends to be recurrent and subsequently require surgical intervention if identified. The recurrence of DNI should alert the physician to explore the possibility of an underlying structural anomaly such as bronchogenic cyst. Prompt imaging studies are helpful to detect such congenital anomalies early and provide adequate treatment.

According to the sites of involvement, DNI can be categorized as retropharyngeal, parapharyngeal, and peritonsillar abscess. The sites of DNI varied among the different age groups. Retropharyngeal abscess is more likely to be found in children younger than 6 year olds, while peritonsillar abscesses occur more frequently in adolescents. Different sites of DNI involved differ in their clinical manifestations. The most common symptoms of peritonsillar abscess are fever, odynophagia, uvular deviation, or asymmetric tonsillar enlargement. On the other hand, along with fever, neck masses, or nuchal pain, are commonly seen in patients with retropharyngeal and parapharyngeal abscesses.

As shown in the illustrated case, a lateral view of neck radiography may be helpful for the initial evaluation of DNI, but a CT scan examination of head and neck, which provides detailed anatomical information and is helpful for surgical planning, remains the most widely used modality for diagnosing DNI. Physicians should consider arranging a head and neck CT for the children with a tentative diagnosis of DNI.

Reports from Taiwan disclosed that most cases of DNI were caused by polymicrobials. The common pathogens identified from pus cultures included *Streptococcus pyogenes* (Group A Streptococcus), *Viridans streptococci*, *Escherichia coli*, *Klebsiella pneumoniae*, coagulase-negative *Staphylococci*, and oropharyngeal anaerobic bacteria. Therefore, empirical antibiotics for DNI should cover both Gram-positive, Gram-negative, and anaerobic pathogens. We suggest amoxicillin-clavulanic acid alone, or third generation of cephalosporins, either alone or in combination with metronidazole, as first-line treatment. Some studies suggest further coverage for methicillin-resistant Staphylococcus aureus (MRSA) because of an increased risk of MRSA infection in DNI, especially in children younger than 2 years of age.

Surgical intervention is not necessary for patients who respond well to medical treatment. Surgical drainage should be reserved for patients with airway compromise, poor response to antibiotic treatment, or patients who are immunosuppressed, or suffer from DNI complications.

Further Reading

Coticchia JM, Getnick GS, Yun RD, Arnold JE. Age-, site-, and time-specific differences in pediatric deep neck abscesses. Arch Otolaryngol Head Neck Surg 2004;130:201-7.

Meier JD, Grimmer JF. Evaluation and management of neck masses in children. Am Fam Physician 2014;89:353-8.

Huang CM, Huang FL, Chien YL, Chen PY. Deep neck infections in children. J Microbiol Immunol Infect. 2017;50:627-633.

Chang L, Chi H, Chiu NC, Huang FY, Lee KS. Deep neck infections in different age groups of children. J Microbiol Immunol Infect 2010;43:47-52.

Grisaru-Soen G, Komisar O, Aizenstein O, Soudack M, chwartz D, Paret G. Retropharyngeal and parapharyngeal abscess in children epidemiology, clinical features and treatment. Int J Pediatr Otorhinolaryngol 2010;74:1016-20

Tan PT, Chang LY, Huang YC, Chiu CH, Wang CR, Lin TY. Deep neck infections in children. J Microbiol Immunol Infect. 2001;34:287-92

Yen CW, Lin CY, Tsao LY, Yang SC, Chen HN, Chang MY. Children's deep neck infections in central Taiwan. Acta Paediatr Taiwan 2007;48:15-9

Millar KR, Johnson DW, Drummond D, Kellner JD. Suspected peritonsillar abscess in children. Pediatr Emerg Care 2007;23: 431-8.

Nagy M, Backstrom J. Comparison of the sensitivity of lateral neck radiographs and computed tomography scanning in pediatric deep-neck infections. *Laryngoscope* 1999;109:775-9.

Meyer AC, Kimbrough TG, Finkelstein M, Sidman JD. Symptom duration and CT findings in pediatric deep neck infection. *Otolaryngol Head Neck Surg* 2009;140:183-6.

Naidu SI, Donepudi SK, Stocks RM, Buckingham SC, Thompson JW. Methicillin-resistant *Staphylococcus aureus* as a pathogen in deep neck abscesses: a pediatric case series. Int J Pediatr Otorhinolaryngol 2005;69:1367-71.

Abdel-Haq N, Quezada M, Asmar BI. Retropharyngeal abscess in children: the rising incidence of methicillin-resistant *Staphylococcus aureus*. Pediatr Infect Dis J 2012;31:696-9.

Bolton M, Wang W, Hahn A, Ramilo O, Mejias A, Jaggi P. Predictors for successful treatment of pediatric deep neck infections using antimicrobials alone. Pediatr Infect Dis J 2013; 32:1034-6.

Osborn TM, Assael LA, Bell RB. Deep space neck infection: Principles of surgical management. *Oral Maxillofac Surg Clin North Am* 2008;20:353-65.

Case 15. A 5-Year-Old Boy with Fever and a Painful Enlarging Erythematous Left Neck Mass: Pyriform Sinus Fistula with Infection

Kuan-Ta Ho and Yhu-Chering Huang

Keywords

Pyriform sinus fistula · Congenital anomaly · Recurrent left neck pyogenic infection · Surgical intervention

Key Points

- Common clinical presentation is recurrent neck mass, repeated episode of infection and suppurative thyroiditis (mostly on the left-sided).
- Being a congenital abnormality of the third or fourth branchial pouch.
- Diagnostic examinations include computed tomography, magnetic resonance imaging, barium esophagography and intra-operative dye injection.
- Treatments are antimicrobial agents, aspiration, incision, and drainage.
- Surgical intervention should be considered.

K.-T. Ho (✉)
Division of Pediatric Infectious Diseases, Department of Pediatrics, Chang Gung Memorial Hospital, Taoyuan, Taiwan

Department of Pediatrics, Chang Gung Memorial Hospital, Keelung, Taiwan

Y.-C. Huang
Pediatrics, Chang Gung Memorial Hospital, Chang Gung University, Taoyuan, Taiwan
e-mail: ychuang@cgmh.org.tw

Case Report

A 5-year-6-month-old healthy boy without history of systemic diseases. He received regular vaccination and had normal development milestone. This time, he presented with a left neck mass for more than 10 days. The mass was enlarging with local erythematous change, swelling, warm sensation, and tenderness. Other associated symptoms included intermittent fever (starting from more than 10 days prior to the appearance of neck mass till 5 days ago, up to 38.5 °C), left ear pain, and mild cough for weeks. There is no dysphagia, shortness of breath, drooling, vomiting, sore throat, abdominal pain, or skin rash. His spirit and appetite were as usual. None of his family members had similar symptoms. He was brought to local clinic and our otolaryngology outpatient department for help, and received oral Augmentin for 10 days. Due to a poor therapeutic response, he was referred to our emergency department for further evaluation and treatment.

At our emergency department, the boy appeared ill-looking. The vital signs were body temperature 37.3 °C, pulse rate 102/min, respira-

Y.-C. Huang et al. (eds.), *Paediatric Infectious Diseases*,
https://doi.org/10.1007/978-981-19-7276-8_15

tory rate 22/min, and blood pressure 107/68 mmHg. Physical examination showed a left neck mass about 2.5 cm × 2.5 cm with unclear boundary, erythematous change of overlying skin, local tenderness, warm sensation and limited rotation of the neck. Besides, he had mildly injected throat, non-enlarged tonsil without exudate, and clear bilateral breath sound. Initial hemogram and biochemistry profile revealed leukocytosis (white blood cell: 12,700/μL) with elevated serum CRP (34 mg/L). The plain chest film showed no active lung lesion or airway deviation. Under the tentative diagnosis of deep neck infection, head and neck computed tomography (CT) scan was arranged and revealed a 2.9 × 2.6 × 2.3 cm irregular rim-enhancing fluid collection in the left neck abutting the left thyroid gland (Fig. 1). A pyriform sinus fistula-related infection with abscess formation was suggested by this image. He was then admitted to our general pediatric ward.

After admission, empiric antibiotics with intravenous amoxicillin-clavulanate (100 mg/kg/day based on amoxicillin component) was given. However, neck swelling with limited range of motion and local tenderness did not improve after 3 days of intravenous amoxicillin-clavulanate therapy. Echo-guided aspiration of the abscess with drainage was performed. His clinical condition improved gradually. There was no more fever, neck swelling, local skin erythematous change, tenderness, and limited range of motion of neck. No pathogen was identified by bacterial culture of the aspirate. Surgical management of pyriform sinus fistula was suggested. However, the parents preferred conservative therapy. Thus, the patient was discharged with a final diagnosis of pyriform sinus fistula-related left neck abscess.

Nine months later, he was hospitalized for the second episode of left neck swelling. The symptoms were almost identical to the first episode, including left neck mass, local erythematous change, swelling, and tenderness. There was no fever this time. Head and neck CT scan revealed a similar picture as previous one (Fig. 2). After echo-guided aspiration and antibiotics treatment, he was discharged after 7 days of hospitalization course. The diagnosis was left pyriform sinus fistula with recurrence of secondary bacterial infection.

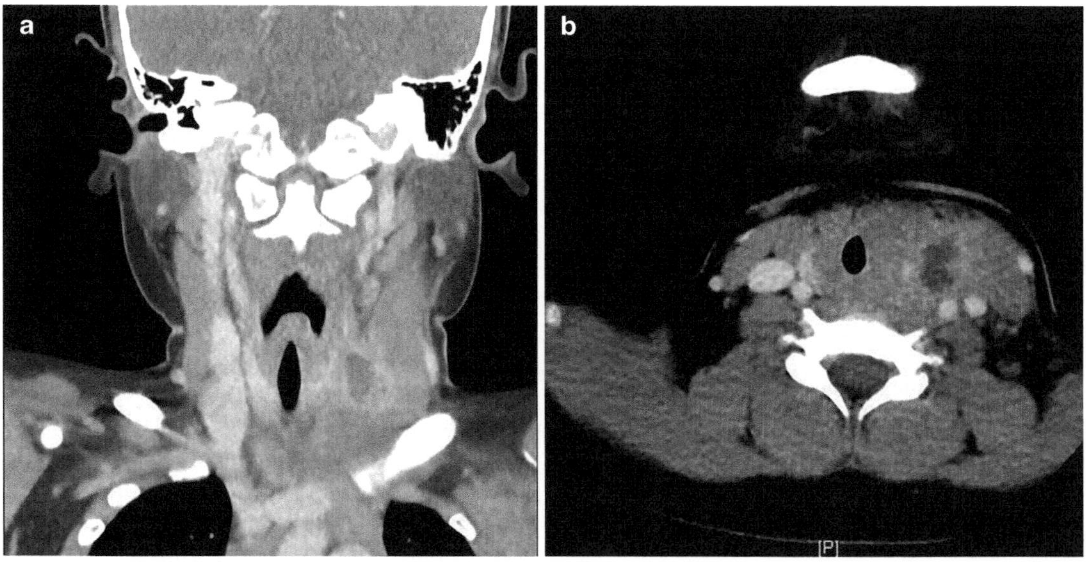

Fig. 1 Head and neck CT scan for the first episode revealed a 2.9 × 2.6 × 2.3 cm irregular rim-enhancing fluid collection in the left neck abutting the left thyroid gland in coronal plane (**a**) and axial plane (**b**)

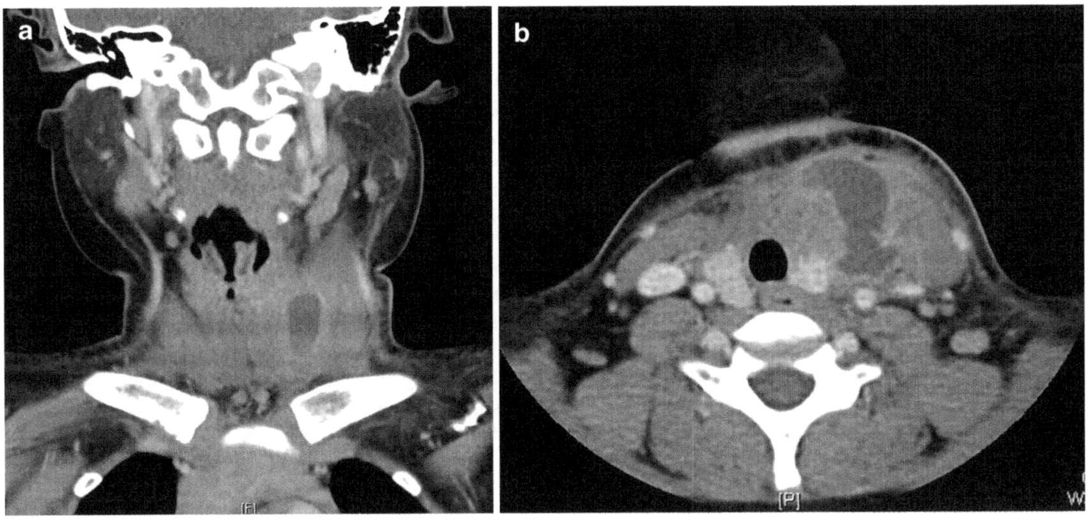

Fig. 2 Head and neck CT scan for the second episode revealed an irregular rim-enhancing fluid collection in the left neck abutting the left thyroid gland in coronal plane (**a**) and axial plane (**b**)

Discussion

Congenital brachial abnormality is an important differential diagnosis of head and neck tumors or recurrent deep neck infection in childhood. The congenital brachial malformation results from a failure to regress or to develop normally during embryogenesis. Various forms of branchial remnants include fistulae, cysts, sinus tracts, and cartilaginous formation. Although these lesions have been present since birth, most of these abnormalities remain asymptomatic until later in life when the first infection episode is encountered. A delay in early diagnosis of congenital brachial malformation may result in recurrent infections with significant morbidities.

The pyriform sinus fistula is recognized as a type of branchial anomaly, which is always located at left side and arise from a failed obliteration of the third or fourth pharyngeal pouches during embryogenesis. Males and females are affected equally. The clinical presentations of pyriform sinus fistula include fever, local erythematous change, unilateral neck swelling (almost always left-sided), local warm sensation, pain, dysphagia, respiratory distress, recurrent acute suppurative thyroiditis, retropharyngeal abscess, and peri-thyroid abscess formation. According to a previous retrospective study by Sheng et al., neck abscess (78.8%), acute thyroiditis (11.4%), neck mass (6.9%), and thyroid lesion (2.8%) were the initial presentations in children with pyriform sinus fistula. As shown in the illustrated case, repeated left neck infectious episodes with abscess formation is the most common and typical mode of presentation.

When a child has repeated episodes of neck infection, we should be alert to arrange necessary image studies to evaluate possible congenital structural abnormality, especially pyriform sinus fistula, particularly when the infection always occurs at left side. There are several diagnostic tools for the detection of pyriform sinus fistula, including CT scan, magnetic resonance imaging, barium esophagography, and intra-operative dye injection. The manifestations on CT scan are sinus tract extending from the pyriform sinus apex through the strap muscle layer to the thyroid or peri-thyroid tissue with abnormal soft tissue swelling, enhancement and/or abscess formation. Barium esophagography may reveal proximal portion of the sinus or fistulous tract, extending from the apex of the pyriform sinus. An accurate imaging diagnosis would facilitate the decision for a complete resection of the fistula and preventing recurrent infections.

The treatment strategy for pyriform sinus fistula can be divided into two steps that include acute infection control and definite surgical resection. Antibiotic treatment is the first line of therapy at acute infectious stage for infection control. Empiric antibiotics should be active against common colonizing bacteria of the mouth. The most common offending organism is α-hemolytic streptococci and *Staphylococcus aureus* followed by gram-negative organisms and anaerobic bacteria. Other pathogens including mycobacteria, fungi, and pneumocystis cause more indolent infection and occur mostly in immunocompromised patients.

Recurrent episodes or detection of mixed bacterial flora suggests that the infection arises from a fistula. Echography/CT guided aspiration with or without tube drainage is helpful for management of patients with massive abscess formation or with a poor therapeutic response to antibiotics. Incision and drainage should be reserved for emergent conditions, e.g., respiratory distress with compromised airway. This is because the incision and drainage procedure may destroy local tissues and result in post-surgery-related tissue adhesion, which makes a subsequent surgery more difficult for a complete fistula excision. The definitive treatment of pyriform sinus fistula remnants is complete surgical excision, because the abnormal structure will not resolve spontaneously. If left unresected or incompletely resected, there is a high risk of recurrent infections. There is not a consensus for the optimum timing for surgical excision. In general, surgical excision may be performed at non-infectious stage.

Further Reading

Waldhausen JH. Branchial cleft and arch anomalies in children. Semin Pediatr Surg. 2006;15:64-9.

Sheng Q, Lv Z, Xu W, Liu J. Differences in the diagnosis and management of pyriform sinus fistula between newborns and children. Sci Rep. 2019 6;9:18497.

Amano H, Uchida H, Sato K, Kawashima H, Tanaka Y, Takazawa S, Jimbo T. Differences in the characteristics and management of pyriform sinus fistula between neonates and young children. Pediatr Surg Int. 2012;28:15-20.

Sheng Q, Lv Z, Xiao X, Zheng S, Huang Y, Huang X, et al. Diagnosis and management of pyriform sinus fistula: experience in 48 cases. J Pediatr Surg. 2014;49:455-9.

Sheng Q, Lv Z, Xu W, Liu J. Reoperation for Pyriform Sinus Fistula in Pediatric Patients. Front Pediatr. 2020; 8:116.

Smith JR, Wassner AJ. Thyroiditis. In: Kliegman RM, St Geme JW, Blum NJ, et al. eds. Nelson Textbook of Pediatrics, 21th edition. Philadelphia: Churchill Livingstone, 2020.

Chen T, Ge G, Chen J, Zhao X, Sheng Q, Zhu L, et al. Pyriform Sinus Fistula in Children: Preferred Imaging Modality and Risk Factors for Diagnostic Delay. Front Pediatr 2020;8:575812.

Pan J, Zou Y, Li L, Yang TY, Yang JL, Hu C. Clinical and imaging differences between neonates and children with pyriform sinus fistula: which is preferred for diagnosis, computed tomography, or barium esophagography? J Pediatr Surg 2017; 52:1878-81.

Chi H, Lee YJ, Chiu NC, Huang FY, Huang CY, Lee KS, Shih SL, Shih BF. Acute suppurative thyroiditis in children. Pediatr Infect Dis J. 2002;21:384-7.

Chang P, Tsai WY, Lee PI, Hsiao PH, Huang LM, Lee JS, Peng SF, Li YW. Clinical characteristics and management of acute suppurative thyroiditis in children. J Formos Med Assoc. 2002;101:468-71.

Case 16. A One-Month-Old Infant with Episodic Upward Gaze and Cyanotic Lips in 1 Day Following a 2-Day Cough: Pertussis with Encephalopathy

Chun Yi Lee and Yhu-Chering Huang

Keywords

Pertussis · Seizure · Encephalopathy · Macrolide

Key Points

- Pertussis is a neglected and underdiagnosed disease in Taiwan and in most Asian countries.
- Young infants are most vulnerable to pertussis and prone to develop severe disease such as encephalopathy.
- "Paroxysmal" cough, vomiting during or after coughing and exhaustion following coughing are hallmark characteristics of pertussis.
- High index of suspicion is crucial to the early diagnosis of pertussis and polymerase chain reaction is the mainstream diagnostic method.
- Macrolides (e.g., Azithromycin, clarithromycin, and erythromycin) are the drugs of choice for pertussis.

C. Y. Lee (✉)
Department of Pediatrics, Chang Bing Show Chwan Memorial Hospital, Changhua, Taiwan

Y.-C. Huang
Pediatrics, Chang Gung Memorial Hospital, Chang Gung University, Taoyuan, Taiwan
e-mail: ychuang@cgmh.org.tw

Case Report

A 1-month-old male infant presented to an emergency room at a local hospital for repeated upward gaze and cyanotic lips in 1 day. The baby was born at the gestational age of 38 weeks with a birth weight of 3560 g via Cesarean section. His inborn error screen was negative and he had received two doses of hepatitis B vaccine. He was noted to have intermittent cough in the past 2 days, but no fever was found. Upon visit at ER, his seizure was still ongoing, and his vital signs were body temperature 36 °C, pulse rate 123/min, respiratory rate 23/min, and blood pressure 86/43 mmHg. Physical examinations were unremarkable. He was referred to a medical center for intensive care. The initial laboratory analysis disclosed marked leukocytosis (WBC 42,300/μL, segmented 36.7%, lymphocytes 54.7%, monocytes 8.6%), hemoglobin 12.9 g/dL, and platelet 544,000/μL. The biochemical profiles were hyperglycemia 546 mg/dL, elevated liver transaminases (ALT 374 U/L and AST 751 U/L), high creatine kinase 1224 U/L, C-reactive protein 0.69 mg/dL, and elevated procalcitonin 44.88 ng/mL (normal, <0.1 ng/mL). Otherwise, his renal function, blood electrolytes, and blood gas analysis were within normal limits. His Brain CT scan and chest film were essentially negative.

The baby was admitted to pediatric intensive care unit and intubated on day 1 due to frequent bradycardia and cyanosis. Spinal tapping was done, and cerebrospinal fluid analysis showed

Y.-C. Huang et al. (eds.), *Paediatric Infectious Diseases*,
https://doi.org/10.1007/978-981-19-7276-8_16

WBC 3/μL, RBC 41/μL, protein 262 mg/dL. He received intravenous immunoglobulin under the suspicion of critical enteroviral infection. He also received broad-spectrum antimicrobial therapy. He was extubated and supported by nasal continuous positive pressure on hospital day 4. At this time point, the attending physician noted unexpectedly that the baby had a "paroxysmal-like" cough and any medical maneuver easily induced apnea and desaturation in this baby. We also noted that his mother had cough for 1 month. Hence, we sent his sputum specimen for the detection of *Bordetella pertussis* by polymerase chain reaction (PCR) and started a 5-day course of oral azithromycin therapy for him.

The baby had no more seizure attack while it stayed in the hospital. The PCR tests targeting enterovirus, herpes simplex virus, respiratory syncytial virus, norovirus, and *Mycoplasma pneumoniae* were all negative, while a positive result for *B. pertussis*.

His respiratory symptoms subsided gradually, and he could tolerate ambient air on day 10. After completing additional course of oral trimethoprim-sulfamethoxazole therapy, he was discharged on day 17.

Discussion

Pertussis, or whooping cough, is a major cause of infantile death worldwide before the introduction of pertussis vaccine in the 1980s. Despite the prevalence of pertussis having dropped significantly after vaccine implementation, this disease is still endemic in all countries and can never be eliminated. Besides the naturally occurring cyclic patterns of disease epidemics, there are several factors contributing the spread and resurgence of pertussis: waning of immunity induced by vaccination since the infancy, lack of awareness, and the adaptation of causative pathogen, *Bordetella pertussis*.

Pertussis is a highly contagious respiratory disease. Infants, and young children are particularly at risk of severe and life-threatening disease. The most severe cases and mortality occur mainly in unprotected infants (aged <1 year old) and young children (aged 1–4 years old). One systemic review focusing on neonatal pertussis in South and Southeast Asian countries revealed that the burden of neonatal pertussis and its complications is substantial. An increase in the number of pertussis cases has been noted since early 2000, ranging from 61 to 92.9% in infants aged 0–3 months. The most common symptoms in infants are cough with or without paroxysms, cyanosis, apnea, tachypnea, difficulty in breathing, and leukocytosis. In addition, it can lead to hospitalization (length of stay: 5–7 days), complications (e.g., pneumonia, seizures), and mortality rate ranging from 5.6 to 14.7%. A population-based study from Taiwan disclosed that infants accounted for the highest proportion of all the cases reported to the Taiwan Centers for Diseases Control (49.8%), with a mean incidence of 16.1 cases per 100,000 people per year during 2009–2015. However, pertussis is a neglected and underdiagnosed disease in Taiwan as well as in most Asian countries. A multinational serosurveillance study in Asia indicated that one in 20 adolescents had serologic evidence of recent pertussis infection regardless of vaccination background. Another multinational study also showed that 5.13% of adults with cough lasting >14 days from Taiwan, Thailand, and Malaysia had serological evidence of pertussis infection within the previous 12 months.

The incubation period of pertussis is seven to 10 days. The clinical course of pertussis is typically described as three stages: catarrhal stage (1–2 weeks), paroxysmal stage (3–8 weeks), and convalescent stage (9–12 weeks). The early symptoms in catarrhal stage are indistinguishable from other respiratory infections. Apnea in baby may be an alarming sign of pertussis. However, during this stage, the disease is highly contagious. In the paroxysmal stage, traditional symptoms may appear and compile of paroxysms of many, rapid ("staccato") coughs followed by a high-pitched "whoop" sound; vomiting during or after coughing fits; and exhaustion after coughing fits. Recovery is gradual, and the whole course lasts around 10–12 weeks. Infants, especially those aged 3 months or less, are the highest risk group of developing severe disease.

According to a retrospective case series study from India, 31 out of 36 children requiring intensive care were infants (86.1%). Sixteen of these 31 infants (61.5%) were partially immunized or unimmunized against pertussis. Rapid breathing (88.9%), paroxysmal cough (86.1%), apnea (41.7%), hypoxemia (97.2%), hyperleukocytosis (61.1%), and encephalopathy (52.8%) were common presenting symptoms and signs, as shown in the illustrated case.

Bordetella pertussis contains at least four major virulent factors: pertussis toxin, filamentous hemagglutinin, pertactin, fimbriae types two and three, which are key components of pertussis vaccine. The duration of immunity developing after natural infection has been estimated for 3.5–30 years. Instead, acellular pertussis vaccines have been estimated to confer a shorter duration of immunity than whole cellular pertussis vaccines (4–7 years vs. 5–14 years, respectively). When the immunity to pertussis wanes, breakthrough infection or re-infection is common thereafter. Effectiveness of administering four doses of pertussis vaccine during infancy decreases with time passed since the fourth dose. This regimen does not protect school-aged children against pertussis. Since infants under the age of 6 months do not receive full vaccinations against pertussis, they are vulnerable to contract pertussis, especially from their household members, it is mandatory to intensify pertussis vaccination on pregnant women. However, the acceptance rate was still as low as 29.7% in Taiwan.

Diagnosis of pertussis depends on the awareness and alertness of clinical physicians. *B. pertussis* is a fastidious pathogen, which means this pathogen is not easy to be cultivated. Currently, molecular diagnosis such as PCR is the mainstream diagnostic method, while serologic testing is not standardized or routinely recommended. Of 1152 pediatric severe pneumonia cases, *B. pertussis* were detected from 34 cases by PCR in one study from the Philippines. Treatment should be started as early as possible not only to eradicate the pathogen but also to stop the transmission to close contact. Several antibiotics are available to treat pertussis and include erythromycin, azithromycin, and clarithromycin. Trimethoprim-sulfamethoxazole could be an alternative choice. However, it is worth noting that macrolide resistance has been recognized increasingly in certain countries, including China.

Though the incidence of pertussis markedly decreased due to universal vaccination, outbreaks have been noted worldwide. Pertussis is a neglected and underdiagnosed disease in Taiwan as well as in most Asian countries. With waning of the immunity under the current immunization program, adolescents and young adults are susceptible to *B. pertussis* infection. Young infants are mostly vulnerable to this disease and prone to develop severe complications, even death. High index of suspicion is crucial to the early diagnosis of pertussis. Early recognition and treatment are vital to prevent complications and stop further transmission. Maternal immunization against pertussis during late stages of pregnancy has proven to be well tolerated and would be the best effective strategy to prevent young infants from pertussis.

Further Reading

Macina D, Evans KE. Bordetella pertussis in School-Age Children, Adolescents, and Adults: A Systematic Review of Epidemiology, Burden, and Mortality in Asia. Infect Dis Ther 2021; 10: 1115-40.

Agrawal A, Singh S, Kolhapure S, Kandeil W, Pai R, Singhal T. Neonatal Pertussis, an Under-Recognized Health Burden and Rationale for Maternal Immunization: A Systematic Review of South and South-East Asian Countries. Infect Dis Ther 2019; 8: 139-53.

Chang IF, Lee PI, Lu CY, Chen JM, Huang LM, Chang LY. Resurgence of pertussis in Taiwan during 2009–2015 and its impact on infants. J Microbiol Immunol Infect 2019; 52: 542-8.

Tuan TA, Xoay TD, Nakajima N, et al. Pertussis Infants Needing Mechanical Ventilation and Extracorporeal Membrane Oxygenation: Single-Center Retrospective Series in Vietnam. Pediatr Crit Care Med 2021; 22: e471-e9.

Kavitha TK, Samprathi M, Jayashree M, Gautam V, Sangal L. Clinical Profile of Critical Pertussis in Children at a Pediatric Intensive Care Unit in Northern India. Indian Pediatr 2020; 57: 228-31.

Kuo CC, Huang YC, Hsieh YC, Huang YL, Huang YC, Hung YT. Seroepidemiology of pertussis among elementary school children in northern Taiwan. J Microbiol Immunol Infect 2017; 50: 327-32.

Ohfuji S, Okada K, Mouri Y, et al. Effectiveness of four doses of pertussis vaccine during infancy diminished in elementary school age: A test-negative case-control study in Japan. Vaccine 2021; 39: 11-7.

Yasui Y, Mitsui T, Nishimura T, et al. School-age children and adolescents suspected of having been to be infected with pertussis in Japan. Vaccine 2018; 36: 2910-5.

Son S, Thamlikitkul V, Chokephaibulkit K, et al. Prospective multinational serosurveillance study of Bordetella pertussis infection among 10- to 18-year-old Asian children and adolescents. Clin Microbiol Infec 2019; 25: 250.e1-e7.

Koh MT, Liu CS, Chiu CH, et al. Under-recognized pertussis in adults from Asian countries: a cross-sectional seroprevalence study in Malaysia, Taiwan and Thailand. Epidemiol Infect **2016**; 144: 1192-200.

Chang YW, Chou FH. Acceptance of Pertussis Vaccination among Pregnant Women in Taiwan. J Community Health Nursing **2021**; 38: 85-102.

Sadiasa A, Saito-Obata M, Dapat C. Bordetella pertussis infection in children with severe pneumonia, Philippines, 2012–2015. Vaccine **2017**; 35(7): 993-6.

Kline JM, Lewis WD, Smith EA, Tracy LR, Moerschel SK. Pertussis: a reemerging infection. American family physician **2013**; 88(8): 507-14.

Feng Y, Chiu CH, Heininger U, Hozbor DF, Tan TQ, von König CW. Emerging macrolide resistance in Bordetella pertussis in mainland China: Findings and warning from the global pertussis initiative. Lancet Region Health Western Pacific **2021**; 8: 100098.

Case 17. A 6-Year-Old Girl with Fever for 1 Week, Productive Cough, Running Nose, Decreased Appetite, and Activity: Severe Lower Respiratory Tract Infection Due to Adenovirus

Ming-Ru Lin and Yhu-Chering Huang

Keywords

Adenovirus · Children · Pneumonia · Pleural effusion

Key Points

- Not uncommon and difficult to be differentiated from bacterial sepsis.
- Can cause fatal outcome, even in immunocompetent children, especially caused by serogenotype 7.
- Currently no approved antiviral agents. Cidofovir may be tried in immunocompromised patients with severe pneumonia or disseminated disease.
- Long-term respiratory sequela such as bronchiectasis and bronchiolitis obliterans may occur in children.

Case Report

A previously healthy 6-year-7-month-old girl, who received vaccination as scheduled according to the expanded vaccination program of Taiwan except pneumococcal conjugated vaccine (PCV-7 or PCV-13), was admitted to the hospital due to fever for 1 week. Accompanied symptoms were productive cough, running nose, and markedly decreased appetite and activity. On admission, she appeared ill-looking and vital signs were body temperature 37.5 °C, pulse rate 120/min, respiratory rate 28/min, and blood pressure 103/70 mmHg. Injected throat without tonsils enlargement or exudative change and crackles over bilateral lung fields were noted. Other physical examinations as well as neurologic assessments were essentially negative. Initial laboratory data showed WBC 7500/μL (immature neutrophils 1%, segmented 81%, lymphocytes 11%, monocytes 5%, eosinophil 2%), platelet 290,000/μL, and hemoglobin (Hb) 12.4 g/dL. Blood biochemistry data showed alanine transaminase (ALT) 18 U/L and C-reactive protein (CRP) 21.46 mg/L (normal, <5 mg/L). A chest plain film revealed patchy consolidation over lateral segment of right middle lobe (Fig. 1a). Empirical antibiotics with amoxycillin-clavulanic acid and azithromycin were prescribed under the impression of community-acquired pneumonia. However, high spik-

M.-R. Lin (✉)
Division of General and Emergency Medicine, Department of Pediatrics, Linkou Chang Gung Memorial Hospital, Taoyuan, Taiwan

Y.-C. Huang
Pediatrics, Chang Gung Memorial Hospital, Chang Gung University, Taoyuan, Taiwan
e-mail: ychuang@cgmh.org.tw

Y.-C. Huang et al. (eds.), *Paediatric Infectious Diseases*,
https://doi.org/10.1007/978-981-19-7276-8_17

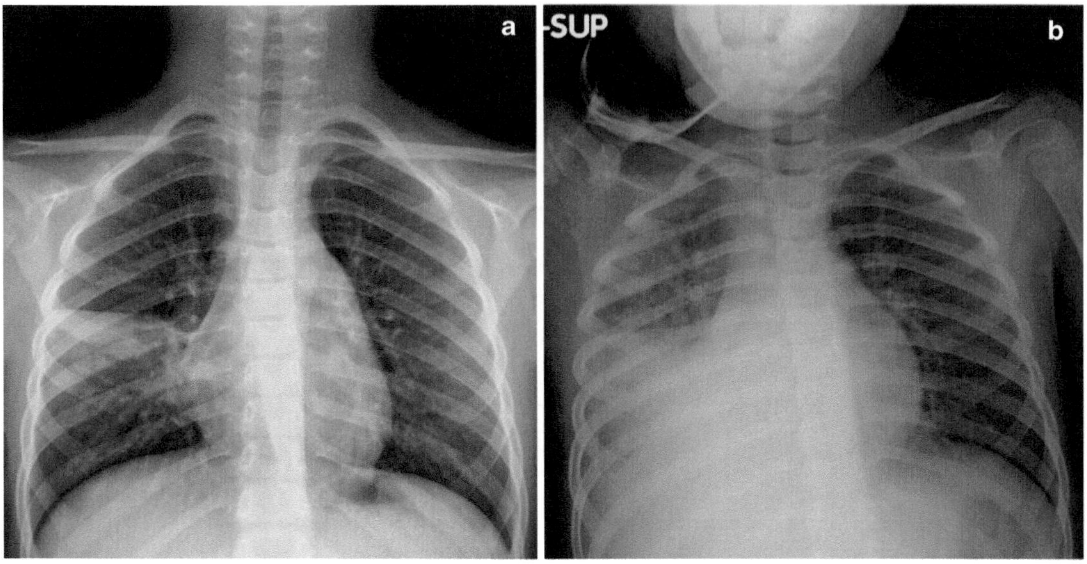

Fig. 1 Patchy consolidation over right middle lobe on chest plain film on admission (**a**) which progressed to lower lobe involvement with parapneumonic effusion and diffused interstitial infiltration over right upper and left lower lobes on hospital day 7 (**b**)

ing fever above 40 °C persisted and follow-up chest plain film revealed progressive consolidation over right middle and lower lobes with para-pneumonic effusion accompanied with diffuse interstitial infiltration over right upper lobe (Fig. 1b), we escalated antibiotics to vancomycin, ceftriaxone, and doxycycline on the 7th day of admission for covering *Streptococcus pneumoniae* serotype 19A and macrolide resistant *Mycoplasma pneumoniae*. Nevertheless, she developed respiratory distress with desaturation (SPO2 85% under room air) on 10th day of admission. Arterial blood gas showed respiratory alkalosis with poor oxygenation (PH 7.44, PCO_2 28 mmHg, PO2 48.8 mmHg, HCO_3 18.8 mm/L). She was transferred to pediatric intensive care units (PICU) with oxygen support by high-flow mask (FiO_2 50%). Computed Tomography (CT) with contrast enhancement of chest (Fig. 2) was done later and disclosed extensive consolidation with air-bronchogram change of right middle and lower lobe with small amount pleural effusion. Small patchy and centrilobular consolidation in right upper lobe and left lower lobe were also observed. Laboratory data showed leukopenia (WBC 2900/μL, immature neutrophils 2%, atypical lymphocyte 3%, segmented 66%, lymphocytes 28%, monocytes 1%), normocytic anemia (Hb 12.4 g/dL, MCV 82.3 fL), elevated aspartate transaminase (AST) 260 U/L, ALT 135 U/L, hypokalemia (potassium 2.2 mEq/L), elevated CRP 46.67 mg/L and procalcitonin 15.89 ng/mL. Analysis of pleural effusion revealed exudative characteristics (serum protein 5.4 g/dL, pleural protein 3.3 g/dL). Her fever gradually subsided on the 12th day (totally 19 days) and she was transferred back to pediatric ward on 15th day of admission. She was discharged on hospital day 25 after antibiotics treatment with improvement of previous lung lesions on chest plain film. She did not develop long term sequelae such as bronchiolitis obliterans or limitation on daily activity.

Bacterial cultures of the specimens obtained from blood, urine, sputum, bronchoalveolar lavage and pleural effusion were all negative. Polymerase chain reaction (PCR) detection for influenza virus A/B and *Mycoplasma pneumoniae* were negative. No growth of mycobacterium was noted on gastric aspiration or sputum samples. Virus isolation of pleural effusion revealed adenovirus serotype 7.

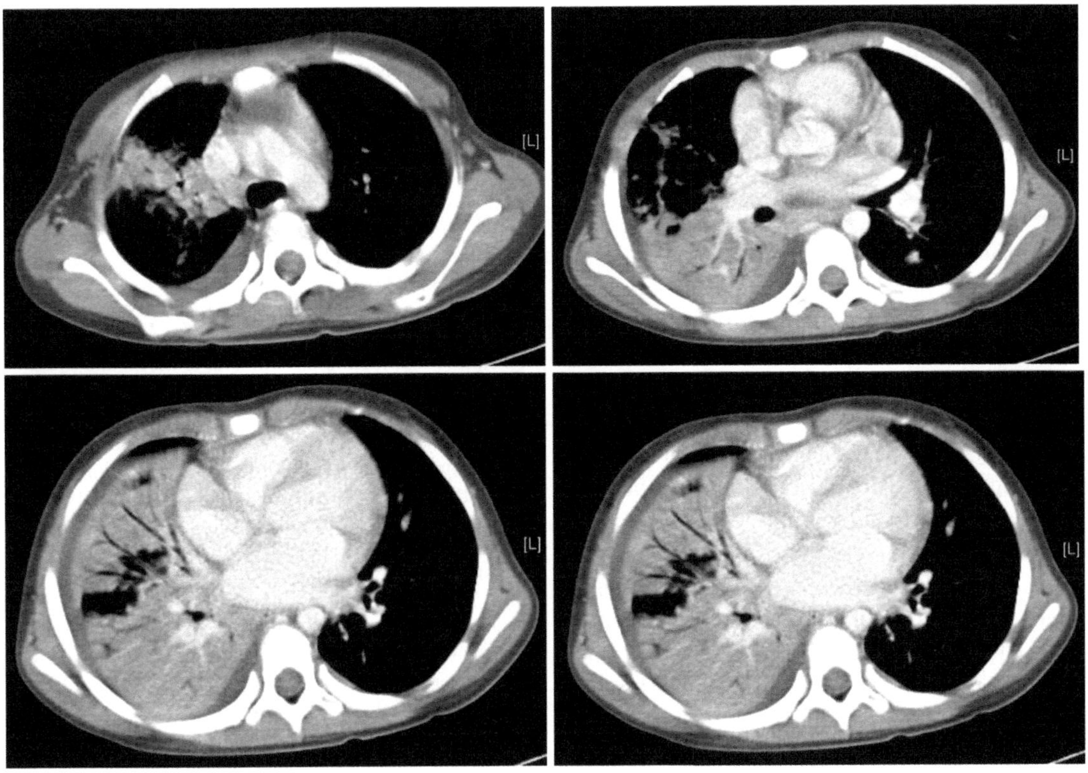

Fig. 2 Extensive consolidation with air-bronchogram change of right middle and lower lobe with small amount pleural effusion on computed tomography with contrast enhancement

Discussion

Human adenovirus (HAdV) is a double-stranded DNA virus and causes diseases more common in children. It usually causes mild illness, including infection of upper and lower respiratory tract, conjunctivitis, gastroenteritis, and cystitis. Typical symptoms of HAdV-related acute respiratory infection (ARI) include fever, cough, and sore throat. In two epidemiological and molecular studies, HAdV, compared to respiratory syncytial virus (RSV), human rhinovirus, and bocavirus (HBoV), tended to infect older children and was more likely to cause leukocytosis, high CRP levels, longer hospital stays, pneumonia, and more frequent antibiotics prescriptions in pediatric ARI inpatients. Therefore, clinically, if a preschool child with acute pharyngitis presents a picture mimicking bacterial infection (but not streptococcus throat), HAdV (particularly type 3) infection should be considered, and antibiotics can be avoided.

Currently, there are at least 88 HAdV serogenotypes in 7 species (HAdV A to G) based on genomic homology. Different serogenotypes may display different tissue tropisms. Some specific serogenotypes, such as 2, 3, 4, 7, 14, 21, and 55, may result in more severe and disseminated diseases, including pneumonia and encephalitis even in immunocompetent patients. In general, Genotype 1–7 predominantly circulate globally and are associated with HAdV infection in infants and children. The predominant serogenotypes differ among countries or regions and change over time. In the United States, Canada, and the United Kingdom, HAdV3 is the most common circulating genotypes, followed by HAdV2 and HAdV1. Whereas, along with HAdV3, which remain the most predominantly circulating genotypes in China and Korea, HAdV7 is the second common genotype, especially in those with severe lower respiratory tract infections. In Taiwan, HAdV-3 has circulated annually since 1999 and remains the dominant circulating serogenotype. A large community outbreak of adenoviral infections was detected in 2011, with the re-emergence of HAdV-7.

As shown in the illustrated case, HAdV7 is believed to be more virulent than other serogenotypes and can cause severe lower respiratory tract infection with resultant fatal outcome, even in immunocompetent children. Clinically, compared with HAdV2 or 3, HAdV7 is significantly associated with pulmonary complications and requiring intensive care, even in otherwise healthy children. Underlying medical problems, especially neurological diseases, are important risk factors associated with development of respiratory failure and subsequent higher mortality rates. Children infected with HAdV7 experience longer durations of fever and hospital stay and are significantly associated with leukopenia, thrombocytopenia, and impaired liver function.

Most HAdV-associated acute respiratory infection are self-limited. Currently, there is no approved antiviral agents for HAdV infection. Cidofovir may be considered for severe HAdV infections in immunocompromised patients and the doses suggested are 1 mg/kg twice per week or 5 mg/kg every 1–2 weeks intravenously.

Long-term respiratory sequela such as long-term small airways dysfunction, bronchiectasis, and bronchiolitis obliterans may occur in children, especially in those infected with genotype 7 and 21.

Further Reading

Ryan MA, Gray GC, Smith B, McKeehan JA, Hawksworth AW, Malasig MD. Large epidemic of respiratory illness due to adeno- virus types 7 and 3 in healthy young adults. Clin Infect Dis 2002; 34(5):577-582

Calvo C, Garcia-Garcia ML, Sanchez-Dehesa R, et al. Eight year prospective study of adenoviruses infections in hospitalized children. Comparison with other respiratory viruses. PloS One 2015; 10: e0132162.

Chen Y, Liu F, Wang C, et al. Molecular identification and epidemiological features of human adenoviruses associated with acute respiratory infections in hospitalized children in southern China, 2012-2013. PloS One. 2016; 11: e0155412.

Robinson CM, Singh G, Lee JY, et al. Molecular evolution of human adenoviruses. Sci Rep. 2013; 3: 1812.

Girouard G, Garceau R, Thibault L, Oussedik Y, Bastien N, Li Y. Adenovirus serotype 14 infection, New Brunswick, Canada, 2011. Emerg Infect Dis. 2013; 19: 119-122.

Hong JY, Lee HJ, Piedra PA, et al. Lower respiratory tract infections due to adenovirus in hospitalized Korean children: epidemiology, clinical features, and prognosis. Clin Infect Dis 2001; 32: 1423-1429.

Huang YC, Huang SL, Chen SP, et al. Adenovirus infection associated with central nervous system dysfunction in children. J Clin Virol. 2013; 57: 300-304.

Lewis PF, Schmidt MA, Lu X, et al. A community-based outbreak of severe respiratory illness caused by human adenovirus serotype 14. J Infect Dis. 2009; 199: 1427-1434.

Xie L, Zhang B, Xiao N, Zhang F, Zhao X, Liu Q, Xie Z, Gao H, Duan Z, Zhong L. Epidemiology of human adenovirus infection in children hospitalized with lower respiratory tract infections in Hunan, China. J Med Virol 2019;91:392-400.

Lee J, Choi EH, Lee HJ. Comprehensive serotyping and epidemiology of human adenovirus isolated from the respiratory tract of Korean children over 17 consecutive years (1991–2007). J Med Virol 2010;82:624-631

Lin KH, Lin YC, Chen HL, et al. A two decade survey of respiratory adenovirus in Taiwan: the reemergence of adenovirus types 7 and 4. J Med Virol 2004;73: 274-279

Tsou TP, Tan BF, Chang HY, et al. Community outbreak of adenovirus, Taiwan, 2011. Emerg Infect Dis. 2012; 18: 1825-1832.

Yamamoto D, Okamoto M, Lupisan S, et al. Impact of human adenovirus serotype 7 in hospitalized children with severe fatal pneumonia in the Philippines. Jpn J Infect Dis 2014;67(2): 105-110

Lin MR, Yang SL, Gong YN, Kuo CC, Chiu CH, Chen CJ, Hsieh YC, et al. Clinical and molecular features of adenovirus type 2, 3, and 7 infections in children in an outbreak in Taiwan, 2011. Clin Microbiol Infect. 2017;23:110-6.

Matthes-Martin S, Feuchtinger T, Shaw PJ, et al.; Fourth European Conference on Infections in Leukemia. European guidelines for diagnosis and treatment of adenovirus infection in leukemia and stem cell transplantation: summary of ECIL-4. Transpl Infect Dis 2012;14:555-563

Yusuf U, Hale GA, Carr J, et al. Cidofovir for the treatment of adenoviral infection in pediatric hematopoietic stem cell transplant patients. Transplantation 2006;81:1398-1404

Case 18. A 9-Year-Old Girl with Fever, Cough Followed by Hemoptysis and Dyspnea: Severe Influenza Virus Infections

Tsung Hua Wu, Chun Yi Lee, and Yhu-Chering Huang

Keywords

Influenza · Pneumonia · Encephalitis

Key Points

- Seasonal influenza virus is a leading cause of acute lower respiratory infection (ALRI) in young children.
- During the influenza season, when a patient presents with an influenza-like illness, a presumptive diagnosis of influenza can be made, regardless of influenza vaccination status.
- Severe respiratory complications are the major cause requiring intensive care, while acute necrotizing encephalitis is the most lethal complication.
- The decision to commence antiviral treatment should also be based on the clinical diagnosis of influenza, not on test results.
- Early use of antiviral agents may shorten the duration of symptoms, interrupt person-to-person viral spread, and reduce the disease severity.

Case 1

A 9-year-old girl without relevant medical history was admitted to pediatric intensive care unit (PICU) due to fever and cough lasting for 6 days. Two of her classmates had influenza A infection, and her father and sister were noted to be febrile within 1 week. She was admitted to a regional hospital initially; however, no antiviral drugs against flu were prescribed because rapid influenza A and B antigen tests were negative. After 5 days of hospitalization, her fever persisted and she had poor activity, decreased appetite, sore throat, hemoptysis, and dyspnea. Then, she was transferred to a medical center and was admitted to PICU.

On admission, the patient appeared ill-looking and had a temperature 39.2 °C, pulse rate 118/min, respiratory rate 42/min, and blood pressure 99/47 mmHg. Physical examination showed bilateral coarse breath sounds. Initial laboratory tests showed leukopenia (WBC 2000/μL, seg-

T. H. Wu
Department of Pediatrics, Show Chwan Memorial Hospital, Changhua, Taiwan

C. Y. Lee (✉)
Department of Pediatrics, Chang Bing Show Chwan Memorial Hospital, Changhua, Taiwan

Y.-C. Huang
Pediatrics, Chang Gung Memorial Hospital, Chang Gung University, Taoyuan, Taiwan
e-mail: ychuang@cgmh.org.tw

Y.-C. Huang et al. (eds.), *Paediatric Infectious Diseases*,
https://doi.org/10.1007/978-981-19-7276-8_18

mented 69%, lymphocytes 28%, monocytes 2%, band 1%), platelet 171,000/μL, and hemoglobin (Hb) 12.1 g/dL. Blood biochemistry data showed sugar 101 mg/dL, blood urea nitrogen (BUN) 10 mg/dL, creatinine 0.48 mg/dL, aspartate transaminase (AST) 86 U/L, alanine transaminase (ALT) 76 U/L, sodium 135 mEq/L, potassium 4.1 mEq/L, chloride 103 mEq/L, calcium 7.7 mg/dL, albumin 3.5 g/dL, C-reactive protein (CRP) 42.69 mg/L (normal, < 5 mg/L), procalcitonin 1.15 ng/mL, creatine kinase 381 U/L, creatine-MB 0.7 ng/mL, and troponin I 0.042 ng/mL. Chest radiography revealed bilateral increased infiltration with haziness over both lung fields (Fig. 1). The etiologic tests for pneumonia, including the rapid influenza A and B antigen test, reverse transcription-polymerase chain reaction (RT-PCR) of influenza and *Mycoplasma pneumoniae*, immunoglobulin G and M of *M. pneumoniae*, and pneumococcal urine antigen test, were negative. No virulent pathogens were detected in the sputum.

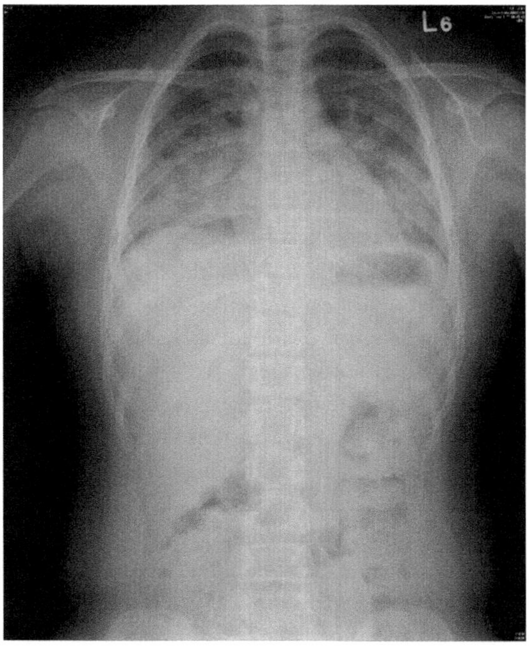

Fig. 1 Chest radiography revealed bilateral increased infiltration with haziness over both lung fields in a 9-year-old girl on admission to pediatric intensive care unit. (Case 1)

In the PICU, broad-spectrum antimicrobial agents, vancomycin plus ceftazidime, were empirically administered for 7 days. Moreover, additional oral oseltamivir 75 mg twice daily for 5 days and doxycycline for 8 days were given. On hospital day 4, the patient was afebrile, and the WBC count rose to 5600/μL. The chest computed tomography on hospital day 10 revealed multiple consolidation patches in bilateral upper and lower lobes without pleural effusion (Fig. 2). In addition, the blood biochemistry profiles all returned to normal limits (AST 22 U/L, ALT 25 U/L, CRP 1.16 mg/L) expect platelet count 455,000/μL. A chest X-ray performed on hospital day 20 showed a significant reduction of the bilateral lung infiltration. Finally, her throat viral culture yielded influenza A H1N1. She was diagnosed as influenza A H1N1 with pneumonia and pleural effusion and was discharged on day 20.

Case 2

A 2-year-old male toddler presented to a regional hospital with a 2-day history of cough, rhinorrhea, and fever. He was admitted under impression of pneumonia and received empirical amoxicillin-clavulanate, gentamicin, and ceftriaxone therapy. After 5-day hospitalization, the patient remained febrile alongside episodic shortness of breath and productive cough. He was referred to a medical center. He denied having any underlying illness or travel history; however, three of his household members (father, mother, and a 3.5-year-old sister) also had symptoms of fever, cough, and rhinorrhea within this week. The older sister was also hospitalized.

On admission, he appeared lethargic, malaise, and pale looking. The physical examination revealed a body temperature 38.5 °C, pulse rate 120/min, respiratory rate 48/min, and blood pressure 113/70 mmHg. Lung auscultation revealed bilateral rales with subcostal retraction, and chest radiography was performed, which was reported as showing consolidation in right upper lobe, right middle lobe, and left upper lobe (Fig. 3). Initial laboratory tests showed WBC 4800/μL (segmented 77%, lymphocytes

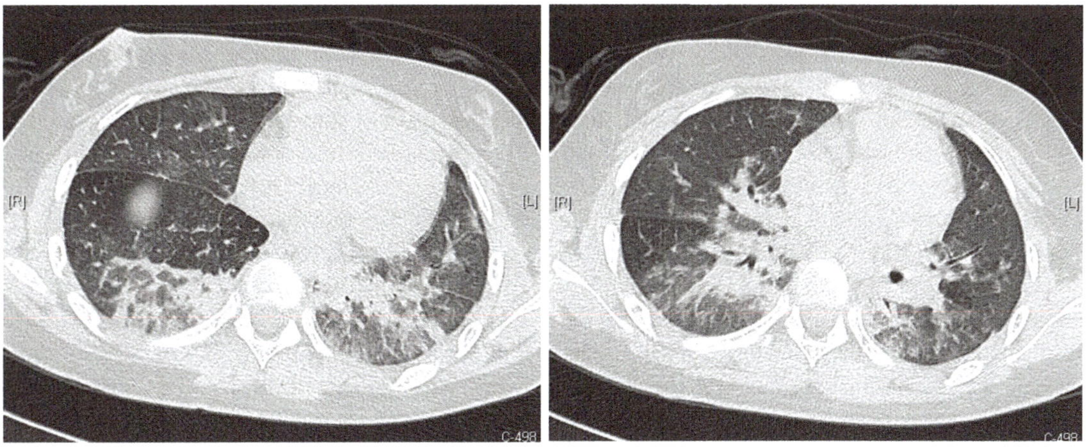

Fig. 2 Chest computed tomography on hospital day 10 revealed multiple consolidation patches in bilateral upper and lower lobes without pleural effusion (Case 1)

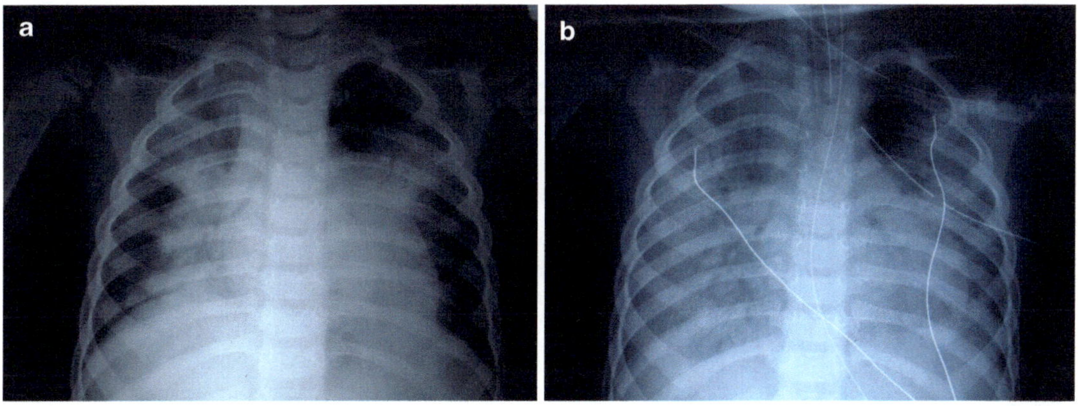

Fig. 3 Chest radiography showed consolidation in right upper lobe, right middle lobe, and left upper lobe in a 2-year-old boy (Case 2) on admission (**a**) to a medical center and on hospital day 8 (**b**)

18%, monocytes 4%, atypical lymphocyte 1%), platelet count 116,000/μL, and hemoglobin 12.3 g/dL. Blood biochemistry data showed sugar 103 mg/dL, creatinine 0.5 mg/dL, aspartate transaminase (AST) 858 U/L, alanine transaminase (ALT) 848 U/L, sodium 137 mEq/L, potassium 4.3 mEq/L, chloride 98 mEq/L, calcium 8.6 mg/dL, albumin 2.7 g/dL, C-reactive protein 42.69 mg/L (normal, <5 mg/L), and an arterial blood gas done in O_2 hood (FiO_2 50%) with a pH 7.4, pCO_2 38.1 mmHg, pO_2 53.8 mmHg, and HCO_3 23.6 mm/L. Coagulation profile reported a prothrombin time of 12.3 s and a partial thromboplastin time of 46.2 s. A lumbar puncture was performed; analysis of the cerebrospinal fluid (CSF) revealed WBC count 0 cells/mm^3, red blood cell count 25 cell/mm^3, and negative result of Gram staining. The etiologic tests for pneumonia, including pneumococcal urine antigen test, *Mycoplasma pneumoniae* immunoglobulin G and M, respiratory syncytial virus antigen test, and adenovirus antigen test, were negative. No virulent pathogens were detected in the sputum, blood, and CSF.

On day 2 of hospitalization (day 8 of illness), the patient was in respiratory distress and he was stuporous, but no seizure was observed. His blood pressure was 110/63 mmHg, and an arterial blood gas in O_2 hood (FiO_2 50%) showed a pH 7.34, pCO_2 40.4 mmHg, pO_2 49.2 mmHg, and HCO_3 21.8 mm/L. He was intubated and received high-frequency oscillatory ventilation (HFOV) support, and broad-spectrum antimicrobial agents: vancomycin plus ceftriaxone therapy. Throat virus isolation from the patient and his sister was positive for influenza A on hospital day 4. He received 2-day course of intravenous immune globulin (IVIG) (1 g/kg/day) and 7-day course of amantadine therapy. His clinical condition stabilized gradually, and his liver enzymes (AST and ALT) declined subsequently. HFOV was discontinued on hospital day 14. A chest X-ray performed 3 days after extubation showed a significant reduction of the bilateral lung infiltration. Although his consciousness recovered, he had complications of involuntary movements and slurred speech. On hospital day 22, the magnetic resonance imaging (MRI) scans of his brain showed diffused cerebral atrophy (Fig. 4). His electroencephalography (EEG) reported diffused cortical dysfunction that focal epileptiform activity over left temporal area was suspected. He was discharged finally with a diagnosis of influenza A virus infection complicated with encephalitis, hepatitis, pneumonia, and acute respiratory distress syndrome.

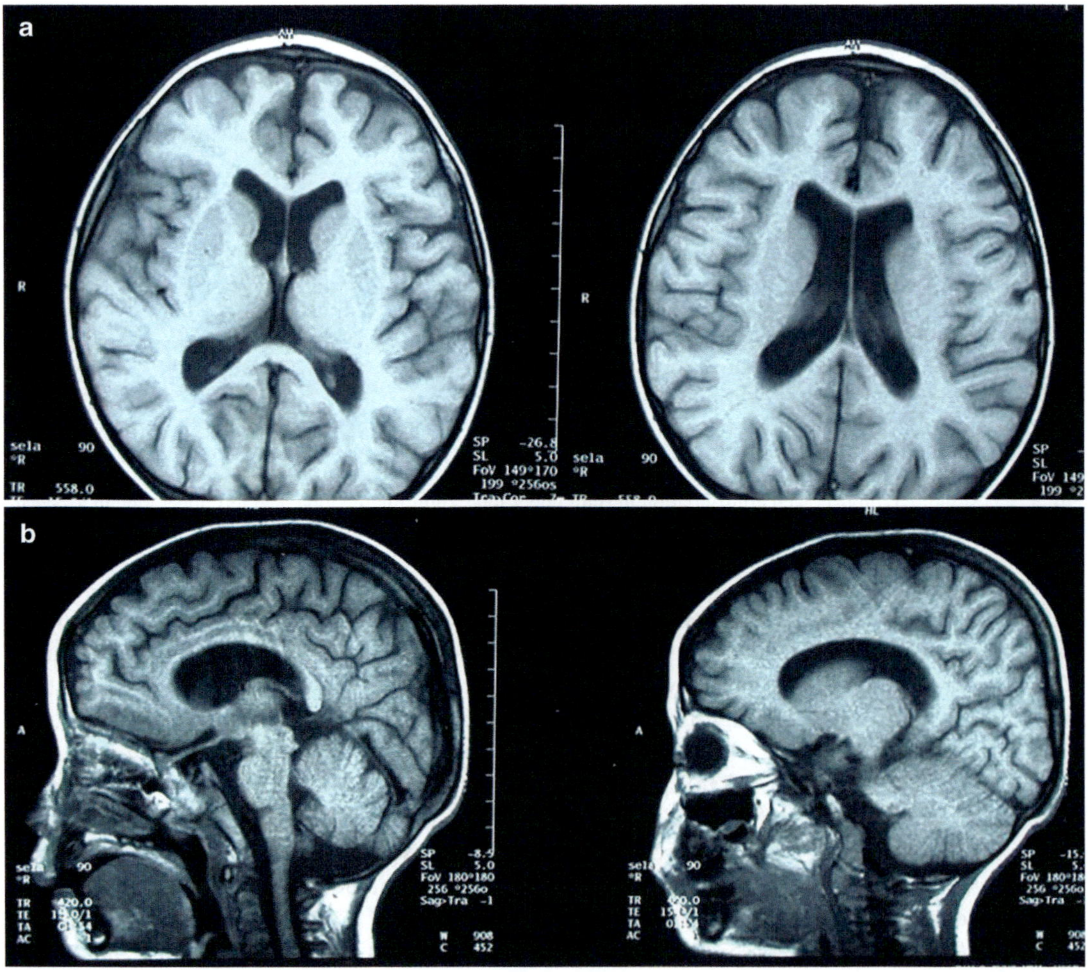

Fig. 4 On hospital day 22, the magnetic resonance imaging (MRI) of brain in Case 2 showed diffused cerebral atrophy in the axial view (**a**) and coronal view (**b**)

Discussion

Seasonal influenza virus is a leading cause of acute lower respiratory infection (ALRI) in young children and produces annual epidemics that affect 5–15% of the world population. Complications and hospitalizations are more frequent in childhood. Wang et al. reviewed 57 published studies worldwide in 2018 to estimate the influenza disease burden among children under 5 years, and there are at least 109.5 million influenza virus episodes, 10.1 million influenza-virus-associated ALRI cases; 870,000 influenza-virus-associated ALRI hospital admissions, 15,300 in-hospital deaths, and up to 34,800 overall influenza-virus-associated ALRI deaths. Overall, influenza virus is responsible for 7% of ALRI cases, 5% of ALRI hospitalization, and 4% of ALRI deaths in children <5 years. Of note, infants under 6 months are particularly vulnerable to influenza infection, and influenza strikes severely in low-income and lower-middle-income countries, with about 82% of in-hospital deaths occurred.

Influenza viruses are segmented, negative strand RNA viruses, and currently divided into four types, type A to type D. Only influenza virus A, B, and C can cause human infections. The mean incubation period of influenza is 2 days, ranging from 1 to 4 days. Influenza usually presents with sudden onset of fever, any constitutional symptoms (such as myalgia, headache, general soreness, malaise, fatigue, weakness), and any respiratory symptoms (such as sore throat, cough, sometimes nasal stuffiness). The symptoms may persist for 2–5 days, and then decrease in severity of discomfort. In infants and younger children, the clinical manifestations are similar to those of common cold. During influenza season, when a patient presents with an influenza-like illness, a presumptive diagnosis of influenza can be made, regardless of influenza vaccination status. The decision to commence antiviral treatment should also be based on the clinical diagnosis of influenza, not on test results.

Influenza virus A and B account for the majority of influenza in humans. Some studies indicated influenza A causes more severe infections than influenza B. The mean age of patients with influenza B was higher than that of patients with influenza A, and myositis was more commonly seen in children with influenza B than influenza A. However, there was no statistically significant difference in disease severity and complications in patients with influenza A and influenza B. Certain influenza strains were linked to develop severe disease: individuals infected by influenza A (H1N1) pdm09 clade 6B/6B.1/6B.2 were at higher risk for influenza-related complications, and B/Yamagata causes more severe illness than B/Victoria.

For pediatric inpatients with influenza, severe respiratory complications are the major cause requiring intensive care. Manifestations of acute lower respiratory infections following influenza may be due to influenza virus itself or secondary bacterial infection. In a medical center in Southern China, between 2013 and 2017, 1770 hospitalized pediatric patients had a laboratory-confirmed influenza, of whom 80 (4.5%) were admitted to the PICU and 13 (0.73%) died. Of 77 patients enrolled for analysis, the median age was 3.0 years, with 83.1% of the patients aged <5 years. Complications occurred in all 77 patients, and included pneumonia (100%), respiratory failure (96.1%), acute respiratory distress syndrome (22.1%), septic shock (15.6%), and influenza-associated encephalopathy (13.0%). Coinfection was detected in 58.7% of the cases, with bacterial coinfections accounting for 36.4%, *M. pneumoniae coinfections* for 11.7%, and viral coinfection for 11.7%. Of the bacterial coinfection cases, *Haemophilus influenzae* (11.7%, 9/77) and *Streptococcus pneumoniae* (7.8%, 6/77) were the predominant typical bacteria identified. The independent risk factors of mortality were oxygen saturation level of <90% at admission and influenza-associated encephalopathy.

Neurologic complications are relatively common among children admitted with influenza and can be life-threatening. In estimate, the rate of influenza-associated neurologic complications were 7.6–8.1% among children receiving intensive care. Seizure with and without fever and encephalitis/encephalopathy are the most common neurologic manifestations associated with influenza while aseptic meningitis is rarely documented. Also, virologic evidence of influenza is rarely identified from the CSF specimen. In a study from Taiwan, Huang et al. reported that between January 1997 and May 2007, a total of 2651 pediatric patients with laboratory-confirmed influenza were identified in a medical center in Northern Taiwan, of whom 1483 (56%) were infected with influenza A viruses and 1168 with influenza B viruses. Seventy-four of the patients (2.8%) had signs or symptoms of CNS dysfunction at presentation to the hospital. Thirty-four patients (45.9%) were infected with influenza A virus and 40 with influenza B virus (54.1%). The 3 most frequently mentioned signs or symptoms of CNS dysfunction were seizure (43.3%), lethargy (20.3%), and altered state of consciousness (13.5%). On admission, the most commonly cited CNS diagnoses were encephalitis (48.6%), seizure disorder (21.6%), encephalopathy (21.6%), febrile convulsion (16.2%), and status epilepticus (6.8%). In a Korean case series study, the most common diagnosis was a simple febrile convulsion (44%), followed by complex febrile convulsion (29%), fever-provoked seizure under pre-existing neurologic disease or afebrile seizure (14%), encephalopathy/encephalitis (8%), and meningitis (5%). For children without chronic neurological condition, the outcome of influenza-associated neurological complication was good, and most of the patients fully recovered. Children with CNS symptoms had nearly seven times higher odds of needing mechanical ventilation and three times higher odds of dying. The most lethal complication was acute necrotizing encephalopathy.

Before the COVID-19 pandemic, influenza virus was the leading respiratory pathogen worldwide. The influenza-associated burden among young children is substantial and can lead to severe respiratory and neurological complication, even death. Clinicians should be aware of influenza infection during the flu season. Influenza-associated neurological complication is not uncommon and could be fatal. Early initiation of antiviral agents is associated with a shorter length of hospital stay. In addition to nonpharmaceutical interventions, vaccination is the best measurement to prevent childhood influenza infection.

Further Reading

Wang X, Li Y, O'Brien KL, et al. Global burden of respiratory infections associated with seasonal influenza in children under 5 years in 2018: a systematic review and modelling study. Lancet Global health **2020**; 8: e497-e510.

Yang JR, Kuo CY, Huang HY, et al. Seasonal dynamics of influenza viruses and age distribution of infected individuals across nine seasons covering 2009-2018 in Taiwan. J Formos Med Assoc **2020**; 119: 850-60.

Oh YN, Kim S, Choi YB, Woo SI, Hahn YS, Lee JK. Clinical similarities between influenza A and B in children: a single-center study, 2017/18 season, Korea. BMC pediatrics **2019**; 19: 472.

Han SB, Rhim JW, Kang JH, Lee KY. Clinical features and outcomes of influenza by virus type/subtype/lineage in pediatric patients. Transl Pediatr **2021**; 10: 54-63.

Shinjoh M, Furuichi M, Narabayashi A, Kamei A, Yoshida N, Takahashi T. Risk factors in pediatric hospitalization for influenza A and B during the seven seasons immediately before the COVID-19 era in Japan. J Infect Chemother **2021**; 27: 1735-42.

Hsieh YC, Tsao KC, Huang CT, Chang KY, Huang YC, Gong YN. Clinical characteristics of patients with laboratory-confirmed influenza A(H1N1)pdm09 during the 2013/2014 and 2015/2016 clade 6B/6B.1/6B.2-predominant outbreaks. Sci Rep **2018**; 8: 15636.

Chen HJ, Su CP, Liu MT, Tsou TP. Comparative epidemiology of influenza B by lineage in intensive care unit-admitted patients with complications: A nationwide study in Taiwan, 2013-2017. Inter J Infect Dis **2019**; 87: 67-74.

Shi T, Nie Z, Huang L, et al. Mortality risk factors in children with severe influenza virus infection admitted to the pediatric intensive care unit. Medicine **2019**; 98: e16861.

Antoon JW, Hall M, Herndon A, et al. Prevalence, risk Factors, and outcomes of influenza-associated neurologic complications in children. Journal Pediatr **2021**; 239: 32-8.

Lin CH, Huang YC, Chiu CH, Huang CG, Tsao KC, Lin TY. Neurologic manifestations in children with influenza virus B infection. Pediatr Infect Dis J 2006; 25: 1081-3.

Huang YC, Li WC, Tsao KC, Huang CG, Chiu CH, Lin TY. Influenza-associated central nervous system dysfunction in Taiwanese childen. Pediatr Infect Dis J 2009; 28: 647-8.

Choi GJ, Park JY, Choi JS, et al. Influenza-associated neurologic complications in hospitalized pediatric patients: A multicenter retrospective study in Republic of Korea. Pediatr Infect Dis J 2021 (online).

Mastrolia MV, Rubino C, Resti M, Trapani S, Galli L. Characteristics and outcome of influenza-associated encephalopathy/encephalitis among children in a tertiary pediatric hospital in Italy, 2017-2019. BMC infectious diseases 2019; 19: 1012.

Case 19. A One-Year-Old Girl with Fever, Cough, and Posttussive Vomiting: Respiratory Syncytial Virus Infection

Hsin Chi and Ping-Ing Lee

Keywords

Coinfection · *Staphylococcus aureus* · Pneumonia · Bronchiolitis · Respiratory syncytial virus

Key Points

- RSV is the most important respiratory tract pathogen of early childhood.
- The most common manifestations are bronchiolitis and pneumonia.
- Risk factors for severe illness are chronic lung disease of prematurity, congenital heart disease, immunodeficiency, and prematurity.
- Bacterial coinfection is associated with more severe disease.
- Composite evidence suggests that bacterial pneumonia may be observed in ≥20% of low-risk infants infected by RSV and the use of empirical antibiotics is justified.

H. Chi (✉)
Division of Pediatric Infectious Diseases, Department of Pediatrics, MacKay College of Medicine, MacKay Children's Hospital, Taipei, Taiwan
e-mail: chi.4531@mmh.org.tw

P.-I. Lee
Pediatrics, National Taiwan University Children's Hospital, National Taiwan University, Taipei, Taiwan
e-mail: pinging@ntu.edu.tw

Case Presentation

Case 1

A 1-year-old girl with no history of known systemic diseases had been well until April 25, 2019, when a spiking high fever of up to 39.5 °C was noted for 4 days. Productive cough, rhinorrhea, and posttussive vomiting were also noted. The symptoms persisted after medications from a primary physician. Thereafter, she was brought to our outpatient department. The influenza and adenovirus rapid antigen test were negative. Symptomatic medications were given, and outpatient department follow-up was arranged. One day before admission, decreased appetite and shortness of breath were noted, so she was brought to our outpatient department again. Respiratory syncytial virus (RSV) rapid antigen test was positive. Then she was admitted to our hospital for further management under the impression of acute RSV bronchiolitis and pneumonia.

On admission, physical examination revealed tachypnea, subcostal retraction, wheezing, and fine crackles in bilateral lung fields. Symptomatic medications, inhalation therapy with O_2 tent and intravenous fluid support were given. Laboratory examinations upon admission revealed leukocytosis (13.9×10^9 cells/L) with lymphocyte predominance (54%) and mildly elevated C-reactive protein (1.096 mg/L). Chest X-ray examination revealed increased infiltrations in bilateral lung fields without obvious pneumonic patch (Fig. 1).

Y.-C. Huang et al. (eds.), *Paediatric Infectious Diseases*,
https://doi.org/10.1007/978-981-19-7276-8_19

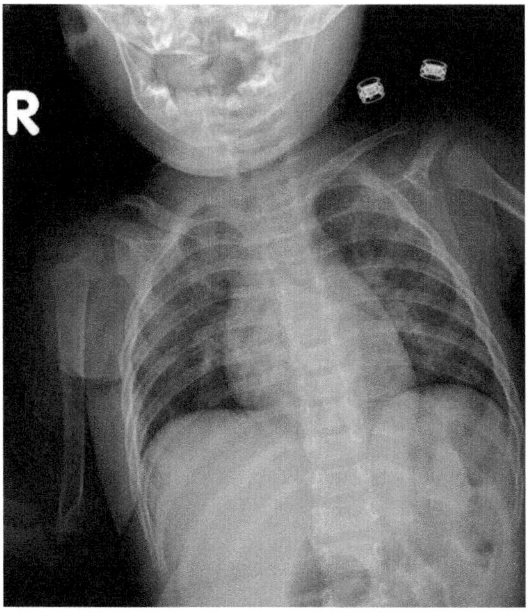

Fig. 1 Chest X-ray of case 1 with respiratory syncytial virus infection. The chest film reveals increased infiltrations in bilateral lung fields

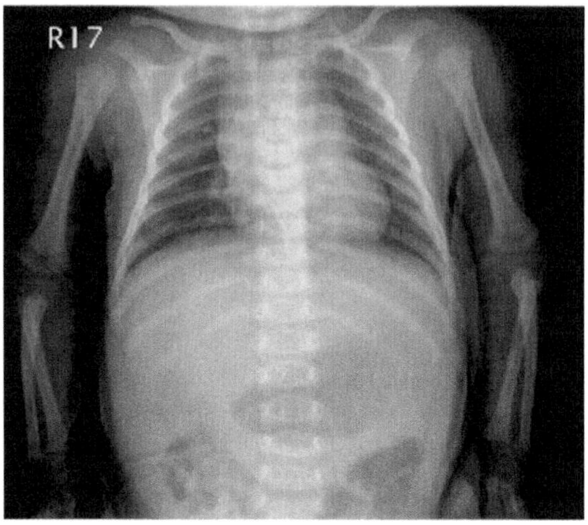

Fig. 2 Chest X-ray of case 2 with respiratory syncytial virus infection. The chest film reveals mild interstitial infiltrations

Fever gradually subsided from hospital day 2. Tachypnea and subcostal retraction were also improving. She was finally discharged in a relatively stable condition.

Case 2

A 1-month-old female baby suffered from cough and diarrhea for 5 days without fever. She was brought to our emergency room where chest radiograph showed mild interstitial infiltrations (Fig. 2). She was tachypneic with a respiratory rate of 50–70/min. Wheezing was audible on chest examination. There were mild subcostal retractions. She was admitted with a diagnosis of acute bronchiolitis. Laboratory data showed a white cell count of 13,960/μL and a normal C-reactive protein level of 0.01 mg/dL. The RSV antigen test of sputum was positive. With supportive care, she was discharged after 5 days. There was no fever during her hospitalization.

She was hospitalized again at the same day of discharge because fever, poor oral intake, and poor activity were noted after returning home. Her respiratory rate was 78/min with suprasternal and subcostal retractions, and bilateral diffuse fine crackles. Sputum RSV antigen test was weakly positive. Empirical ampicillin and gentamicin were given. Blood culture yielded no bacteria. Progressive tachypnea and chest wall retractions, persistent fever, and feeding cyanosis developed 3 days after admission. Chest X-ray showed haziness of the left lung with pneumothorax and pleural effusion (Fig. 3).

She was transferred to intensive care unit where thoracocentesis yielded air and bloody exudative fluid. Culture of pleural fluid grew methicillin-resistant *Staphylococcus aureus* (MRSA). Computed tomography showed consolidation of the right upper lobe and left lung with abscess, and left hydropneumothorax (Fig. 4).

The antibiotics were changed to vancomycin and cefotaxime. Decortication of empyema with chest tube insertion was performed at the seventh day of hospitalization. Fever subsided gradually after the operation. Chest film on the eighteenth day of hospitalization showed pneumatocele in the left lung (Fig. 5), and she was extubated the next day. Follow-up chest film on the 31st day of hospitalization showed resolution of the pneumatocele (Fig. 5). She was discharged in a stable condition.

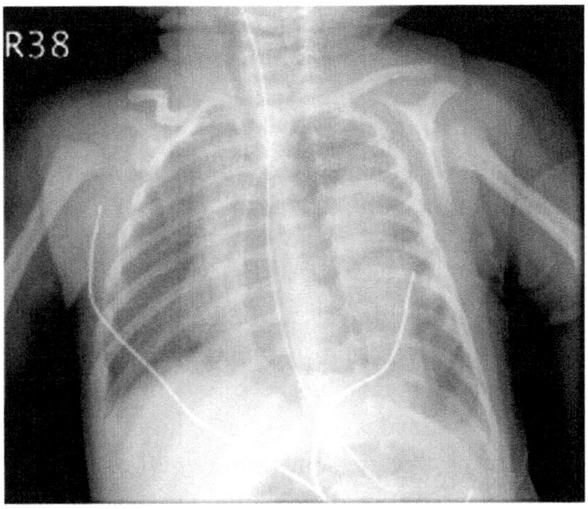

Fig. 3 Chest X-ray of case 2 at the fourth day during the second hospitalization. The CXR reveals haziness of the left lung with pneumothorax and pleural effusion

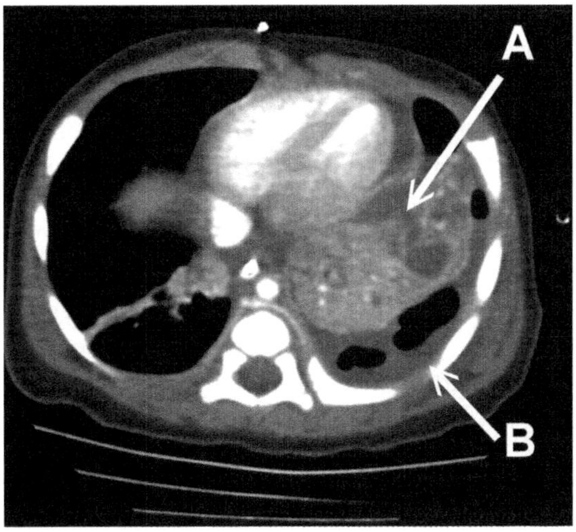

Fig. 4 Chest computed tomography of case 2 shows consolidation in the right upper lobe and left lung with (**a**) abscess and (**b**) left hydropneumothorax in the left lung

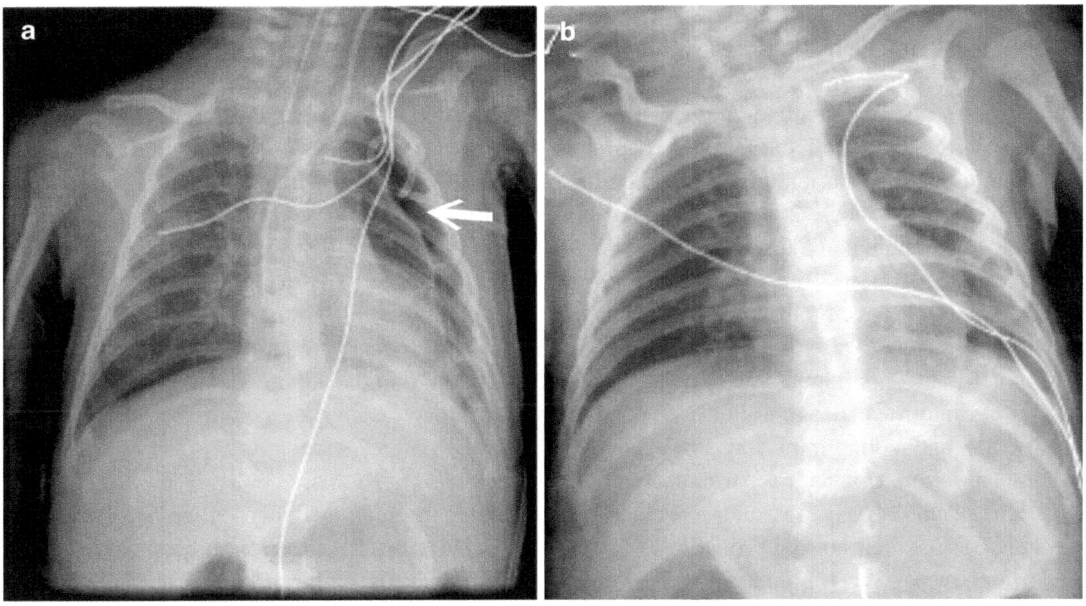

Fig. 5 Chest radiography of case 2 showed (**a**) a pneumatocele (arrow) in the left upper lung on the eighteenth day of hospitalization and (**b**) resolution of the pneumatocele on hospital day 3

Discussion

Respiratory syncytial virus (RSV) is the major cause of bronchiolitis and viral pneumonia in children younger than 2 years of age and is the most important respiratory tract pathogen of early childhood (Shi et al. 2017). RSV infection in infants younger than 6 months have a substantial impact on child mortality in low-income and middle-income countries.

RSV is an enveloped RNA virus with a single-stranded negative-sense genome, and belongs to family *Pneumoviridae* and genus *Orthopneumovirus*. There are two antigenic subgroups of RSV (subgroups A and B), based primarily on sequence and antigenic variations of the G glycoprotein. The peak incidence of severe lower respiratory tract disease and hospitalization is in infants aged about 6 weeks. All RSV diseases of the lower respiratory tract (excluding croup) have their highest incidence in infants aged 6 weeks to 7 months and decrease thereafter. The highest medical risk factors in infants are chronic lung disease of prematurity, congenital heart disease, immunodeficiency, and prematurity.

RSV infections can cause respiratory epithelium necrosis, thick mucus secretions from the respiratory tract, and immune cell accumulation, leading to respiratory tract obstruction. Infants are the most vulnerable to RSV infection, possibly because of their short respiratory tracts, immature immune systems, and a tendency toward Th_2 cell immunity.

The incubation period from exposure to first symptoms is approximately 3–5 days. RSV is probably introduced into most families by young schoolchildren experiencing reinfection. Typically, in a few days, 25–50% of older siblings and one or both parents acquire upper respiratory tract infections, but infants are more severely ill with fever, otitis media, or lower respiratory tract disease.

Typically, the first sign of RSV infection in infants is rhinorrhea. Bronchiolitis is caused by obstruction and collapse of the small airways during expiration. Infants are particularly apt to experience small airway obstruction because of the small size of their normal bronchioles.

The treatment of uncomplicated cases of bronchiolitis is symptomatic. Intravenous or tube feeding is helpful when sucking is difficult because of tachypnea. Humidified oxygen and suctioning usually are indicated for hospitalized infants who are hypoxic. High-flow nasal cannula therapy is used for respiratory distress and is mostly useful for pressure support. Nasal continuous positive airway pressure is used in the intensive care unit for infants who have increased work of breathing, and mechanical ventilation is used for respiratory failure. There is disagreement regarding the usefulness of aerosolized saline or hypertonic saline, epinephrine, or β2-agonists in RSV bronchiolitis. Corticosteroid therapy is not indicated except in children with a diagnosis of asthma that usually run a prolonged and recurrent course.

The true incidence of pulmonary bacterial coinfection in infants and children hospitalized with a viral respiratory infection is difficult to ascertain, but can vary widely from under 1–44%. Evidences show that coinfection with bacteria may be present in patients infected by RSV, especially in those with severe illness. In contrast to case 1 who had a mild RSV infection, lung infection with MRSA complicated RSV infection in case 2 in about 1 week. This illustrates that such a coinfection may not be uncommon. Although it is suggested that "In nearly all instances of bronchiolitis, antibiotics are not useful. (Nelson's Textbook of Pediatrics, 21st ed.), superimposed bacterial pneumonia should be considered in severe RSV pneumonia, and bacterial coinfection is not uncommon for RSV infection in young children". Children with RSV complicated by *S. aureus* infection have also been reported. RSV may cause functional changes in the cells of the respiratory tract that facilitate the initiation of bacterial infections with *S. aureus*, similar to what has been seen with RSV and the adherence of other pathogenic respiratory bacteria including *Streptococcus pneumoniae*, *Pseudomonas aeruginosa*, and *Bordetella pertussis*.

One indirect evidence of an RSV-bacterial association is the reduction in hospitalized RSV-pneumonia in children who have received a 9-valent pneumococcal conjugate vaccine in the context of a vaccine trial in South Africa. In a report from Mexico, postmortem lung tissue samples from children younger than 2 years of age who died of RSV pneumonia showed that 25% was complicated by bacteria infection. Composite evidence suggests that bacterial pneumonia may be present in ≥20% of low-risk infants infected by RSV and thus the use of empirical antibiotics is justified.

The monoclonal antibody palivizumab is licensed for prophylaxis in high-risk infants during the RSV season and does prevent about half of the expected hospitalizations in that population. Six-monthly intramuscular administration of palivizumab is effective for prevention of RSV hospitalization in regions with no single seasonal peak of RSV infection such as Taiwan. Next-generation monoclonal antibodies that are more potent and have longer duration are in clinical trials for preventing RSV infection in premature babies.

Candidate RSV vaccines in development generally contain the highly conserved surface fusion (F) protein of the virus, which is considered essential in disease pathogenesis. There is no licensed vaccine against RSV at present.

Further Reading

Shi T, McAllister DA, O'Brien KL, Simoes EAF, Madhi SA, Gessner BD, et al. Global, regional, and national disease burden estimates of acute lower respiratory infections due to respiratory syncytial virus in young children in 2015: a systematic review and modelling study. *Lancet* 2017;**390**:946–58.

Scheltema NM, Gentile A, Lucion F, Nokes DJ, Munywoki PK, Madhi SA, et al. Global respiratory syncytial virus-associated mortality in young children (RSV GOLD): a retrospective case series. *Lancet Glob Health* 2017;**5**:e984-e91.

Sung CC, Chi H, Chiu NC, Huang DT, Weng LC, Wang NY, et al. Viral etiology of acute lower respiratory tract infections in hospitalized young children in Northern Taiwan. *J Microbiol Immunol Infect* 2011;**44**:184-90.

Chi H, Chang IS, Tsai FY, Huang LM, Shao PL, Chiu NC, et al. Epidemiological study of hospitalization associated with respiratory syncytial virus infection in Taiwanese children between 2004 and 2007. *J Formos Med Assoc* 2011;**110**:388-96.

Rima B, Collins P, Easton A, Fouchier R, Kurath G, Lamb RA, et al. ICTV Virus Taxonomy Profile: Pneumoviridae. *J Gen Virol* 2017;**98**:2912-3.

Collins PL, Graham BS. Viral and host factors in human respiratory syncytial virus pathogenesis. *J Virol* 2008;**82**:2040-55.

Vu HT, Yoshida LM, Suzuki M, Nguyen HA, Nguyen CD, Nguyen AT, et al. Association between nasopharyngeal load of Streptococcus pneumoniae, viral coinfection, and radiologically confirmed pneumonia in Vietnamese children. *Pediatr Infect Dis J* 2011;**30**:11-8.

Chi H, Hsu CH, Chang JH, Chiu NC, Hung HY, Kao HA, et al. A novel six consecutive monthly doses of palivizumab prophylaxis protocol for the prevention of respiratory syncytial virus infection in high-risk preterm infants in taiwan. *PLoS One* 2014;**9**:e100981.

Griffin MP, Yuan Y, Takas T, Domachowske JB, Madhi SA, Manzoni P, et al. Single-dose nirsevimab for prevention of rsv in preterm infants. *N Engl J Med* 2020;**383**:415-25.

Weinberger DM, Klugman KP, Steiner CA, Simonsen L, Viboud C. Association between respiratory syncytial virus activity and pneumococcal disease in infants: a time series analysis of US hospitalization data. PLoS Medicine 2015; 12:e1001776.

Thorburn K, Riordan A. Pulmonary bacterial coinfection in infants and children with viral respiratory infection. Expert Rev Anti Infect Ther 2012;10:909-16.

Stockman LJ, Reed C, Kallen AJ, Finelli L, Anderson LJ. Respiratory syncytial virus and *Staphylococcus aureus* coinfection in children hospitalized with pneumonia. Pediatr Infect Dis J 2010;29:1048-50.

Bustamante-Calvillo ME, Velázquez FR, Cabrera-Munõz L, et al. Molecular detection of respiratory syncytial virus in postmortem lung tissue samples from Mexican children deceased with pneumonia. Pediatr Infect Dis J 2001;20:495-501.

Crowe JE. Respiratory syncytial virus. In: Kliegman RM, St Geme JW, Blum NJ, et al. eds. Nelson Textbook of Pediatrics, 21th edition. Philadelphia: Churchill Livingstone, 2020.

Levin D, Tribuzio M, Green-Wrzesinki T, et al. Empiric antibiotics are justified for infants with respiratory syncytial virus lower respiratory tract infection presenting with respiratory failure: A prospective study and evidence review. Pediatr Crit Care Med 2010; 11:390-5.

Madhi SA, Klugman KP. A role for *Streptococcus pneumoniae* in virus associated pneumonia. Nat Med. 2004;10:811-3.

Case 20. A 4-Month-Old Male Infant with Dry Cough, Progressive Shortness of Breath: Cytomegalovirus Pneumonitis

Ting-Yu Yen and Yhu-Chering Huang

Keywords

Cytomegalovirus · Pneumonitis · Intravenous immunoglobulin · Ganciclovir · Fibrosis · Immunocompetent · Infant

Key Points

- Not uncommon and difficult to be differentiated from other viral pneumonia in immunocompetent children.
- Manifestations range from mild to severe and life-threatening diseases, including bronchopulmonary dysplasia, cystic lung disease, persistent pulmonary hypertension of the newborn, and pulmonary fibrosis.
- CMV pneumonitis should be suspected in a patient who presents with a discrepancy between the severity of hypoxemia and the distribution of infiltrates on the chest radiograph.
- Diagnosis should integrate clinical, virological, radiological, laboratory, and pathological evidence. Detection of viral DNA by PCR in respiratory samples has emerged as the most sensitive predictor of CMV pneumonitis.
- Patients with severe CMV pneumonitis should be evaluated for immunodeficiency when no other underlying cause is identified.
- Early ganciclovir or valganciclovir treatment and adjunctive immunoglobulin may help reduce morbidity and mortality from severe disease.

Case Report

A 4-month-old male infant was admitted to the pediatric intensive care unit (PICU) due to dyspnea and decreased appetite and activity for 2 days. The infant was born at full-term with a birth weight of 2900 g via normal spontaneous delivery. The current body weight was 5 kg and the body height was 56 cm, both below the third percentile. A dry cough, progressive shortness of breath, decreased oral intake, decreased activity, and decreased urine output occurred within 2 days. On admission, the baby appeared in respiratory distress and with cyanosis, and vital signs were body temperature 37.5 °C, pulse rate 157/min, respiratory rate 50/min, blood pressure

T.-Y. Yen (✉)
Division of Pediatric Infectious Diseases, Department of Pediatrics, National Taiwan University Hospital, and College of Medicine, National Taiwan University, Taipei, Taiwan

Y.-C. Huang
Division of Pediatric Infectious Diseases, Department of Pediatrics, Chang Gung Memorial Hospital, and College of Medicine, Chang Gung University, Taoyuan, Taiwan
e-mail: ychuang@cgmh.org.tw

Y.-C. Huang et al. (eds.), *Paediatric Infectious Diseases*,
https://doi.org/10.1007/978-981-19-7276-8_20

117/70 mmHg, and oxygen saturation 80–85%. Acutely ill appearance, cyanotic lips, subcostal retractions, and coarse breathing sound were found. Other physical examinations and neurologic assessments were within normal limit. Initial laboratory data showed leukocytosis with lymphocyte predominant (WBC 33,500/μL, neutrophils 23%, lymphocytes 66%), normal platelets (359,000/μL), and hemoglobin levels (Hb, 13.5 g/dL). C-reactive protein (CRP) was 0.8 mg/L (normal, <5 mg/L), other blood biochemical data such as glucose, blood urea nitrogen (BUN), creatinine, total bilirubin, aspartate aminotransferase (AST), alanine aminotransferase (ALT), and electrolytes were within normal limits. Arterial blood gas showed moderate hypoxemia (PaO_2 53 mmHg). Chest X-Ray revealed increased infiltration over bilateral lung fields (Fig. 1). Under the impression of bronchopneumonia, favor viral infection, with suspected secondary bacterial infection, intravenous amoxicillin-clavulanic acid was administered.

However, worsening shortness of breath and respiratory distress developed on the hospital day 5. Laboratory data showed markedly leukocytosis with lymphocyte predominant (WBC 69,400/μL, neutrophils 20.8%, lymphocytes 62.5%, atypical lymphocyte 1.8%, eosinophil 10%) and normal level of CRP (2.5 mg/L). Arterial blood gas

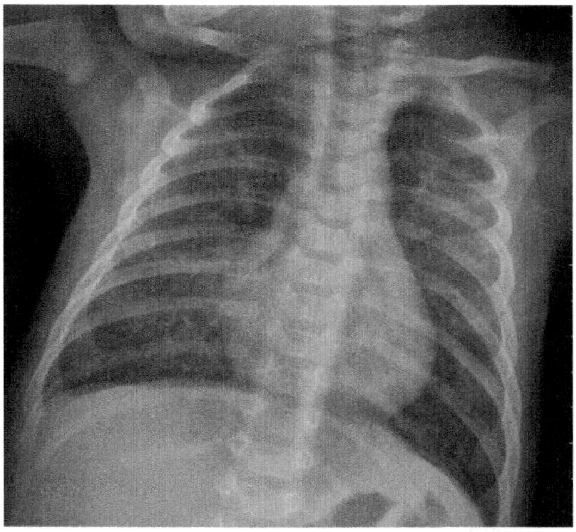

Fig. 1 Chest X-Ray on admission revealed increased infiltration over bilateral lung fields

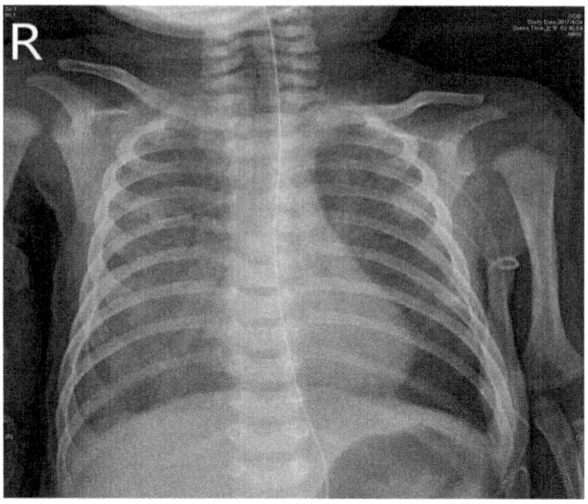

Fig. 2 Chest X-ray showed progressive ground glass opacity on hospital day 5

showed severe hypoxemia (PaO_2, 32 mmHg). Progressive ground glass opacity (GGO) was shown on chest X-ray (Fig. 2). Azithromycin was prescribed to cover potential pertussis infection. Unfortunately, subcostal retraction, suprasternal retraction, tachypnea, and intermittent desaturation remained exacerbated over the following week. Endotracheal intubation and ventilator support were given for acute respiratory distress syndrome (ARDS), and bronchoscope was performed for bronchoalveolar lavage (BAL) study on hospital day 8. High-resolution computed tomography (HRCT) of the chest showed large area of peribronchial patchy ill-defined consolidations at bilateral upper lobes and diffuse ground glass opacities at bilateral lower lobes, consistent with viral pneumonia. Sputum respiratory syncytial virus antigen test, pertussis polymerase chain reaction (PCR), and bacterial culture were all negative findings. Cytomegalovirus (CMV) shell vial culture revealed positive finding from urine (70–90 cells/200×) and BAL (15 cells/slide). Both blood CMV IgG and IgM showed positive results, and blood CMV quantitative PCR (qPCR) revealed 1760 copies/mL. Viral isolations from throat swab and BAL both yielded CMV subsequently. Indirect ophthalmoscopy revealed negative finding for CMV retinitis. Therefore, ganciclovir (6 mg/kg/dose Q12H) was prescribed, and intravenous immune globulin (IVIG, 0.6 g/kg/dose) was administered at this point and

3 weeks later, respectively. Immune profile survey, including lymphocyte subsets and immunoglobulins (IgG, IgG subclasses, IgA, IgM, and IgE), were within normal limits. In the following days, the condition gradually stabilized. Extubation was performed smoothly on admission day 25. One month later, chest CT revealed diffuse ground glass opacities in bilateral lungs and patchy consolidations at right middle lobe with mild bronchiectasis and focal interlobar interstitial thickening, which were consistent with residual bilateral viral pneumonia and mild fibrotic change at right middle lobe. After 6 weeks of ganciclovir treatment, oral valganciclovir (16 mg/kg/day QD) was prescribed for continuous therapy. The baby was discharged on day 60 with a final diagnosis of CMV pneumonitis complicated with ARDS and pulmonary fibrosis.

Discussion

Human cytomegalovirus (CMV), belonging to beta herpesviruses, is the largest human herpesvirus with 230 kb double-stranded DNA genome and is prevalent in the human population [1]. A systematic survey estimated the global seroprevalence of CMV to be 83%, 86%, and 86% in the general population, women of reproductive age, and blood or organ donors, respectively [2].

CMV can persist for life in infected individuals, with intermittent replication and viral shedding from mucosal surfaces, such as saliva, urine, and genital secretions. CMV shedding is relatively frequent in seropositive infants, young children, young adults, and pregnant women [1, 3]. In neonates and early infancy, common routes of transmission include transplacentally vertical transmission, aspiration of infected cervical secretion at birth, ingestion of CMV-containing breast milk, and transfusion with CMV-seropositive blood [4]. Transplacental vertical transmission of CMV to the fetus occurs in approximately 40% of primary seropositive mothers and 1–2% of reactivated pregnant women, and the risk of fetal harm from primary infection in the first trimester is highest. The congenital infection rate is approximately 0.4–2% [1]. However, perinatally acquired pulmonary CMV infection is even more common than transplacental acquisition, ranging from 10% to 15%. The range of incubation periods for perinatal cytomegalovirus infection is between 4 and 12 weeks [4].

Compared with immunocompetent individuals, CMV is a significant cause of morbidity and even mortality in immunocompromised hosts, such as neonates, preterm infants, HIV-infected hosts, and patients receiving immunosuppressive therapy or allogeneic hematopoietic stem cell transplantation. In normal hosts, primary CMV infection rarely causes severe disease, usually manifesting as a mononucleosis syndrome. Some cases of primary infection manifested as arthritis, colitis, pneumonitis, hepatitis, encephalitis, and myocarditis [1]. CMV pneumonitis has varying degrees of severity, with most presenting as mild disease that may be overlooked or present as a self-limited respiratory infection. However, premature or immunocompromised infants may develop diffuse severe interstitial pneumonia that can be life-threatening, as shown in the illustrated case. Significantly, infants with CMV-infected pneumonia required more mechanical ventilation support and longer hospital stays. As a result, it is also associated with adverse chronic respiratory outcomes, including bronchopulmonary dysplasia, cystic lung disease, persistent pulmonary hypertension of the newborn, and pulmonary fibrosis [5]. CMV pneumonitis should be suspected in a patient who presents with a discrepancy between the severity of hypoxemia and the distribution of infiltrates on the chest radiograph.

CMV pneumonitis can be diagnosed by detecting the presence of the virus in serum and/or respiratory samples. Polymerase chain reaction (PCR) assays have been shown to be more sensitive for the detection of CMV than other measurements, such as serology, viral phosphoprotein 65 (pp65), and CMV cultures [5]. Therefore, PCR detection of viral DNA from respiratory samples, obtained by bronchoscopy or tracheal aspiration, has been the most predictive method for CMV pneumonitis due to its high sensitivity and direct detection in the respiratory tract [6]. Radiological examinations of CMV pneumonitis reveal ground-glass and airspace opacities, reduced lung volume, pulmonary nodules, and interstitial infiltrates on chest X-ray or chest computed tomography [7]. For pathological findings, lung biopsy with cytomegalovirus inclusion bodies or immunostaining for viral antigens remains the gold standard for diagnosis of CMV pneumonitis, but it was not routinely performed due to its high invasiveness [5].

CMV pulmonary infection has been defined in adults with signs and symptoms of pulmonary infection, serum CMV isolation, evidence of CMV in sputum or bronchoalveolar lavage (BAL) fluid, or detection of cytomegalic inclusions in bronchoalveolar lavage cells or lung tissues. However, diagnostic criteria for childhood CMV pneumonitis remain challenging. Latent CMV infection can intermittently shed virus on mucosal surfaces, which makes even CMV isolated in BAL and sputum still not always defining the presence of acute CMV pulmonary disease, especially at a young age [5]. Second, there is no clear threshold for viral load in serum, urine, or respiratory samples to differentiate between asymptomatic and clinically relevant infections. Third, the clinical manifestations of pulmonary CMV infection may be indistinguishable from other common viral lung diseases. In other words, the diagnosis and treatment decisions of children with suspected pulmonary CMV involvement should incorporate clinical, virological, radiological laboratory, and pathological findings. Besides, patients with pulmonary or other tissue-invasive CMV infections should be evaluated for immunodeficiency when no other underlying cause has been identified.

Currently, licensed antiviral drugs available for the treatment and/or prevention of CMV infection include ganciclovir, valganciclovir, foscarnet, cidofovir, maribavir, and letermovir [8]. Intravenous ganciclovir (pediatric dosage: induction, 5 mg/kg q12h for 14–21 days; maintenance, 5 mg/kg qd or 6 mg/kg qd for 5 days/week) or oral valganciclovir (pediatric dosage: 7 × body surface are × creatinine clearance; maximum: 900 mg/day) are primary regimen for use off-label for CMV pneumonitis, and ganciclovir use limited due to potential renal and bone marrow toxicity and antiviral resistance [5]. Alternatives for the treatment of pulmonary CMV also include foscarnet, maribavir, cidofovir, and letermovir; however, significant side effects and toxicity might occur with these medications [9]. Intravenous immunoglobulin or CMV hyperimmune globulin is recommended as adjunctive therapy in immunocompromised patients and possibly in cases of severe CMV disease and hypogammaglobulinemia [5].

In conclusion, although CMV pneumonitis is common in immunocompromised hosts, it can occur in immunocompetent patients, with an increasing number of reported cases. Especially in infants, it may be associated with a complex disease course, increased ventilator requirements, and lead to significant morbidity. Therefore, CMV pneumonitis should be considered in a patient who presents with a discrepancy between the severity of hypoxemia and the distribution of infiltrates on the chest radiograph. To overcome diagnostic challenges in childhood, clinicians should promptly integrate clinical, virological, radiological laboratory, and pathological evidences. For severe cases, timely and appropriate use of antiviral therapy and adjuvant immunoglobulin should be considered, and patients should be evaluated for immunodeficiency when no other underlying cause has been identified.

References

1. Britt WJ. Cytomegalovirus. In Nelson's Textbook of Pediatrics. 21th ed. Philadelphia, PA: Elsevier. 2019:1718-23.e1.
2. Zuhair M, Smit GSA, Wallis G, et al. Estimation of the worldwide seroprevalence of cytomegalovirus: A systematic review and meta-analysis. Rev Med Virol. 2019 May;29(3):e2034.
3. Barbosa NG, Yamamoto AY, Duarte G, et al. Cytomegalovirus shedding in seropositive pregnant women from a high-seroprevalence population: The Brazilian cytomegalovirus hearing and maternal secondary infection study. Clin Infect Dis. 2018 Aug 16;67(5):743-750.

4. Coclite E, Di Natale C, Nigro G. Congenital and perinatal cytomegalovirus lung infection. J Matern Fetal Neonatal Med. 2013 Nov;26(17):1671-5.
5. Restrepo-Gualteros SM, Gutierrez MJ, Villamil-Osorio M, et al. Challenges and clinical implications of the diagnosis of cytomegalovirus lung infection in children. Curr Infect Dis Rep. 2019 May 30;21(7):24.
6. Govender K, Jeena P, Parboosing R. Clinical utility of bronchoalveolar lavage cytomegalovirus viral loads in the diagnosis of cytomegalovirus pneumonitis in infants. J Med Virol. 2017 Jun;89(6):1080-1087.
7. Kunihiro Y, Tanaka N, Matsumoto T, et al. The usefulness of a diagnostic method combining high-resolution CT findings and serum markers for cytomegalovirus pneumonia and pneumocystis pneumonia in non-AIDS patients. Acta Radiol. 2015 Jul;56(7):806-13.
8. Al-Eyadhy AA, Hasan G, Bassrawi R, et al. Cytomegalovirus associated severe pneumonia, multi-organ failure and Ganciclovir associated arrhythmia in immunocompetent child. J Infect Chemother. 2017 Dec;23(12):844-847.
9. Acosta E, Bowlin T, Brooks J, et al. Advances in the Development of Therapeutics for Cytomegalovirus Infections. J Infect Dis. 2020 Mar 5;221(Suppl 1):S32-S44.

Case 21. A 4-Year-Old Boy with Fever, Aggravated Cough, and Persistent Abdominal Pain: Pneumonia Presenting as Acute Abdomen

Ping-Ing Lee

Keywords

Lung consolidation · *Streptococcus pneumoniae* · Abdominal pain · Acute abdomen · Peritonitis

Key Points

- Pneumonia with severe inflammatory response may be associated with signs of peritoneal irritation, such as muscle guarding and rebound pain of the abdomen. Therefore, pneumonia may mimic acute abdomen in children, especially those with lung consolidation.
- There may be no or scanty symptoms and signs relating to respiratory tract in children with pneumonia.
- Lung consolidation may appear suddenly on chest film within a few hours or within 1 day. Given that the radiological features of early pneumonia may be subtle and thus be missed in children, repeated chest X-ray may be necessary, if indicated.

Case Report

A previously healthy 4-year-old boy had cough and rhinorrhea for 6 days. Because of the presence of wheezing on auscultation, attending physician prescribed some anti-asthma medications, including inhaled steroid. Fever up to 39.2 °C with aggravated cough and persistent abdominal pain appeared on the day of his arrival at the emergency room. The pulse rate was 91/min, the respiratory rate was 26/min, and the systolic and diastolic blood pressure was 106 mmHg and 56 mmHg, respectively. He appeared acutely ill. The consciousness was clear. The throat was not injected. Chest auscultation revealed occasional wheezing. The abdominal wall was guarded on palpation with diffuse rebound pain. The liver and the spleen were not palpable. Laboratory data showed a white blood cell count of 28,000/μL with 83% segmented neutrophils. The C-reactive protein value was 0.93 mg/dL. Lactic acid level increased to 5.1 mmol/L. Chest X-ray examinations showed interstitial infiltration of the lungs with unremarkable plain abdominal film (Figs. 1 and 2).

Because of the presence of severe persistent abdominal pain with peritoneal sign, exploratory laparoscopy was performed immediately. Diffuse reddish change of bowel walls and diffuse bowel distension was noted during the operation without a specific focus of infection. Normal saline irrigation and ascites culture were done. The chest film on the next day showed consolidation

P.-I. Lee (✉)
Department of Pediatrics, National Taiwan University Children's Hospital, National Taiwan University, Taipei, Taiwan
e-mail: pinging@ntu.edu.tw

Y.-C. Huang et al. (eds.), *Paediatric Infectious Diseases*,
https://doi.org/10.1007/978-981-19-7276-8_21

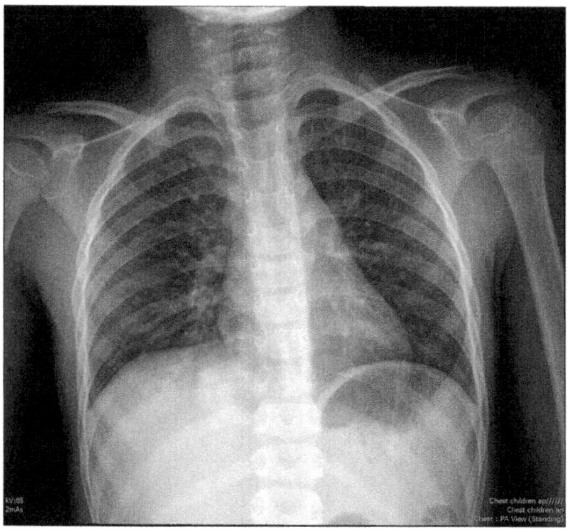

Fig. 1 Chest film on arrival at emergency room

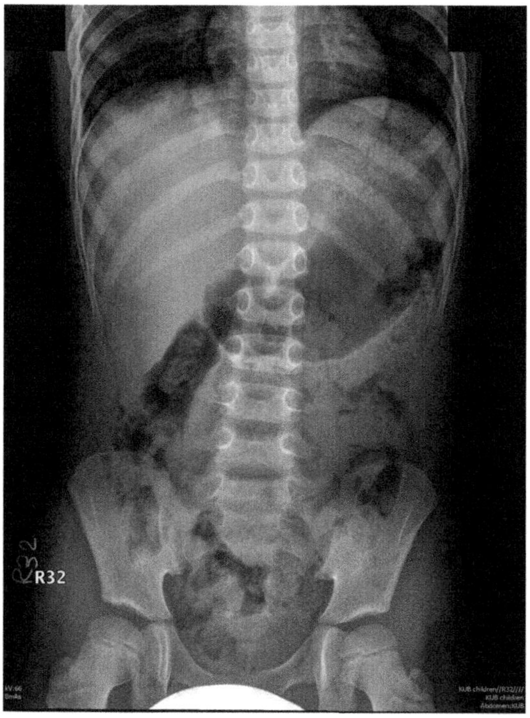

Fig. 2 Plain abdominal X-ray on arrival at emergency room

at right lower lung field (Fig. 3). Blood culture and ascites culture showed no growth. The sputum culture yielded *Streptococcus pneumoniae*. The urinary antigen test for *S. pneumoniae* was

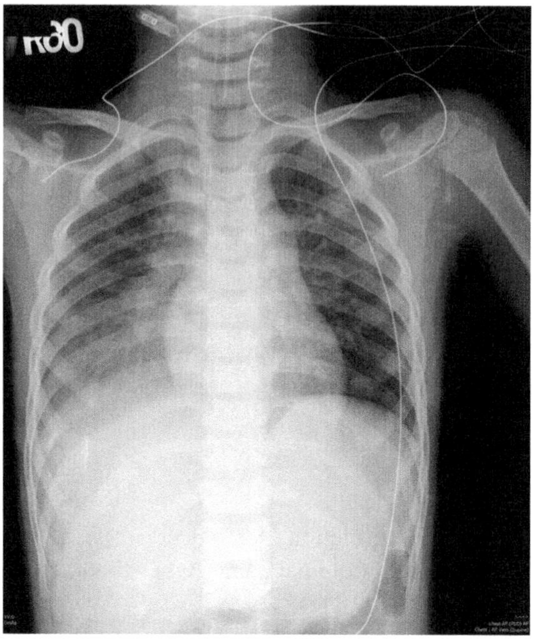

Fig. 3 Chest film on the next day after arrival at emergency room

positive. He recovered after appropriate antibiotic treatment for pneumococcal pneumonia.

Discussion

Pneumonia is a known cause of abdominal pain and may mimic acute abdomen in cases of pediatric patients. However, the general practitioner tends to associate community acquired pneumonia only with chest symptoms. The possibility of pneumonia may be ignored by the unapparent symptoms/signs of respiratory tract. As illustrated by this case, he had cough for some duration due to bronchial asthma, and wheezing was the only finding on chest auscultation. The possibility of pneumonia cannot be excluded for children without typical symptoms/signs related to respiratory tract.

Typical manifestations of pneumonia are cough, production of sputum, tachy-dyspnea, chest discomfort, fever or hypothermia, fine crackles on auscultation, diminished breath sound, bronchial sound, and percussion dullness on sites of consolidation. Pneumonia may present with nonspecific symptoms like fatigue, myalgia, anorexia, headache, as well as abdominal pain. Physical findings of the chest are frequently obscure in young children because of a poor cooperation. Pneumonia is in fact considered as the most frequent extra-abdominal cause of acute abdominal pain in children. A prompt correct diagnosis may avoid unnecessary delay in the diagnosis and administration of appropriate antibiotics.

Although it has been well known that persistent abdominal pain may be the presenting symptom of pneumonia in children, the underlying mechanism is obscure. It was thought that the abdominal pain may be referred from irritation of the diaphragmatic pleura. However, many children with abdominal pain have pneumonia affecting upper or middle lobes, and one-sided pneumonia may be associated with abdominal pain on the contralateral side.

The referred pain theory cannot explain associated peritoneal irritation, as shown by the presence of muscle guarding and rebound pain of the abdomen in present case. Most pneumonia-associated peritoneal irritations involve the whole abdomen. A few reports showed that the abdominal finding may sometimes be localized. It has been suggested that the abdominal pain may arise from a mechanism similar to that of mesenteric adenitis. A severe systemic inflammatory response may sometimes induce mesenteric adenitis and peritoneal irritation. One example is typhoid fever-associated severe persistent abdominal pain that may also be associated with mesenteric adenitis with signs of peritoneal irritation. Because of peritoneal irritation, it is not uncommon that these infections be mistakenly treated by laparotomy initially.

Pneumonic changes on chest films are frequently overlooked by reports of children with pneumonia presenting as acute abdomen. Chest radiography should be performed in a child with fever and abdominal pain without obvious focus. The present case also illustrates that lung consolidation may appear suddenly on chest film within a few hours or within 1 day. Given that the radiological features of early pneumonia may be subtle and be missed in children, repeated chest X-ray examinations within a short time may be necessary, if indicated.

S. pneumoniae is the single most common cause of pyogenic bacterial pneumonia in children beyond the first few weeks of life. Diagnosis of pneumococcal pneumonia is a difficult challenge to pediatricians, because the normal upper respiratory tract flora frequently contains *S. pneumoniae* and sputum collection may be difficult in young children. Pneumococcal urinary antigen test is an acceptable test to augment diagnostic methods for *S. pneumoniae* infection. The sensitivity ranged between 50% and 80%, and the specificity is about 90% in adults. Studies involving children have documented the lack of specificity. Nevertheless, the test has a high sensitivity and a good negative predictive value for the diagnosis of pneumococcal pneumonia in children. The growth of *S. pneumoniae* in the sputum and the positive pneumococcal urinary test in this case suggest that the most possible offending pathogen was *S. pneumoniae*.

Further Reading

Ravichandran D, Burge DM. Pneumonia presenting with acute abdominal pain in children. Br J Surg 1996;83:1707-8.

Gongaware RD, Weil 3rd R, Santulli TV. Right-lower-lobe pneumonia and acute appendicitis in childhood: a therapeutic disorder. J Pediatr Surg 1973;8:33-5.

Kanegaye JT, Harley JR. Pneumonia in unexpected locations: an occult cause of pediatric abdominal pain. J Emerg Med 1995;13:773-9.

Armeni E, Mylona V, Karlis G, Makrygiannisa E. Pneumonia presenting with lower right abdominal pain and migratory polyarthritis. Respir Med Case Rep 2012; 5: 29-30.

Vendargon S, Wong PS, Tan KK. Pneumonia presenting as acute abdomen in children: a report of three cases. Med J Malaysia 2000;55:520–3.

Tsalkidis A, Gardikis S, Cassimos D, et al. Acute abdomen in children due to extra-abdominal causes. Pediatr Int 2008;50:315-8.

Osterwalder I, Özkan M, Malinovska A, Nickel CH, Bingisser R. Acute abdominal pain: missed diagnoses, extra-abdominal conditions, and outcomes. J Clin Med 2020;9:899.

Arjunan M, Al-Salamah AA. Typhoid fever with severe abdominal pain: diagnosis and clinical findings using abdomen ultrasonogram, hematology-cell analysis and the Widal test. J Infect Dev Ctries 2010;4:593-6.
Lee PI, Chiu CH, Chen PY, Lee CY, Lin TY, Taiwan Pediatric Working Group for "Guideline on the management of CAP in children." Guidelines for the management of community-acquired pneumonia in children. Pediatr Neonatol 2007;28:167-80.
Isaacs D. Problems in determining the etiology of community-acquired childhood pneumonia. Pediatr Infect Dis J 1989;8:143-8.
Ramsey BW, Marcuse EK, Foy HM, et al. Use of bacterial antigen detection in the diagnosis of pediatric lower respiratory tract infections. Pediatrics 1986;78:1-9.

Case 22. A 2-Year-Old Girl with Community-Acquired Pneumonia Followed by Thrombocytopenia and Anemia: *Streptococcus pneumoniae* Associated with Hemolytic Uremic Syndrome

Wan-Chun Lai, Yu-Chia Hsieh, and Yhu-Chering Huang

Keywords

Community-acquired pneumonia · *Streptococcus pneumoniae* · Hemolytic uremic syndrome · Thomsen-Friedenreich antigen

Key Points

- Hemolytic uremic syndrome is a complication in 0.4–0.6% of IPD cases, which is characterized by microangiopathic hemolytic anemia, thrombocytopenia, and acute kidney injury.
- The symptoms of HUS typically developed 3–13 days (most at 7–9 days) after the onset of the symptoms related to pneumococcal infection.
- In the circumstance of HUS, the fibrinogen level, prothrombin time, and partial thromboplastin times are usually normal or slightly elevated and active bleeding is rare.
- Blood transfusion with washed blood product and avoiding the plasma transfusion remains an important concept because these procedures are thought to reduce the exposure to T antigen.
- Renal placement therapy is indicated for anuria and deteriorated renal function.

W.-C. Lai (✉) · Y.-C. Hsieh
Division of Pediatric Infectious Diseases, Department of Pediatrics, Chang Gung Memorial Hospital at Linkou, Taoyuan, Taiwan

Y.-C. Huang
Pediatrics, Chang Gung Memorial Hospital, Chang Gung University, Taoyuan, Taiwan

Case Report

A previously healthy 2-year-9-month-old girl was admitted after 5 days of fever, productive cough, and rhinorrhea. A chest radiograph revealed segmental consolidation in right lower lobe of lung, consolidation with air-bronchogram over left lower lobe of lung (Fig. 1). Hemogram disclosed leukocyte count 5000/μL (normal range: 6000–10,400), with elevated band form of 27%, hemoglobin 11.0 g/dL (normal range: 11.6–13.7), platelet count 100,000/μL (normal range: 150–400), and elevated C-reactive protein (CRP): 322.57 mg/L (normal range: <5 mg/L) on

Y.-C. Huang et al. (eds.), *Paediatric Infectious Diseases*,
https://doi.org/10.1007/978-981-19-7276-8_22

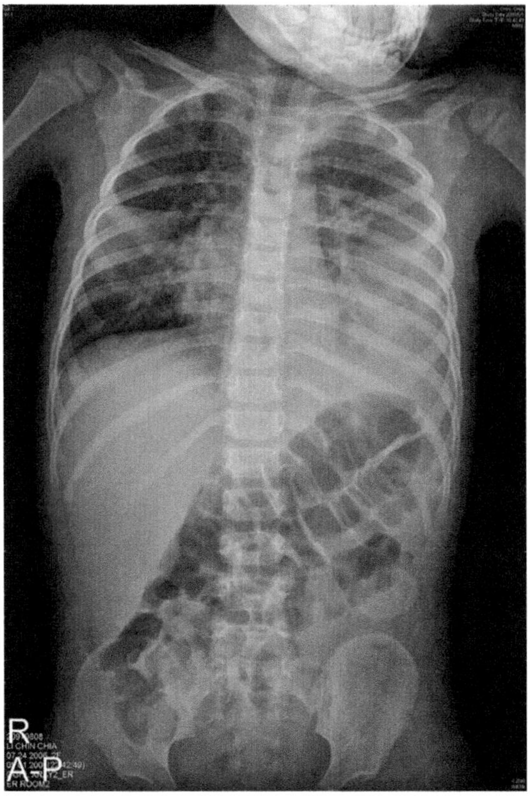

Fig. 1 On the day of admission, the chest plain film disclosed consolidation with air-bronchogram over left lower lobe and segmental consolidation in right lower lobe

admission. Urine pneumococcal antigen test (Binax NOW) showed a positive result. Empiric ceftriaxone (75 mg/kg/day) and azithromycin (10 mg/kg/day) were prescribed for severe community-acquired pneumonia. The patient was then transferred to pediatric intensive care unit (PICU) on the day of admission because of increased respiratory distress and oliguria. She was intubated for ventilator support. Leukopenia (3800/μL) with bandemia (band form 34%), anemia (hemoglobin: 10.5 g/dL) and thrombocytopenia (platelet count: 37,000/μL) was found on hospital day 2. Antibiotics were adjusted to vancomycin (~60 mg/kg/day) and ceftriaxone (100 mg/kg/day). A chest ultrasound examination reported lobar pneumonia in right middle lobe and left lower lobe with suspicious necrotic change over left lower lobe. Bilateral parapneumonic effusion was visualized. A pleural effusion specimen from left side after a chest tube insertion showed cloudy, leukocyte count 3760/μL with 97% neutrophils and 3% lymphocytes, red blood cell 3120 per microliter, and gram stain disclosed gram positive cocci +++. Both blood culture and pleural effusion culture subsequently yielded *Streptococcus pneumoniae,* serotype 14. On hospital day 3, there was progressive anemia (hemoglobin: 7.7 g/dL) and thrombocytopenia (7000/μL). Coagulation profiles showed prothrombin time 15.9 s (normal range: 10.0–13.0), partial thromboplastin time 48.4 s (normal range: 24.0–31.0), and fibrinogen level 687 mg/dL (normal range: 190–380). Peripheral blood smear disclosed fragmented red blood cells and Burr cells. Oliguria with daily urine output 0.25 mL/kg/h and elevated serum creatinine level (1.57 mg/dL) were also noted. The Thomsen-Friedenreich antigen was positive. Pneumococcal pneumonia with hemolytic uremic syndrome (HUS) was impressed. Blood was seen in the endotracheal tube, and thus washed red blood cell and leukocyte-poor platelet were transfused. Anuria then developed and continuous renal replacement therapy (CRRT) was applied. Anuria improved and the CRRT was discontinued on day 7. Anemia and thrombocytopenia also improved. Fever continued during hospitalization. Non-enhanced computed tomography of chest was performed on hospital day 8 and disclosed lobar pneumonia over left lower lobe and empyema (Fig. 2). The chest tube was removed on day 13 and the endotracheal tube was extubated on day 14. A pneumatocele was found on the chest plain film on day 15, further chest computed tomography revealed necrotizing pneumonia over left lower lobe and hydropneumothorax, suggestive of bronchopleural fistula. An operation of decortication and lobectomy of left lower lobe by video-assisted thoracoscope was performed by the pediatric surgeon. Meropenem was ever substituted for ceftriaxone between day 8 to day 18 and vancomycin was discontinued on day 12. After fever subsided on day 18, ceftriaxone was substituted for Meropenem and then shifted to oral form of amoxicillin (100 mg/kg/day) on day 23–29. The pathology report disclosed necrosis and abscess, suggesting acute necrotizing pneumonia. A follow-up CXR film showed significant improvement (Fig. 3). She was discharged on day 27.

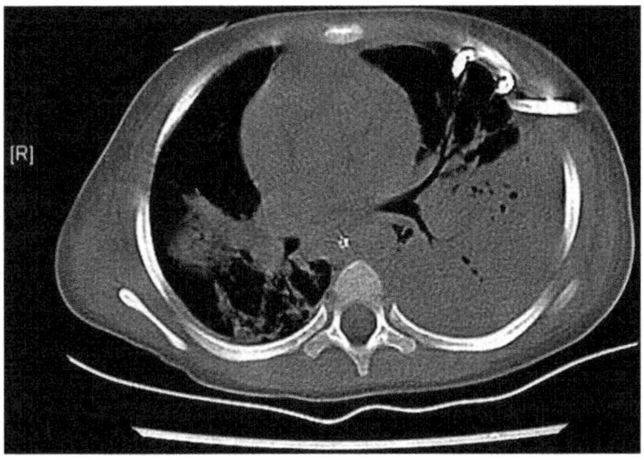

Fig. 2 Chest computed tomography without contrast (concerning acute renal failure) on day 8 of admission reports consolidation with air-bronchogram in left lower lobe, left site empyema status post pigtail catheter drainage and segmental consolidation in right upper lobe and right lower lobe

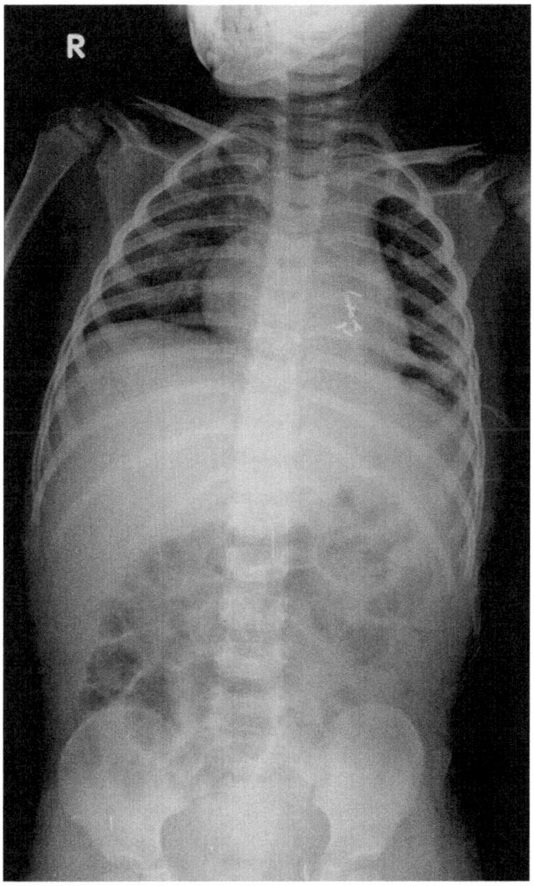

Fig. 3 Before discharge (admission day 21), chest plain film disclosed minimal consolidation over left lower lobe and post-operative metallic clips

Discussion

Streptococcus pneumoniae (*S. pneumoniae*) is a gram-positive, facultative anaerobic bacteria. There are over 90 known serotypes for different capsular expression. *S. pneumoniae* can colonize at respiratory tract at all ages among humans, and children bear higher colonization rate than adults. *S. pneumoniae* can cause diseases as well. Manifestations of pneumococcus infection range from upper and lower respiratory tract infection, sepsis, bacteremia to meningitis. The confirmatory diagnosis of invasive pneumococcal disease (IPD) is defined as isolation of *S. pneumoniae* from a normally sterile site of body. IPD causes morbidity and mortality in clinical practice. After introducing the pneumococcal conjugate vaccine (PCV), the rate of IPD has decreased. In the children, the major serotypes causing IPD were serotype 14, 19F, and 6B before the vaccine era, while these serotypes declined in the post-vaccine era. In Taiwan, IPD was most frequently seen in patients aged between 2 and 5 years. Taiwan introduced PCV7 in 2006 and PCV10 in 2010 used in the private sector in children aged under 5 years. However, IPD caused by serotype 19A gradually increased. Therefore, Taiwan Centers for Disease Control started to introduce PCV13 in children age 2–5 years first and then shifted to national immunization program during infancy. The incidence of IPD decreased thereafter. IPD caused by serotype 19A declined as well. Instead, serogroup 15 became the leading serotypes of IPD in pediatric group aged under 5 years.

Hemolytic uremic syndrome (HUS) is a complication in 0.4–0.6% of IPD cases, which is characterized by microangiopathic hemolytic anemia, thrombocytopenia, and acute kidney injury. Traditionally, most of the HUS cases are caused by Shiga-like toxin producing *Escherichia coli* (STEC); however, *S. pneumoniae* infection, complement pathway dysregulation, and inborn errors of metabolism also contribute to the occurrence of HUS. In the non-STEC HUS cases, pneumococcal infection-associated HUS accounted for 40%. The pathophysiology of HUS is now believed to be associated with TF antigen activation. The Thomsen-Friedenreich antigen

(T antigen) is a structure on the surface of erythrocytes, platelets, and glomerular endothelial cells. The T antigen is normally shielded by neuraminic acid. Pneumococcus produce neuraminidase which is capable of exposing the normally hidden T antigen by cleaving the N-acetylneuraminic acid. The unmasked T antigen subsequently bound to the anti-T IgM antibodies and resulted in the HUS. In addition, the role of the alternate pathway of complement's contribution to the HUS is under investigation. *S. pneumoniae* associated HUS (P-HUS) was first reported in the 1970s. Empyema and meningitis are mostly seen in P-HUS. Decades after the first case had been reported, high mortality rate to 50% and the development of chronic kidney disease or hypertension in two-third of the survivors were reported. The prognosis dramatically improved in the following years, possibly related to the advanced technique in critical care skill. All serotypes of *S. pneumoniae* have the neuraminidase, but the activity varied. Thus, theoretically, different activities and likelihood also differ among serotypes. In the pre-vaccine era, it is not surprising that serotype 14 was the most associated serotype; other attributable serotypes were 6B, 9 V, 19, 3, 8, 7, and 23F. In the post 7-valent pneumococcal conjugate vaccine era, 19A became the most frequently seen serotype. Clinically, the symptoms of HUS typically developed 3–13 days (most at 7–9 days) after the onset of the symptoms related to pneumococcal infection. The accurate diagnosis of P-HUS is still under debate. In most cases, the diagnosis is made in the combination of clinical and laboratory features and evidence of pneumococcal infection. According to the Canadian Pediatric Society, the P-HUS is defined in two categories. Definite cases are those with a thrombotic microangiopathy on renal pathology, in addition to clinical features of HUS and evidence of pneumococcal infection. Some experts considered the positive Coombs test instead of the pathology report is enough for diagnosis. Possible cases are those difficult to distinguish between severe infection-related end organ failure or HUS. The European Pediatric Study Group for HUS recommended the diagnosis of P-HUS made by a HUS combined with a proven or suspected invasive pneumococcal infection. The detection of T-antigen also plays a role in the diagnosis by many experts, using the direct Coombs test, polyagglutination test, and peanut lectin agglutination test. The detection of P-HUS is a dilemma to differentiate HUS from disseminated intravascular coagulation (DIC). Both of these conditions may occur in severe infection and presented with anemia, thrombocytopenia, and renal failure. However, in the circumstance of HUS, the fibrinogen level, prothrombin time, and partial thromboplastin times are usually normal or slightly elevated and active bleeding is rare.

The management goal for P-HUS is supportive care. Adequate fluid supplement, maintaining the electrolytes balance, nutrition support, and appropriate antibiotics prescription are the gold standard. The American Academy of Pediatrics suggests non-critically ill and previously healthy children with nonmeningeal invasive pneumococcal disease be treated with penicillin or ampicillin empirically. In critically ill patients, Vancomycin plus a third generation of cephalosporin were suggested. Blood transfusion with washed blood product and avoiding the plasma transfusion remains an important concept because these procedures are thought to reduce the exposure to T antigen. In some circumstances, renal placement therapy is indicated for anuria and deteriorated renal function.

Further Reading

David W. Kimberlin M, FAAP; Michael T. Brady, MD, FAAP; Mary Anne Jackson, MD, FAAP; Sarah S. Long, MD, FAAP. Red Book® 2018 Committee on Infectious Diseases; American Academy of Pediatrics.

Poehling KA, Talbot TR, Griffin MR, Craig AS, Whitney CG, Zell E, et al. Invasive pneumococcal disease among infants before and after introduction of pneumococcal conjugate vaccine. Jama. 2006;295(14):1668–74. Epub 2006/04/13. https://doi.org/10.1001/jama.295.14.1668. PubMed PMID: 16609088.

Browall S, Backhaus E, Naucler P, Galanis I, Sjöström K, Karlsson D, et al. Clinical manifestations of invasive pneumococcal disease by vaccine and non-vaccine types. European Respiratory Journal. 2014;44(6):1646–57. https://doi.org/10.1183/09031936.00080814.

Whitney CG, Farley MM, Hadler J, Harrison LH, Bennett NM, Lynfield R, et al. Decline in invasive pneumococcal disease after the introduction of protein-polysaccharide conjugate vaccine. N Engl J Med. 2003;348(18):1737–46. Epub 2003/05/02. https://doi.org/10.1056/NEJMoa022823. PubMed PMID: 12724479.

Copelovitch L, Kaplan BS. *Streptococcus pneumoniae*–Associated Hemolytic Uremic Syndrome: Classification and the Emergence of Serotype 19A. Pediatrics. 2010;125(1):e174-e82. https://doi.org/10.1542/peds.2007-2017.

Scobell RR, Kaplan BS, Copelovitch L. New insights into the pathogenesis of *Streptococcus pneumoniae*-associated hemolytic uremic syndrome. Pediatr Nephrol. 2020;35(9):1585–91. Epub 2019/09/14. https://doi.org/10.1007/s00467-019-04342-3. PubMed PMID: 31515631.

Lu CY, Chiang CS, Chiu CH, Wang ET, Chen YY, Yao SM, et al. Successful Control of *Streptococcus pneumoniae* 19A Replacement With a Catch-up Primary Vaccination Program in Taiwan. Clin Infect Dis. 2019;69(9):1581–7. Epub 2019/03/30. https://doi.org/10.1093/cid/ciy1127. PubMed PMID: 30923808.

Pneumococcal Disease, Centers for Disease Control and Prevention. https://www.cdc.gov/pneumococcal/clinicians/diagnosis-medical-mgmt.html.

Waters AM, Kerecuk L, Luk D, Haq MR, Fitzpatrick MM, Gilbert RD, et al. Hemolytic uremic syndrome associated with invasive pneumococcal disease: the United kingdom experience. J Pediatr. 2007;151(2):140–4. Epub 2007/07/24. https://doi.org/10.1016/j.jpeds.2007.03.055. PubMed PMID: 17643764.

Loupiac A, Elayan A, Cailliez M, Adra AL, Decramer S, Thouret MC, et al. Diagnosis of *Streptococcus pneumoniae*-associated hemolytic uremic syndrome. Pediatr Infect Dis J. 2013;32(10):1045–9. Epub 2013/09/27. https://doi.org/10.1097/INF.0b013e31829ee872. PubMed PMID: 24067551.

Case 23. A Cluster of Community-Acquired Pneumonia in Two Siblings of School Age: Macrolide-Resistance *Mycoplasma pneumoniae* Infection

Huei-Min Hung, Yu-Chia Hsieh, and Yhu-Chering Huang

Keywords

Pneumonia · *Mycoplasma pneumoniae* · Macrolide-resistance

Key Points

- *M. pneumoniae* becomes the most common bacterial pathogen responsible for community-acquired pneumonia in the era of pneumococcal conjugate vaccines.
- Polymerase chain reaction and serologic tests are two common diagnostic tools for detection of *Mycoplasma pneumoniae* infection; however, they cannot differentiate *M. pneumoniae* infection from carriage.
- Measurement of *Mp*-IgM-antibody secreting cells by enzyme-linked immunospot (ELISpot) assay can be a promising test for diagnosing pneumonia *caused by M. pneumoniae.*
- Macrolide-resistant *Mycoplasma pneumoniae* emerged in Japan, prevailed in Eastern Asian countries, and then spread worldwide.
- With the increasing rate of macrolide-resistance, the choice of antibiotic therapy for severe community-acquired pneumonia caused by *M. pneumoniae* should be reappraised.

Case 1

A previously healthy 7-year-old boy was admitted with a 5-day history of fever, cough, and rhinorrhea. A chest radiograph revealed consolidation over the left lower lobe (Fig. 1). Laboratory investigations showed a white blood cell count of 7300/μL (normal range: 6000–10,400), while differential count revealed 60% segmented and 2% band neutrophils. An elevated C-reactive protein concentration of 96.64 mg/L (normal range: <5 mg/L) was noted. Therapy with intravenous amoxicillin/clavulanic acid (amoxicillin 100 mg/kg/day) plus azithromycin (10 mg/kg/day) was prescribed. Fever (40–41 °C) was still noted and we even changed amoxicillin/

H.-M. Hung · Y.-C. Hsieh (✉)
Division of Pediatric Infectious Diseases, Chang Gung Memorial Hospital at Linkou, Taoyuan, Taiwan

Y.-C. Huang
Pediatrics, Chang Gung Memorial Hospital, Chang Gung University, Taoyuan, Taiwan
e-mail: ychuang@cgmh.org.tw

Y.-C. Huang et al. (eds.), *Paediatric Infectious Diseases*,
https://doi.org/10.1007/978-981-19-7276-8_23

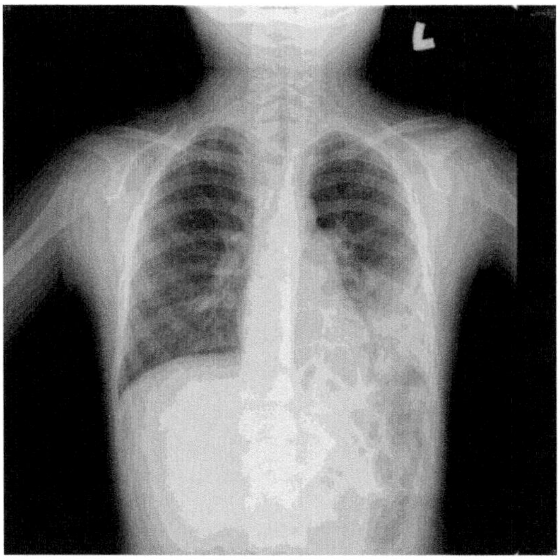

Fig. 1 A chest radiograph revealed consolidation over the left lower lobe in a previously healthy 7-year-old boy

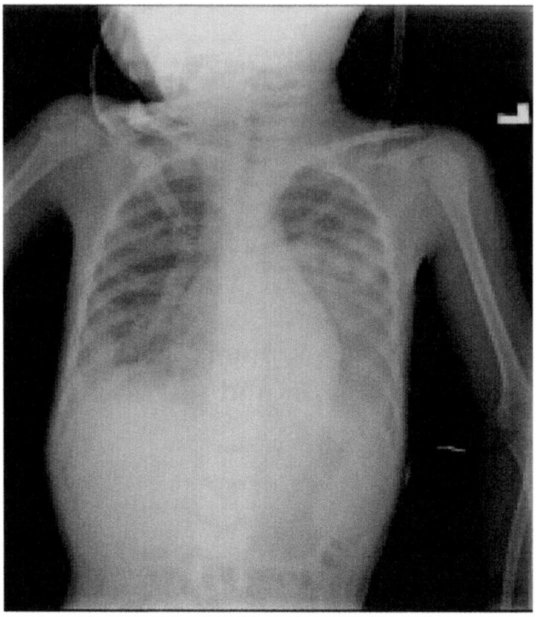

Fig. 2 A chest radiography revealed patchy opacity over the left upper lobe and right lower lobe in a previously healthy 6-year-old girl

clavulanic acid to ceftriaxone (75 mg/kg/day) and added oseltamivir. Serologic investigations performed on the first day of hospitalization were negative for IgM and IgG (Savyon Diagnostics, Ashdod, Israel) against *M. pneumoniae,* but IgM against *M. pneumoniae* was positive (55 BU/mL) 6 days later. Doxycycline (4.4 mg/kg/day) was then added. After treatment with doxycycline, the fever decreased to 38–39 °C. On the ninth day of hospitalization, the patient underwent lung biopsy for definite diagnosis. Oral prednisolone (1 mg/kg/day) was used to reduce the low grade fever on the twelfth day of hospitalization, and the patient became afebrile on the thirteenth day. He was discharged on day 17 after admission.

Case 2

On the same day, the 6-year-old sister of case 1 was also admitted with a 7-day history of fever, cough, and rhinorrhea. A chest radiography revealed patchy opacity over the left upper lobe and right lower lobe (Fig. 2). Laboratory investigations showed a white blood cell count of 15,400/mm^3 with 88% segmented and 3% band neutrophils. The C-reactive protein level was 149 mg/L. Empiric treatment with vancomycin, ceftriaxone, azithromycin, and oseltamivir were initiated. On the second day of hospitalization, she was intubated because of hypoxemia. On the fourth day of hospitalization, she developed acute respiratory distress syndrome (ARDS) ($PaO_2/FiO_2 < 200$ mmHg). Extracorporeal membrane oxygenation (ECMO) therapy was undertaken. Serologic tests performed on the first day of hospitalization was positive for IgM (24 BU/mL) and negative for IgG against *M. pneumoniae*; IgM increased to 72 BU/mL and IgG remained negative 4 days later. Doxycycline was added on the seventh day of hospitalization. After use of doxycycline, oxygenation improved gradually and gas flow of ECMO could be decreased. The patient was successfully decannulated from ECMO after 12 days and received conventional ventilator support for an additional 3 days. High-resolution computed tomography (HRCT) revealed multiple cystic lesions with ground glass appearance in both lung fields (Fig. 3). Systemic steroid (methylprednisolone 3.5 mg/kg/day) therapy was initiated for persistent tachypnea and fever. The patient was discharged on day 40 (Hsieh et al. 2012).

M. pneumoniae real-time PCR assay from nasopharyngeal aspirate, lung tissue, and pleural

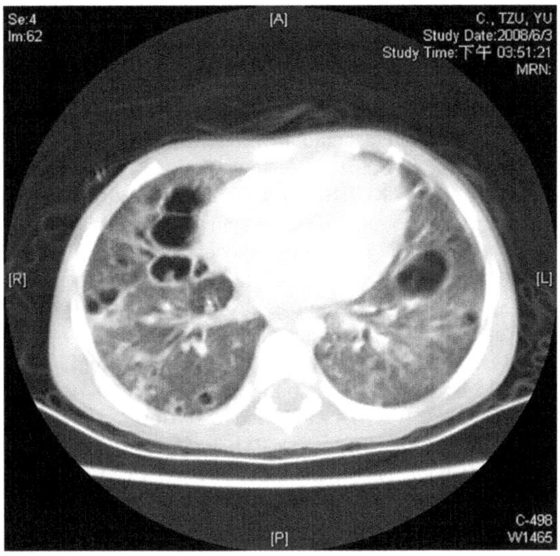

Fig. 3 High-resolution computed tomography (HRCT) revealed multiple cystic lesions with ground glass appearance in both lung fields

fluid of the brother and nasopharyngeal aspirate of the sister were all positive. Sequencing of the 23S rRNA in both cases identified an A2064G transition in domain V, which is indicative of a macrolide-resistant phenotype.

Discussion

Mycoplasma pneumoniae (*M. pneumoniae*) is a bacterium which lacks a rigid cell wall. In both children and adults, it is a major cause of respiratory diseases such as pharyngitis, tracheobronchitis, and community-acquired pneumonia. Pneumonia caused by *M. pneumoniae* is sometimes referred to as "walking pneumonia" since symptoms are generally mild. Occasionally, *M. pneumoniae* can cause other severe respiratory illnesses such as bronchiolitis obliterans, chronic interstitial fibrosis, and acute respiratory distress syndrome. *M. pneumoniae* has also been linked to reactive airway disease, asthma, and a broad range of extrapulmonary manifestations such as encephalitis, erythema multiforme, Steven-Johnson syndrome, and hemolytic anemia. In general, 8–35% of cases with community-acquired pneumonia was caused by *M. pneumoniae* in different countries. In Taiwan, *M. pneumoniae* is responsible for 38% of childhood community-acquired pneumonia and is the second most common bacterial pathogen before the use of pneumococcal conjugate vaccine. *M. pneumoniae* becomes the most frequent bacterial cause of pediatric community-acquired pneumonia in Taiwan after the widespread implementation of pneumococcal conjugate vaccine. It is transmitted from person-to-person contact by respiratory droplets and the incubation period varies from 1 to 4 weeks. Epidemiologic data show that epidemic peaks of *M. pneumoniae* occur every 3–7 years, as indicated by three outbreaks in 2011–2012, 2014–2015, and 2015–2016 in Japan and Europe. Genotype shifts from one P1 adhesin subtype to another occurred repeatedly at an interval of 10 years. Diagnostic tests with polymerase chain reaction (PCR) and serology cannot differentiate *M. pneumoniae* infection from carriage. Measurement of *Mp*-IgM-antibody secreting cells (ASCs) by enzyme-linked immunospot (ELISpot) assay can be a promising test for diagnosing *pneumonia caused by M. pneumoniae*.

Most people can recover from an infection caused by *M. pneumoniae* without antibiotics. However, someone who develops pneumonia caused by *M. pneumoniae* would be prescribed the antibiotics to help the patient recover from the infection. There are several types of antibiotics (macrolide, tetracycline, or fluoroquinolone) available to treat pneumonia caused by *M. pneumoniae*. Macrolides are the empirical choice of treatments in individuals with *M. pneumoniae* infection, especially the children. However, macrolide-resistant strain was identified from children with pneumonia for the first time in Japan in 2000. Afterwards the macrolide-resistant strain spread to other Asian countries and the macrolide-resistant rate was ever up to 90% in some regions of Japan and China. Macrolide resistance was also reported in the United States and the European countries. In Taiwan, 24% of patients with pneumonia were caused by macrolide-resistant *M. pneumoniae* in 2010, and the macrolide-resistant rate increased to 77% between 2017 and 2019.

The major cause of macrolide resistance in *M. pneumoniae* is the loss of binding ability of the macrolides to the 23S rRNA components of the bacterial ribosome, which involves mutations at positions A2063G/C/T, A2064G/C, and C2617G in 23S rRNA. Compared with macrolide-sensitive strains, macrolide-resistant *M. pneumoniae* infection has been associated with a longer febrile period, a longer duration of cough illness, and a longer course of antibiotic therapy. In the United States, 12% of hospitalized children with *M. pneumoniae* infection were ever admitted to the intensive care unit. Macrolide-resistant *M. pneumoniae* is associated with more complications and makes treatment more challenging. It is helpful to understand the epidemiology and outbreaks of *M. pneumoniae* infections by analyzing the molecular characteristics of clinical isolates. Several methods for molecular typing of *M. pneumoniae* isolates have been developed, including multilocus sequence typing (MLST), multilocus variable-number tandem-repeat analysis (MLVA), and P1 typing. MLST scheme displays a highly discriminative method to know the epidemiology and outbreaks of *M. pneumoniae* infection.

The high rate of macrolide resistance in Taiwan attributed to co-dissemination of sequence type 3 (ST3) and sequence type 17 (ST17) resistant clone. ST3 constitutes the majority of both macrolide susceptible and resistant strains in Japan, South Korea, and Moscow. The resistance rate in South Korea increased from 54.1% to 84.4% during 2010–2016 after the emergence of macrolide-resistant ST3 lineages. The ST17 lineage was not frequently observed in Japan and South Korea. On the contrary, the dissemination of macrolide-resistant ST17 linkage was noticed in Taiwan. Clonal dominance of macrolide resistance was observed in Asia where the prevalence of macrolide-resistant *M. pneumoniae* is high. In contrast, the low prevalence of macrolide-resistant *M. pneumoniae* in the United States and Europe was reported as polyclonal origin of macrolide resistance. It is imperative to continuously monitor spread and evolution of macrolide-resistant strains to obtain additional perspectives on macrolide resistance.

Further Reading

Waites KB, Xiao L, Liu Y, Balish MF, Atkinson TP. Mycoplasma pneumoniae from the Respiratory Tract and Beyond. Clin Microbiol Rev 2017;30:747-809.

Hsieh YC, Tsao KC, Huang CG, Tong S, Winchell JM, Huang YC, et al. Life-threatening pneumonia caused by macrolide-resistant Mycoplasma pneumoniae. Pediatr Infect Dis J 2012;31:208-9.

Jain S, Williams DJ, Arnold SR, Ampofo K, Bramley AM, Reed C, et al. Community-acquired pneumonia requiring hospitalization among U.S. children. N Engl J Med. 2015;372(9):835-45. Epub 2015/02/26. doi: 10.1056/NEJMoa1405870. PubMed PMID: 25714161; PubMed Central PMCID: PMCPMC4697461.

Yang TI, Chang TH, Lu CY, Chen JM, Lee PI, Huang LM, et al. Mycoplasma pneumoniae in pediatric patients: Do macrolide-resistance and/or delayed treatment matter? J Microbiol Immunol Infect. 2019;52(2):329-35.

Lai WC, Hsieh YC, Chen YC, Kuo CY, Chen CJ, Huang YC, et al. A potent antibody-secreting B cell response to Mycoplasma pneumoniae in children with pneumonia. J Microbiol Immunol Infect. 2021. https://doi.org/10.1016/j.jmii.2021.08.010.

Meyer Sauteur PM, Seiler M, Truck J, Unger WWJ, Paioni P, Relly C, et al. Diagnosis of Mycoplasma pneumoniae Pneumonia with Measurement of Specific Antibody-Secreting Cells. Am J Respir Crit Care Med. 2019;200(8):1066-9.

Hung HM, Chuang CH, Chen YY, Liao WC, Li SW, Chang IY, et al. Clonal spread of macrolide-resistant Mycoplasma pneumoniae sequence type-3 and type-17 with recombination on non-P1 adhesin among children in Taiwan. Clin Microbiol Infect. 2021;27(8):1169 e1-e6.

Kutty PK, Jain S, Taylor TH, Bramley AM, Diaz MH, Ampofo K, et al. Mycoplasma pneumoniae Among Children Hospitalized With Community-acquired Pneumonia. Clin Infect Dis. 2019;68(1):5-12.

Degrange S, Cazanave C, Charron A, Renaudin H, Bebear C, Bebear CM. Development of multiple-locus variable-number tandem-repeat analysis for molecular typing of Mycoplasma pneumoniae. J Clin Microbiol. 2009;47(4):914-23.

Brown RJ, Holden MT, Spiller OB, Chalker VJ. Development of a Multilocus Sequence Typing Scheme for Molecular Typing of Mycoplasma pneumoniae. J Clin Microbiol. 2015;53(10):3195-203.

Hsieh YC, Li SW, Chen YY, Kuo CC, Chen YC, Chang IY, et al. Global Genome Diversity and Recombination in Mycoplasma pneumoniae. Emerg Infect Dis. 2022;28(1):111-7.

Lee JK, Lee JH, Lee H, Ahn YM, Eun BW, Cho EY, et al. Clonal Expansion of Macrolide-Resistant Sequence Type 3 Mycoplasma pneumoniae, South Korea. Emerg Infect Dis. 2018;24(8):1465-71.

Ando M, Morozumi M, Adachi Y, Ubukata K, Iwata S. Multilocus Sequence Typing of Mycoplasma pneumoniae, Japan, 2002-2016. Emerg Infect Dis. 2018;24(10):1895-901.

Voronina EN, Gordukova MA, Turina IE, Mishukova OV, Dymova MA, Galeeva EV, et al. Molecular characterization of Mycoplasma pneumoniae infections in Moscow from 2015 to 2018. Eur J Clin Microbiol Infect Dis. 2020;39(2):257-63.

Qu J, Chen S, Bao F, Gu L, Cao B. Molecular characterization and analysis of Mycoplasma pneumoniae among patients of all ages with community-acquired pneumonia during an epidemic in China. Int J Infect Dis. 2019;83:26-31.

Diaz MH, Benitez AJ, Winchell JM. Investigations of Mycoplasma pneumoniae infections in the United States: trends in molecular typing and macrolide resistance from 2006 to 2013. J Clin Microbiol. 2015;53(1):124-30.

Case 24. A 13-Year-Old Girl with Fever for 13 Days and Cough and Dyspnea for 7 Days: Miliary Tuberculosis

Ping-Ing Lee

Keywords

Miliary tuberculosis · Immune reconstitution inflammatory syndrome · Anti-tuberculous therapy · Tuberculin skin test

Key Points

- Miliary TB is a severe form of TB that is thought to be a consequence of hematogenous dissemination of *M. tuberculosis*.
- Miliary infiltrates on a chest radiograph or computed tomography images are characteristic and probably diagnostic finding for miliary TB.
- Many patients with miliary TB manifest tuberculin anergy. A negative tuberculin skin test cannot exclude the possibility of TB.
- Miliary tuberculosis is uniformly fatal if not treated. Treatment should be initiated immediately based on strong clinical suspicion, because mortality from miliary TB is most often due to delays in treatment.

P.-I. Lee (✉)
Department of Pediatrics, National Taiwan University Children's Hospital, National Taiwan University, Taipei, Taiwan
e-mail: pinging@ntu.edu.tw

Case Report

A 13-year-old girl had fever up to 39 °C for 13 days. Cough and dyspnea developed 7 days ago. She has received one dose of Bacillus Calmette–Guérin (BCG) shortly after birth. She was treated with azithromycin with a tentative diagnosis of mycoplasma pneumonia because the *Mycoplasma pneumoniae* IgM test was positive. The chest film was described as "interstitial pneumonia." Oxygen desaturation and progression of chest X-ray lesions occurred and she was transferred to our hospital for admission. Physically, she was tachypneic with chest wall retractions. The breath sound was clear. The liver could be palpated 4 cm below right costal margin. One oral ulcer was noted on the uvula. The white count was 7780/μL with 74.9% segmented neutrophil. Liver enzyme levels were elevated, including alanine transaminase of 100 U/L and aspartate transaminase of 127 U/L. C-reactive protein value was 1.49 mg/dL. Empirical tetracycline, vancomycin, and cefotaxime were given.

Microbiological tests for influenza, adenovirus, enterovirus, cytomegalovirus Epstein-Barr virus, and *M. pneumoniae* were all negative in results. Tuberculin skin test was negative. Hypotension was noted for two times after admission. Isoniazid, rifampin, pyrazinamide, and levofloxacin were given because chest radiograph showed infiltrates compatible with military tuberculosis (TB) (Fig. 1). Chest computed tomogra-

Y.-C. Huang et al. (eds.), *Paediatric Infectious Diseases*,
https://doi.org/10.1007/978-981-19-7276-8_24

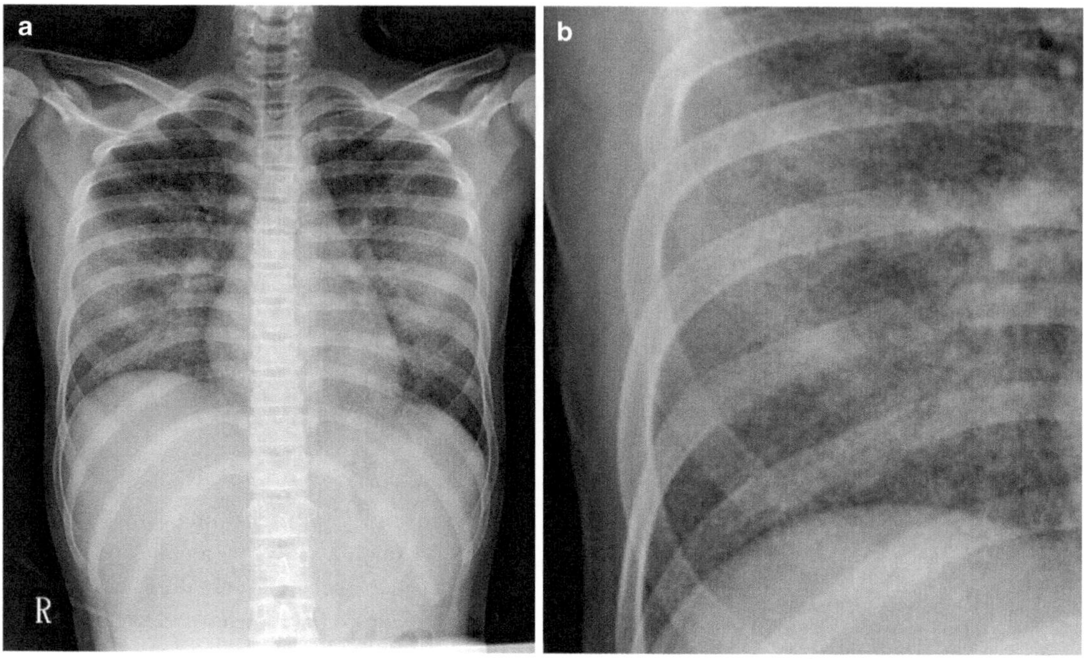

Fig. 1 Chest X-ray taken at admission. (**a**) The chest film shows bilateral interstitial infiltration; (**b**) Magnified image of right lower lung field of the same chest film shows "military" lesions

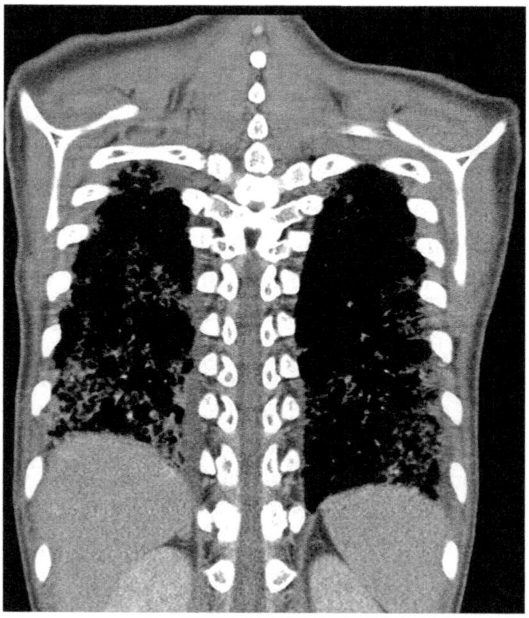

Fig. 2 Chest computed tomography showed diffuse, multiple small nodules over bilateral lungs

phy (CT) showed diffuse, multiple small nodules over bilateral lungs (Fig. 2) with osteolytic lesions on the fourth and the eighth thoracic spin. T2-weighted image of brain magnetic resonance imaging (MRI) showed a high-intensity lesion at right interhemispheric region (Fig. 3).

Blood desaturation and impending respiratory failure occurred shortly after the start of anti-tuberculous therapy and the follow-up chest film revealed progressive bilateral infiltrations with consolidation (Fig. 4). Methylprednisolone was given for possible immune reconstitution inflammatory syndrome.

Laboratory tests showed the presence of acid-fast bacilli in sputum specimen. *Mycobacterium tuberculosis*, that was susceptible to all anti-tuberculous agents tested, was isolated from the sputum. Ophthalmology consultation found numerous choroidal tubercles on bilateral sub-retinal regions by fundoscopic examination. The clinical condition improved a few days later with gradual resolution of lesions on chest film (Fig. 5). Pyrazinamide and levofloxacin were used for 2 months. Isoniazid and rifampin were used for 12 months. Follow-up visits showed that the infection had been resolved completely without sequel.

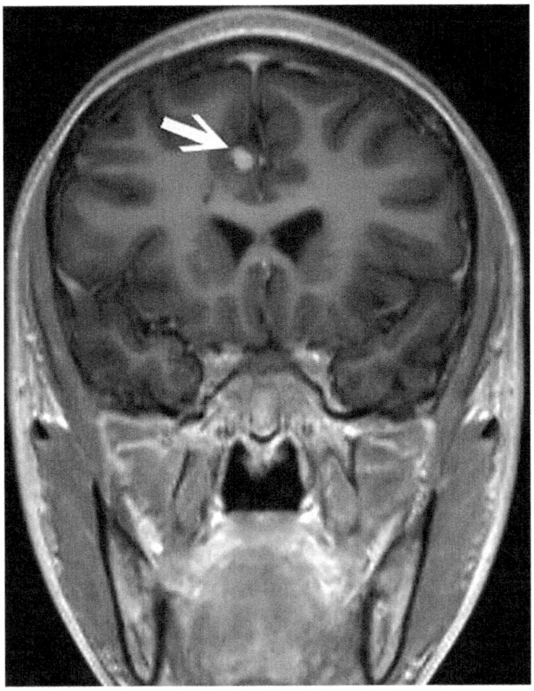

Fig. 3 T2-weighted image of brain magnetic resonance imaging showed a high-intensity lesion at right interhemispheric region (arrow)

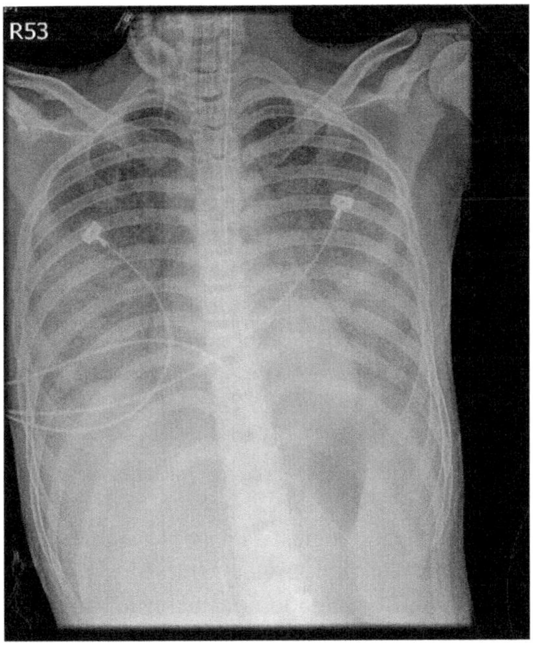

Fig. 4 Chest X-ray taken 2 days after admission showed progression of lung lesions

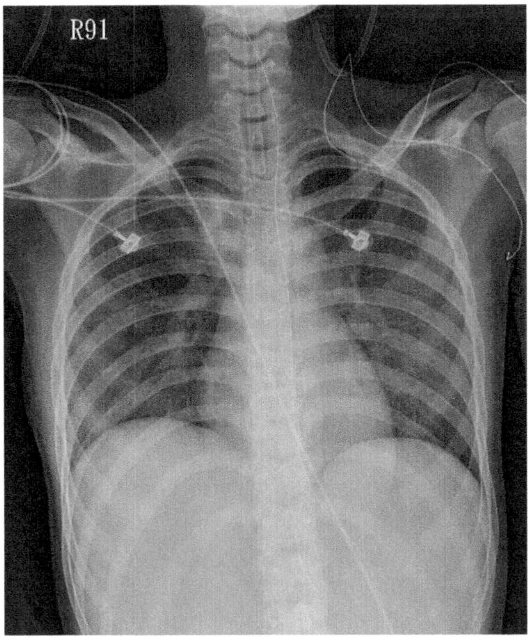

Fig. 5 Lesions on chest film taken 13 days after admission showed gradual resolution

Discussion

Miliary TB is a severe form of TB that is thought to be a consequence of hematogenous dissemination of *M. tuberculosis*. The term miliary TB is used to describe its gross pathological resemblance to millet seeds. It tends to occur in the very young or individuals with T-cell immunodeficiency. It may occasionally be observed in persons with no apparent immunocompromised conditions, as illustrated by the present case. The incidence of miliary TB is increasing in some populations, such as human immunodeficiency virus (HIV)-infected persons and those receiving chemotherapy.

Miliary TB occurred either soon after primary infection in children or as a terminal event in untreated TB. Miliary tuberculosis in children usually complicates the primary infection, occurring within 2–6 months of the initial infection. In children, the illness is usually in an acute form with nonspecific symptoms, such as intermittent fevers, anorexia, weakness, weight loss, headache, and abdominal pain. Pleural effusion, peritonitis, and meningitis are frequently observed.

As illustrated by the present case, miliary infiltrates on a chest radiograph are characteristic and probably diagnostic finding for miliary TB. Classic miliary pattern is defined as a collection of tiny, discrete pulmonary opacities with diffuse distribution, each of which measures <2–3 mm in diameter. However, data from published studies suggest that the classic miliary pattern may not be evident in up to 50% of patients with miliary tuberculosis. High-resolution CT scans have considerably improved diagnostic sensitivity for miliary tuberculosis and reveal classic miliary pattern even when the chest radiograph looks apparently normal.

Cultures of sputum, gastric contents, urine, and cerebrospinal fluid are positive in some combination in patients. However, no more than one-third of sputum smears are positive for acid-fast bacilli. A higher proportion of patients with miliary TB manifest tuberculin anergy than those with pulmonary TB or extrapulmonary TB. Because of tuberculin anergy, the tuberculin skin test is not useful as a diagnostic test in patients with miliary tuberculosis. The negative tuberculin skin test in present case cannot exclude the possibility of TB.

Bacillus Calmette-Guérin (BCG) vaccine, used to prevent TB, is a live-attenuated vaccine derived from a strain of *M. bovis*. BCG vaccination of children results in a 60–80% decrease in the incidence of TB, while efficacy has varied widely in different reports. Although BCG vaccine does not always prevent infection, it prevents progression to severe illness, including miliary TB.

Miliary tuberculosis is uniformly fatal if not treated. The mortality related to miliary tuberculosis is about 15–20% in children and 25–30% in adults. Treatment should be initiated immediately based on strong clinical suspicion, because mortality from miliary TB is most often due to delays in treatment. The resolution of miliary tuberculosis is slow, even with proper therapy. Fever usually declines within 2–3 weeks of starting chemotherapy, but the chest radiographic abnormalities might not resolve for many months.

Although anti-tuberculous treatment is the cornerstone of management, there is no consensus regarding the optimum duration of treatment. In the absence of associated meningeal involvement, the American Thoracic Society, the Centers for Disease Control and Prevention, the Infectious Disease Society of America, and the British Thoracic Society recommend that 6 months of treatment (2-month intensive phase with isoniazid, rifampicin, pyrazinamide, and ethambutol or streptomycin, followed by a 4-month continuation phase with isoniazid and rifampicin) is adequate in miliary TB, whereas the American Academy of Pediatrics advocates 9 months of treatment. In the presence of associated TB meningitis, treatment needs to be given for at least 12 months. According to the World Health Organization guidelines, miliary TB is included under treatment category I and patients receive 6 months of treatment. Taiwan Guidelines for TB Diagnosis and Treatment, published in 2017, recommends 2-month intensive phase with isoniazid, rifampicin, pyrazinamide, and ethambutol, followed by a continuation phase with isoniazid and rifampicin for 7–10 months for the treatment of miliary TB in children. TB meningitis should be treated for at least 12 months, and one of levofloxacin, moxifloxacin, aminoglycoside, and prothionamide should be used instead of ethambutol in the intensive phase.

Although several trials have been conducted in patients with various forms of extrapulmonary TB, including meningitis, pericarditis, and pleurisy, the role of adjunct corticosteroid treatment in patients with miliary tuberculosis remained controversial. For the present case, steroid therapy is necessary because the clinical condition deteriorated rapidly after the start of anti-tuberculous therapy. The clinical pictures are compatible with immune reconstitution inflammatory syndrome (IRIS) or paradoxical reaction that is identified in 6–30% of patients receiving anti-tuberculous therapy.

Immunopathological damage is suggested as a possible explanation for the paradoxical worsening of TB after initiation of treatment, in which an abnormal, excessive immune response arises against alive or dead *M. tuberculosis* after the start of chemotherapy. It is generally defined as a clinical or radiological worsening of pre-existing

TB lesions or the development of new lesions in a patient who initially improves with antituberculous therapy. Although IRIS is more frequently observed in HIV-positive patients, it may also occur in individuals without underlying conditions. In HIV-infected patients, it may occur after initiation of antiretroviral therapy independently of an effective suppression of HIV viremia. Systemic corticosteroid administration for 4–6 weeks may improve the outcome of IRIS.

Further Reading

Mangtani P, Abubakar I, Ariti C, et al. Protection by BCG vaccine against tuberculosis: a systematic review of randomized controlled trials. Clin Infect Dis 2014;58:470-80.

Sharma SK, Mohan A, Sharma A, Mitra DK. Miliary tuberculosis: new insights into an old disease. Lancet Infect Dis 2005;5:415-30.

Cheng VC, Ho PL, Lee RA, et al. Clinical spectrum of paradoxical deterioration during antituberculosis therapy in non-HIV-infected patients. Eur J Clin Microbiol Infect Dis 2002; 21:803-9.

Mert A, Arslan F, Kuyucu T, et al. Miliary tuberculosis: Epidemiological and clinical analysis of large-case series from moderate to low tuberculosis endemic Country. Medicine 2017;96:e5875.

Trunz BB, Fine P, Dye C. Effect of BCG vaccination on childhood tuberculous meningitis and miliary tuberculosis worldwide: a meta-analysis and assessment of cost-effectiveness. Lancet 2006;367:1173-80.

Fitzgerald DW, Sterling TR, Haas DW. *Mycobacterium tuberculosis*. In: Mandell GL, Bennett JE, Dolin R, eds. Mandell, Douglas, and Bennett's Principles and Practices of Infectious Diseases, 9th edition. Philadelphia: Churchill Livingstone, 2020.

Cameron LH, Starke JR. Tuberculosis (*Mycobacterium tuberculosis*). In: Kliegman RM, St Geme JW, Blum NJ, et al. eds. Nelson Textbook of Pediatrics, 21th edition. Philadelphia: Churchill Livingstone, 2020.

Kim JH, Langston AA, Gallis HA. Miliary tuberculosis: epidemiology, clinical manifestations, diagnosis, and outcome. Rev Infect Dis 1990; 12: 583-90.

Lanzafame M, Vento S. Tuberculosis-immune reconstitution inflammatory syndrome. J Clin Tuberc Other Mycobact Dis 201611;3:6-9.

Part IV

Heart Infection

Case 25. A 12-Year-Old Female Adolescent with Fever, Vomiting, Abdominal Pain, Right-Hand Purpura, and Headache: Infective Endocarditis

Wan-Chun Lai and Yhu-Chering Huang

Keywords

Infective endocarditis · *Staphylococcus aureus* · Bacteremia · Heart murmur

Key Points

- In the pediatric population, the incidence is relatively low and infants and adolescents are the mostly affected groups.
- Gram positive organism (*Staphylococci*, *Streptococci* and enterococcus species) are the majority of microorganisms, with *Staphylococcus aureus* the most frequently seen.
- Fever and heart murmur are the two most crucial clinical features, seen in approximately 90% and 80% of cases, respectively.
- Clinical suspicion of infective endocarditis should be raised in a patient with prolonged fever, bacteremia, predisposing risk factors and preexisting cardiac disease.
- Antimicrobial treatment for infective endocarditis should be started immediately after completion of blood culture collection.
- As empirical therapy, an anti-staphylococcal regimen (oxacillin or vancomycin) plus gentamicin as synergic effect is recommended.

Case Report

A 12-year-old female, who was previously healthy but obese (Body Mass Index 34 kg/m^2, >97th percentile), suffered from acute onset of fever to 40 °C for 1 day. Associated symptoms included vomiting, abdominal pain, right hand purpura, and headache. She ever visited a local medical clinic where symptomatic treatment was given. Later, sudden onset of right upper limb weakness, blurred vision, and disorientation of place and people were noted; therefore, she was sent to a local hospital. There was no cough, rhinorrhea, shortness of breath, or diarrhea. Four weeks before the illness, there was a ruptured acne over her right eyelid which healed without any specific medical therapy subsequently. The patient denied relevant travel or contact history recently. Hypotension (blood pressure 83/75 mmHg) was

W.-C. Lai (✉)
Division of Pediatric Infectious Diseases, Chang Gung Memorial Hospital at Linkou, Taoyuan, Taiwan

Y.-C. Huang
Pediatrics, Chang Gung Memorial Hospital, Chang Gung University, Taoyuan, Taiwan
e-mail: ychuang@cgmh.org.tw

Y.-C. Huang et al. (eds.), *Paediatric Infectious Diseases*,
https://doi.org/10.1007/978-981-19-7276-8_25

noted at the hospital and improved after normal saline challenge. Then, she was transferred to a tertiary medical center.

Upon arrival at the tertiary medical center, the patient was admitted to pediatric intensive care unit immediately. Her vital signs were body temperature 37.4 °C, pulse rate 105 beats/min, respiratory rate 22 times/min, and blood pressure 118/74 mmHg. Physical examination revealed acute-illness, conscious level of E4V5M6 but disoriented, neck stiffness with positive Brudzinski sign, muscle power 2/5 at right upper limb and otherwise full, bilateral Babinski signs withdrawn and incapability of counting fingers. Auscultation revealed grade II systolic murmur at left middle sternal border and normoactive bowel sound. Furthermore, multiple petechiae-like purpura were noted over right palm, dorsal aspect of bilateral feet, and digits (Fig. 1). A chest radiologic film revealed no active lung lesion or cardiomegaly. An abdominal plain film showed non-specific bowel gas distribution. Blood tests reported leukocytosis (WBC 15,800/μL), mild anemia (Hb 10.4 g/dL), elevated serum C-reactive protein (183.88 mg/L; normal, <5 mg/L) and procalcitonin (0.87 ng/mL) and coagulopathy with disseminated intravascular coagulation (prolonged prothrombin time 18 s, activated partial thromboplastin time 35.1, INR 1.7, elevated d-Dimer 4107 FEU ng/mL, high FDP 14.7 μg/mL, and fibrinogen 531 mg/dL); while, aspartate transaminase, alanine aminotransferase, electrolytes, creatinine, lactate, troponin I, and creatine kinase levels in sera were within normal limits. Computed tomography of brain disclosed no obvious intracranial abnormality. Under the tentative diagnosis of sepsis, suspect central nervous system infection, or infective endocarditis, the patient was treated with vancomycin and ceftazidime initially. Cerebrospinal fluid analysis revealed pleocytosis (leukocyte count 41/μL), but no elevated protein level and subsequently negative for either bacterial culture or viral etiology survey. Several hypointense lesions over bilateral frontal lobes and right cerebellum, with hemorrhagic change were shown in T2 and fluid-attenuated inversion recovery (FLAIR) of magnetic resonance imaging (MRI) of brain (Fig. 2a). Transthoracic echocardiography (TTE) disclosed pericardial effusion (5 mm thickness). Electrocardiogram (ECG) reported first degree atrioventricular block and ST-T change.

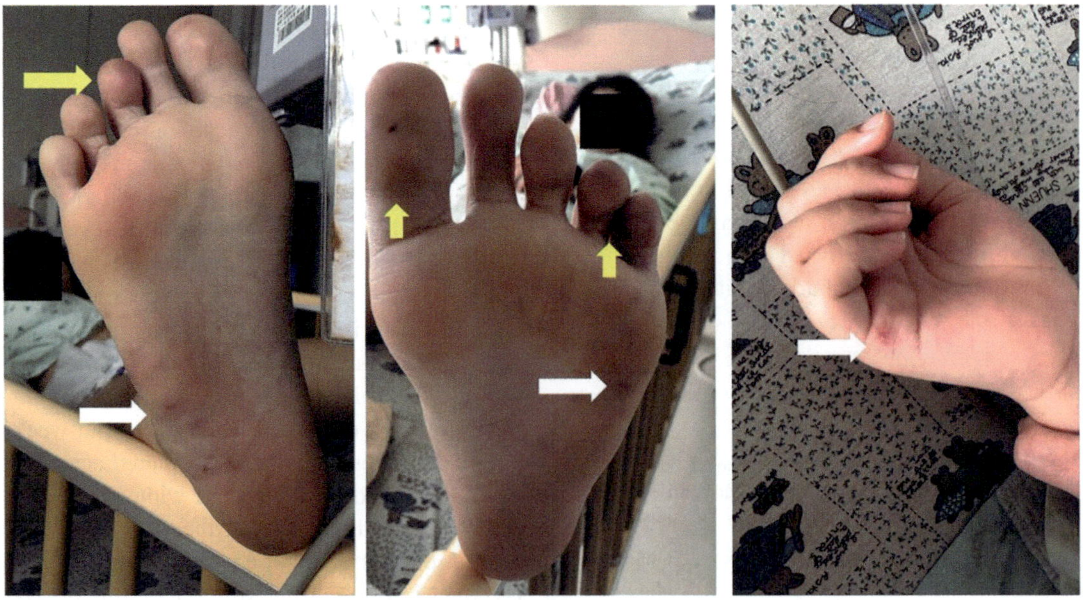

Fig. 1 Multiple non-tender, petechiae-like purpura over palms and soles (white arrowhead) and several small tender lumps over digits (yellow arrowhead)

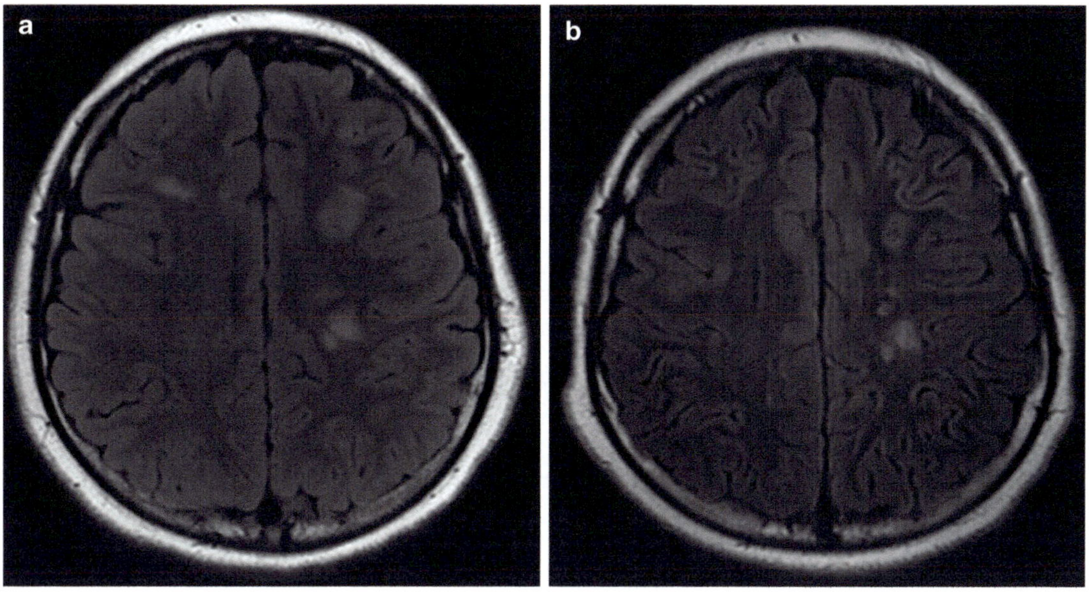

Fig. 2 Magnetic resonance imaging (MRI) of brain in T2 and fluid-attenuated inversion recovery (FLAIR) sequence reported multiple hyperintense lesions over bilateral frontal area initially (**a**). The lesion regressed after 6 weeks (**b**)

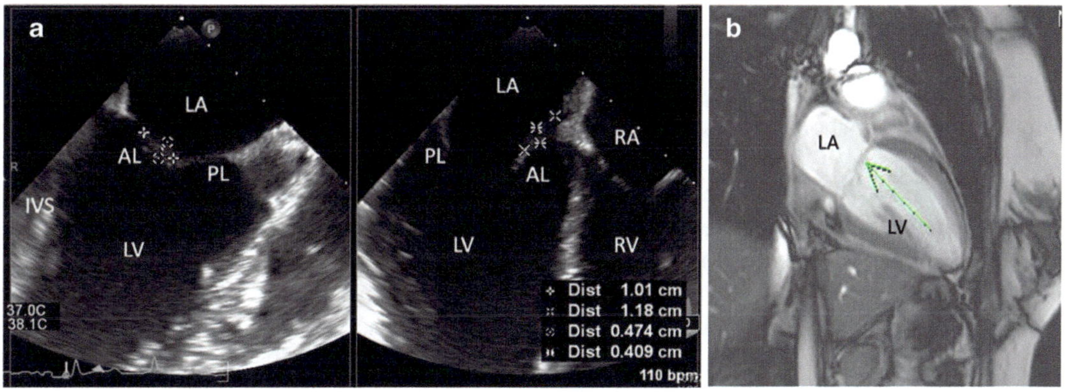

Fig. 3 Transesophageal echocardiography disclosed a flat non-mobile mass 1.1 × 0.3 cm, on atrial side of anterior mitral leaflet (**a**). Cardiac MRI reported a Vegetation at anterior leaflet of mitral valve (**b**)

Blood cultures obtained at the local hospital and at admission yielded methicillin-resistant *Staphylococcus aureus* (MRSA) for a total of three sets of specimens obtained more than 12 h apart. According to the modified Duke criteria of infective endocarditis, the diagnosis of definite infective endocarditis was made by fulfilling one major and three minor criteria. Multidisciplinary consultations were arranged. The Cardiologist arranged transesophageal echocardiography (TEE) which disclosed a 1.1 × 0.3 cm flat non-mobile mass on atrial side of anterior mitral leaflet (Fig. 3a). No dental caries was found after dental examination. However, a funduscopy revealed a yellowish lesion with central hemorrhage at retina over right eye, which suggested MRSA-related subretinal abscess. Vancomycin monotherapy continued and the target trough level was kept between 15 to 20 μg/mL. In order to survey the source of infection, gallium inflammatory scan was arranged and disclosed multiple lesions over nasopharynx, lymph nodes, left leg,

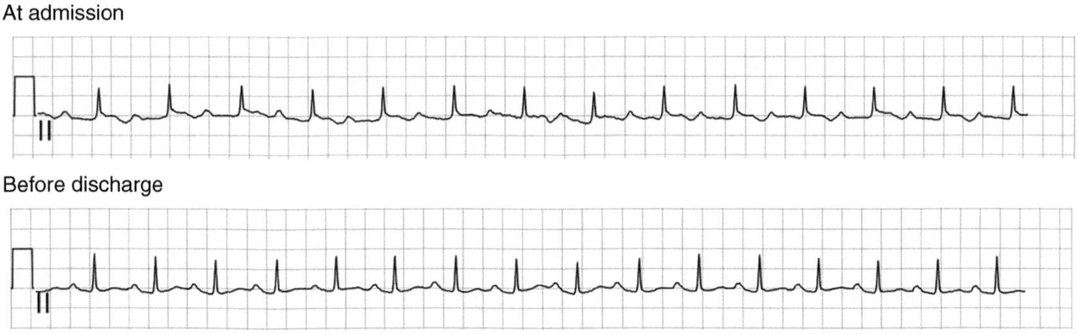

Fig. 4 Electrocardiogram (ECG) at admission disclosed first degree AV block and ST-T changes. Before discharge, the ECG showed first degree AV block

indicating systemic inflammatory responses or septic emboli. Further cardiac MRI confirmed myocardial injury at upper portion of interventricular septum, which possibly attributed to interfere the conduction system, and a vegetation at anterior leaflet of mitral valve (Fig. 3b). After 19 days of vancomycin treatment, fever was still noted occasionally, and daptomycin was added in addition to vancomycin. Fever subsided since then and the followed-up MRI of brain showed regression of the brain lesions (Fig. 2b). An ophthalmologic examination disclosed resolution of retinal abscess over right eye. First degree atrioventricular block was also noted on electrocardiogram (Fig. 4). After more than 7 weeks of vancomycin and 4 weeks of daptomycin, the patient was discharged with oral form of linezolid for additional 8 days. Her muscle power of right upper limbs was 4+/5 and the blurred vision improved. Some desquamation change was found over previous skin lesions (Osler's nodes and Janeway lesions). The final diagnosis was MRSA-related native valve infective endocarditis with mitral valve vegetation, complicated with cerebral septic emboli, and first degree atrioventricular block.

Discussion

Infective endocarditis (IE) is a life-threatening situation in which the infection involves the endocardium or valve of heart. The disease pathogenesis is thought to begin with the injured endothelium of heart followed by the denuded subendothelial layer which is prone to the formation of either bacterial colonization or platelet-fibrin thrombotic vegetation. The bacteria can grow in situ on the damaged endocardium or thrombotic lesion, causing the infected vegetation. Intracardiac devices, prosthetic valves, sclerotic valvular disease, indwelling vascular catheters are the most common cardiac condition for endocardium damage in an adult. In contrast, rheumatic heart disease was once the most common cause in children in the developing countries. In the developed countries, congenital heart disease, high velocity jet of blood flow (ventricular septal defect, endocardial cushion defects) and permanent indwelling intravascular catheter in the preterm neonates had taken up the role. Other risk factors include previous history of endocarditis, poor dental sanity, intravenous drug user, immunocompromised and recent dental or other surgical procedures.

The incidence of infective endocarditis varied in different age groups. The overall incidence is approximately 2–10 per 100,000 person-year. In the pediatric population, the incidence is relatively low, approximately 0.34–0.64 cases per 100,000 person-year. Infant period and late adolescence are the mostly affected groups.

Infective endocarditis is a complex disease with various disease spectrum, management, and prognosis in different situations. The classifications of infective endocarditis should include the location of the infection involved (right-sided versus left sided, which valve or device, native or prosthetic), the type of acquisition (community-associated or healthcare-associated), and the causative microorganism.

Gram positive organism (*Staphylococci*, *Streptococci* and enterococcus species) are the majority of microorganisms which account for 80% of infective endocarditis. *Staphylococcus aureus* is the most frequently seen microorganism, accounted for 30–40% of cases. Coagulase-negative staphylococci colonizes the skin and is characterized by biofilm formation, which more frequently causes prosthetic valve endocarditis than native valve endocarditis. *Streptococci* accounted for about 30% of cases. *Viridans Streptococci* group are abundant in mouth, which was the substantial species of streptococci in infective endocarditis. Enterococcus species accounted for approximately 10% of the cases. Besides the gram-positive cocci, the HACEK species (*Haemophilus species, Aggregatibacter species, Cardiobacterium species, Eikenella corrodens*, and *Kingella species*) are gram negative microorganisms which slowly grow and colonize in human oropharynx, accounting for about less than 5% of cases of IE.

Fever and heart murmur are the two most crucial clinical features of infective endocarditis, which are seen in approximately 90% and 80% of cases, respectively. Severe sepsis with or without shock, heart failure, and embolic events may rapidly develop and progress to a fatal outcome. Non-specific and subacute somatic complaints, including low grade fever, chills, lethargy, fatigue, weight loss, arthralgias, and diaphoresis could also develop for weeks or months Those well-known phenomena, including Janeway lesions (non-tender, hemorrhagic skin lesion on palms and soles), Osler's nodes (purple-red, tender lumps on fingers or toes) and Roth spot (retinal hemorrhage), are rare, and present in less than 10% of patients. The extracardiac manifestations are considerably less common in pediatric population than in adults.

Neurological complications may present symptomatically in 15–30% of IE. Stroke-like presentation is the most common symptom upon diagnosis, as shown in the illustrated case. Most of them are the consequence of embolic events from vegetations. Presence of neurological events increases the risk of mortality and sequelae.

Clinical suspicion of infective endocarditis should be raised in a patient with prolonged fever, bacteremia, predisposing risk factors and preexisting cardiac disease. The diagnosis is made by integrating multiple clinical presentations. According to the Modified Duke criteria, the definite diagnosis should meet two major criteria, five minor criteria, or one major plus three minor criteria. Possible endocarditis can be diagnosed based on three minor criteria or one major plus one minor criteria. Briefly, the two major criteria are (1) blood culture positive for IE: typical microorganisms (as described above) consistent with IE for 2 separate blood cultures or from persistently positive blood cultures; (2) evidence of endocardial involvement: echocardiogram positive for IE or new valvular regurgitation. The five minor criteria include predisposition, predisposing heart condition, or injection drug use; fever; vascular phenomena: major arterial emboli, septic pulmonary infarcts, mycotic aneurysm, intracranial hemorrhage, conjunctival hemorrhages, and Janeway lesions; immunologic phenomena: glomerulonephritis, Osler's nodes, Roth's spots, and rheumatoid factor; and microbiological evidence: positive blood culture but does not meet a major criterion as noted above or serological evidence of active infection with organism consistent with IE.

Positive blood culture is important for the microbiologic evidence of diagnosis of IE. Three sets of blood culture from separated peripheral sites, obtained 30 min apart and before antibiotic administration are recommend in all patients with suspected IE. Nevertheless, blood culture-negative endocarditis accounted for about 10% of IE.

Every patient in clinical suspicion of infective endocarditis should undertake transthoracic echocardiography (TTE) immediately. Transesophageal echocardiography (TEE) is mandatory in patients with high suspicion of infective endocarditis, but with negative TTE report. The sensitivity and specificity of detecting vegetations is both higher for TEE comparing to TTE. If needed, a repeated TTE or TEE is recommended within 5–7 days.

Antimicrobial treatment for infective endocarditis should be started immediately after completion of blood culture collection. Several considerations should be taken into the initial treatment regimen, including prior antibiotic exposure or not, native valve or prosthetic valve, community-associated or healthcare-associated and local microbial epidemiology. As empirical therapy, an anti-staphylococcal regimen (ampicillin, oxacillin, or vancomycin) plus gentamicin as synergic effect is recommended. The regimen should be adjusted once the antibiogram result is available. In general, combination therapy is recommended, except for *Staphylococcal* endocarditis, for which monotherapy is sufficient. Daptomycin is an alternative therapy for methicillin-resistant *Staphylococcal* endocarditis. However, short course of combination of anti-staphylococcal agent (oxacillin or vancomycin) plus rifampicin and gentamicin are standard in *Staphylococcus aureus*-related prosthetic valve endocarditis. The duration of antibiotics treatment is generally 4–6 weeks in exception of uncomplicated native valve endocarditis caused by methicillin susceptible *Streptococci* (treatment for 2 weeks). During the treatment courses, monitoring for serum drug level and nephrotoxicity is necessary.

Surgical intervention for IE is indicated in selective situations. The three main indications are heart failure caused by valvular dysfunction, uncontrolled infection despite appropriate antibiotics treatment, and infection source control and prevention of systemic embolic event when a large size of vegetation (usually >10 mm) persists.

Further Reading

Cahill TJ, Prendergast BD. Infective endocarditis. Lancet. 2016;387:882-93.

Chambers HF, Bayer AS. Native-Valve Infective Endocarditis. N Engl J Med. 2020;383:567-76.

Day MD, Gauvreau K, Shulman S, Newburger JW. Characteristics of children hospitalized with infective endocarditis [published correction appears in Circulation. 2010;122: e560]. Circulation. 2009;119:865-870.

Johnson JA, Boyce TG, Cetta F, Steckelberg JM, Johnson JN. Infective endocarditis in the pediatric patient: a 60-year single-institution review. Mayo Clin Proc 2012;87:629-35.

Shah ASV, McAllister DA, Gallacher P, et al. Incidence, Microbiology, and Outcomes in Patients Hospitalized With Infective Endocarditis [published correction appears in Circulation. 2020;141(25):e960]. Circulation. 2020;141(25):2067-77.

García-Cabrera E, Fernández-Hidalgo N, Almirante B, et al. Neurological complications of infective endocarditis: risk factors, outcome, and impact of cardiac surgery: a multicenter observational study. Circulation. 2013;127:2272-2284.

The 2015 ESC Guidelines for the management of infective endocarditis. Eur Heart J. 2015;36:3036-3037.

Baddour, L. M., Wilson, W. R., Bayer, A. S., et al. Infectious Diseases Society of America. Infective endocarditis: diagnosis, antimicrobial therapy, and management of complications: a statement for healthcare professionals from the Committee on Rheumatic Fever, Endocarditis, and Kawasaki Disease, Council on Cardiovascular Disease in the Young, and the Councils on Clinical Cardiology, Stroke, and Cardiovascular Surgery and Anesthesia, American Heart Association: endorsed by the Infectious Diseases Society of America. Circulation, 2005;111: e394-e434.

Lee JH, Kwak JG, Cho S, et al. Surgical outcomes of infective endocarditis in children: should we delay surgery for infective endocarditis? Eur J Cardiothorac Surg. 2021;ezab149. https://doi.org/10.1093/ejcts/ezab149

Kang DH, Kim YJ, Kim SH, et al. Early surgery versus conventional treatment for infective endocarditis. N Engl J Med. 2012;366(26):2466-2473.

Wilson W, Taubert KA, Gewitz M, et al. Prevention of infective endocarditis: guidelines from the American Heart Association: a guideline from the American Heart Association Rheumatic Fever, Endocarditis, and Kawasaki Disease Committee, Council on Cardiovascular Disease in the Young, and the Council on Clinical Cardiology, Council on Cardiovascular Surgery and Anesthesia, and the Quality of Care and Outcomes Research Interdisciplinary Working Group [published correction appears in Circulation. 2007 Oct 9;116(15):e376-7]. Circulation. 2007;116(15):1736-1754. https://doi.org/10.1161/CIRCULATIONAHA.106.183095

Asgeirsson H, Thalme A, Weiland O. *Staphylococcus aureus* bacteraemia and endocarditis - epidemiology and outcome: a review. Infect Dis (Lond). 2018;50:175-192.

Case 26. A 7-Year-Old Girl with General Weakness, Fatigue, and a Feeling of Discomfort Following Influenza: Influenza Associated Myocarditis and Pericarditis

Yi-Ching Chen and Yhu-Chering Huang

Keywords

Influenza virus · Myocarditis · Pericarditis

Key Points

- While influenza viruses are zoonoses, only influenza virus A, B, and C can cause human infections.
- Potential lethal complications of influenza include secondary bacterial infection, influenza associated encephalopathy, and acute myopericarditis.
- For a patient with "a feeling of not doing well," syncope or even symptoms of circulatory collapse following influenza, the occurrence of influenza-associated cardiac complication should be considered.
- Early use of antiviral agents may shorten the duration of symptoms, interrupt person-to-person viral spread, and reduce the disease severity.
- Due to the risk of potentially lethal complications, every effort to prevent influenza virus infection, including annual influenza vaccination, cannot be overemphasized.

Case Report 1

A previously healthy 7-year-old girl visited our emergency department (via outpatient department for admission) with the chief complaint of general weakness, fatigue, and "a feeling of not doing well" for 2 days. She was in her usual state of health until 7 days prior to hospitalization, when fever developed. Non-productive cough, clear rhinorrhea, and lethargic appearance were also observed. She was an elementary school student and had no recent contact history of sick persons. She was taken to a local clinic initially where an influenza rapid antigen test showed positive for influenza B. After taking four doses of oral oseltamivir, the fever subsided on the fourth day of illness. However, intermittent epigastric pain developed 1 day after the fever subsided, associated with nausea, vomiting, persistent dizziness, and myalgia. Due to progressive discomfort, she was taken to the emergency department for help.

Y.-C. Chen (✉)
Division of Pediatric Infectious Diseases, Department of Pediatrics, Chang Gung Memorial Hospital, Taoyuan, Taiwan

Y.-C. Huang
Division of Pediatric Infectious Diseases, Department of Pediatrics, Chang Gung Memorial Hospital, Chang Gung University, Taoyuan, Taiwan
e-mail: ychuang@cgmh.org.tw

Y.-C. Huang et al. (eds.), *Paediatric Infectious Diseases*,
https://doi.org/10.1007/978-981-19-7276-8_26

Upon arrival, vital signs were temperature 36.8 °C, pulse rate 112 beats/min, respiratory rate 20 times/min, and blood pressure 82/62 mm of mercury. On examination, she looked acutely ill and lethargic. Chest auscultation revealed bilateral clear breathing sound; heart beat was regular but tachycardiac, with distant heart sounds. The abdomen was soft without a specific tender point or peritoneal sign. Initial laboratory data showed leukocytes count 11,000/μL, segmented 76%, lymphocytes 17%, monocytes 5%, basophil 1%, normal platelet count (200,300/μL), and hemoglobin (18.8 g/dL) level. Blood biochemistry data showed sugar 101 mg/dL, elevated liver enzyme (aspartate transaminase 125 U/L, alanine transaminase 77 U/L), hyponatremia (132 mEq/L), hypochloremia (96 mEq/L), hypokalemia (3.4 mEq/L), and normal C-reactive protein level (<0.2 mg/L). Furthermore, significant elevated CK-MB (120.3 ng/mL), CK (2461 U/L), and troponin-I (0.964 ng/mL) levels were also observed with high serum lactate (20.1 mg/dL) and N-terminal pro-brain natriuretic peptide (NT-proBNT 5295 pg/mL) levels. Electrocardiogram revealed pre-cordial lead (V3–V6) ST-segment elevation. Chest X-ray showed borderline cardiomegaly (cardiothoracic ratio [C/T ratio] 0.58) (Fig. 1a). Under the impression of myocarditis, suspected influenza infection-related, she was admitted to the pediatric intensive care unit (PICU) for intensive care.

During the hospitalization, continuous infusion of milrinone and dopamine were given due to cardiogenic shock. Echocardiogram performed upon admission (Fig. 1b) revealed inadequate ejection fraction (60%), decreased inferior vena cava collapsibility index (33.5%), which indicates cardiac tamponade and a moderate amount of pericardial effusion (19 mm). Therefore, a pericardial pig-tail catheter was inserted immediately. Immunoglobulin (0.5 mg/kg/day, 4 days), oseltamivir, colchicine, and ibuprofen were all given for treating influenza B infection and anti-inflammatory effect. Pericardiocentesis was performed, which showed transudate pericardial effusion (Specific gravity 1.031, leukocyte 78/μL, neutrophil 68%, lymphocyte 9%, macrophage 21%, RBC 4975/μL). The virus isolation of pericardial effusion was negative. After 1 week of hospitalization, the ejection fraction improved gradually by a follow-up echocardiogram. Inotropic agents also tapered smoothly and were discontinued on the seventh day of ICU stay. The pericardial drainage tube was also removed on the same day. Due to a generally improved condition, she was transferred to the ordinary ward on the eighth day of hospitalization and was discharged from the hospital soon after. Follow-up chest X-ray at the outpatient department showed a normal heart shadow without increased C/T ratio (Fig. 1c). The final diagnosis was influenza B-associated myocarditis and pericarditis with cardiac tamponade.

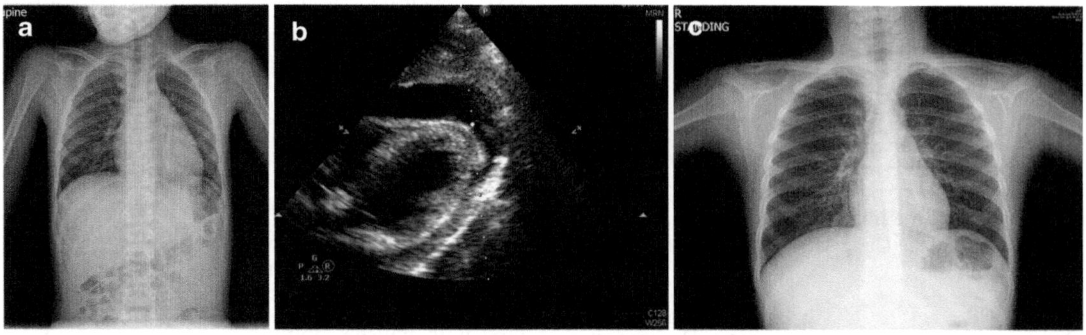

Fig. 1 (**a**) Chest X-ray upon admission in a 7-year-old girl (case 1) with myopericarditis showed borderline cardiomegaly (cardiothoracic ratio [C/T ratio] 0.58). (**b**) Echocardiogram upon admission in a 7-year-old girl (case 1) with myopericarditis showed a moderate amount of pericardial effusion (19 mm). (**c**) Chest X-ray follow-up in a 7-year-old girl (case 1) with myopericarditis showed an essentially normal film

Case Report 2

A 16-year-old girl visited our emergency department due to nearly syncope. She had fever, a mild cough, and rhinorrhea for 2 days and influenza B infection was diagnosed at a local clinic by an influenza rapid antigen test. However, fever persisted despite oral oseltamivir use and severe lethargy was also mentioned. Due to a nearly syncope happened suddenly, she was sent to emergency department for help where tachycardia and undetectable blood pressure was noted initially. After emergent resuscitation, she was admitted to PICU for management.

At PICU, she looked acutely ill with drowsy consciousness, and hypotension persisted despite continuous inotropic agent infusion. Initial laboratory data showed leukocytes count 11,100/μL, segmented 79%, lymphocytes 13%, monocytes 6%, atypical lymphocyte 1%, normal platelet count (230,000/μL), and hemoglobin (13.4 g/dL) level. Blood biochemistry data reveal no abnormal findings. Chest X-ray showed normal C/T ratio (0.4) (Fig. 2a). Echocardiogram showed pericardial effusion. Emergent pericardiocentesis was performed due to cardiogenic shock and blood pressure further stabilized after 140 mL of pericardial effusion was drained out. Under the impression of influenza B related pericarditis, oral ibuprofen, colchicine, and oseltamivir were given. Intravenous peramivir was also administered due to relapsing fever during hospitalization. After 4 days of intensive care, the blood pressure improved gradually and inotropic agents were discontinued smoothy on the same day. Analysis of pericardial effusion was transudate (Specific gravity 1.034, leukocyte 5/μL, neutrophil 1.6%, lymphocyte 49.2%, macrophage 49.2%, RBC 22/μL) with negative for viral culture. Due to improved hemodynamic status, she was transferred to ward 7 days after admission and echocardiogram showed normal ejection fraction without regional wall hypokinesia. A follow-up chest X-ray on hospital day 11 (Fig. 2b) showed an essentially normal film. She was then discharged from the hospital smoothly. The final diagnosis was influenza B-associated pericarditis with cardiac tamponade.

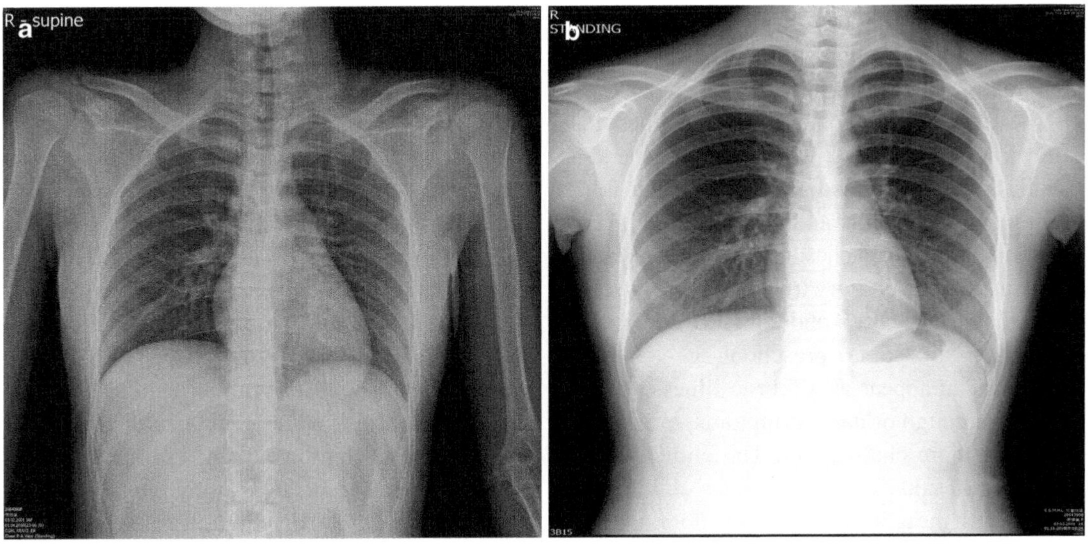

Fig. 2 (**a**) Chest X-ray upon admission in a 16-year-old female adolescent (case 2) with pericarditis showed a normal cardiothoracic ratio (0.4). (**b**) Follow up chest X-ray in a 16-year-old female adolescent (case 2) with pericarditis showed a normal film (on hospital day 11)

Discussion

Belonging to orthomyxoviridae, influenza viruses are segmented, negative strand RNA viruses, and currently divided into four types, type A to type D, according to the divergence of nucleotide sequences. All influenza viruses are zoonoses, arising in the animal reservoir and spilling over into the human populations. However, only influenza virus A, B, and C can cause human infections. With antigenic drift, influenza viruses may cause seasonal epidemics frequently, even year by year, and with rare antigenic shift (genetic reassortment) may cause pandemic infection. The annually cumulative incidence of seasonal influenza infection is 8–10%, and may rise to 20% in the pandemic. Influenza virus is mainly transmitted person to person through large-particle respiratory tract droplets. Indirect transmission route comes from fomite transmission that the infectee's hand exposes to the virus contaminated surface, and further contact their mucosal area (autoinoculation). During the community outbreaks, children are considered to be the main amplifiers of the virus and the primary source for transmission due to their high social contact rate at schools. Secondary spread to adults and other children within the households is common.

The mean incubation period of influenza is 2 days, ranging from 1 to 4 days. The patients usually begin with sudden onset of high fever, accompanied by chills and constitutional symptoms, including headaches, malaise, and myalgia. Subsequently, respiratory tract symptoms such as rhinorrhea, sore throat, and cough become more prominent. In some preschool-age children, influenza can appear as a febrile illness without prominent cough or nasal symptoms, making the diagnosis more challenging. The clinical manifestations in adolescents and older children are similar with those in adults and are dominated by the triad of fever, cough, and myalgia. Laboratory exam had limitations with unsatisfied sensitivity for the diagnosis. Most children with influenza have a normal white blood cell count, but both leukopenia and leukocytosis can be seen. Inflammatory biomarkers are usually not elevated except the development of secondary bacterial infection. The point-of-care antigen rapid test provides variable sensitivity ranging from 20 to 70%. Though the molecular diagnostic method such as RT-PCR or rapid cell culture provides high sensitivity, it is time-consuming and not cost-effective in the clinical setting. Clinically, during influenza season, a patient presents with an influenza-like illness (ILI) (including fever, any constitutional symptoms and any respiratory symptoms), a presumptive diagnosis of influenza should be made, regardless of influenza vaccination status. The decision to commence antiviral treatment should also be based on the clinical diagnosis of influenza, not on test results.

Potential lethal complications, including secondary bacterial infection, influenza-associated encephalitis/encephalopathy, and myopericarditis, are major concerns in patients with influenza. Neurologic manifestations associated with influenza range from simple febrile seizures to fatal immune-mediated encephalitis. Acute necrotizing encephalopathy (ANE) of childhood, first described in Japan in 1995, is one of the most severe forms of neurologic complications triggered by the influenza virus. It typically manifests sudden onset of high fever, generalized convulsions, rapidly disorientated consciousness, and is at high risk of mortality. Cardiac complications such as myocarditis and pericarditis, as shown in the illustrated cases, rarely occur. The clinical symptoms vary and are usually nonspecific, including fever, acute onset chest discomfort, friction rub, weakness, fatigue, nausea, epigastric pain, and even only "a feeling of not doing well." Manifestations of myopericarditis may range from mild symptoms only to severe cardiac failure with or without cardiac tamponade. Pericarditis without myocarditis usually develops days after the influenza symptoms onset and is more associated with post-infectious immune response than direct virus invasion. A high index of suspicion is the key to an early diagnosis of myocarditis or pericarditis in children. For a patient with "a feeling of not doing well," syncope, or even symptoms of circulatory collapse following an ILI, the occurrence of influenza-associated cardiac complication should be considered, and the diagnostic modalities including EKG, laboratory tests of CK-MB, and troponin-I and even an echocardiography examination should be applied. Once diagnosed, cardiac supportive care should be implemented immediately.

Several antiviral agents have been developed against influenza viruses and currently include neuraminidase (NA) inhibitors and baloxavir marboxil. Currently, neuraminidase (NA) inhibitors are still the most commonly used antiviral agents and include oseltamivir (oral form), zanamivir (inhalational administration), peramivir (intravenous administration). If administered within 48 h of disease onset, NA inhibitors can shorten the duration of symptoms, interrupt person-to-person viral spread and reduce the disease severity, viral titers, and the frequency of antibiotic prescriptions for lower respiratory complications. Recently, a novel oral antiviral agent, baloxavir marboxil, was developed and licensed. It is a selective inhibitor of influenza cap-dependent endonuclease, and blocks proliferation of the influenza virus by inhibiting the initiation of mRNA synthesis. Baloxavir showed promising clinical benefit against the influenza virus. Not only they have similar clinical efficacy in the large randomized, non-inferior trial compared to the existing NA inhibitor, but they also offer a single-dose regimen that may have better medication compliance.

Vaccination is the most effective method for prevention of influenza and is recommended for all population older than 6 months of age, particularly for those at high risk of developing complications such as the elderly, the immunosuppressed, underlying chronic disorders (pulmonary diseases, cardiovascular diseases, kidney diseases, etc.), pregnant women, and so on.

In summary, influenza is among the most common respiratory viruses causing a significant disease burden in the seasonal epidemic. Clinical physicians should be familiar with the virus as well the diseases, including the incubation period, clinical symptoms, diagnosis pitfalls, and potential complications. Due to the risk of potentially lethal complications, every effort to prevent influenza virus infection, including annual influenza vaccination, cannot be overemphasized.

Further Reading

Tokars JI, Olsen SJ, Reed C. Seasonal Incidence of Symptomatic Influenza in the United States. Clin Infect Dis. 2018;66(10):1511-1518.

Sridhar S, Begom S, Bermingham A, et al. Incidence of influenza A(H1N1)pdm09 infection, United Kingdom, 2009-2011. Emerg Infect Dis. 2013;19(11):1866-1869.

Miller E, Hoschler K, Hardelid P, Stanford E, Andrews N, Zambon M. Incidence of 2009 pandemic influenza A H1N1 infection in England: a cross-sectional serological study. Lancet. 2010;375(9720):1100-1108.

Paules C, Subbarao K. Influenza. Lancet. 2017;390:697-708.

Gaitonde DY, Moore FC, Morgan MK. Influenza: Diagnosis and Treatment. Am Fam Physician. 2019;100:751-758.

Shah S, Keil A, Gara K, Nagarajan L. Neurologic complications of influenza. J Child Neurol. 2014;29(9):NP49-NP53.

Huang YC, Li WC, Tsao KC, Huang CG, Chiu CH, Lin TY. Influenza-associated central nervous system dysfunction in Taiwanese children. Pediatr Infect Dis J 2009; 28: 647-8

Ukimura A, Izumi T, Matsumori A; Clinical Research Committee on Myocarditis Associated with 2009 Influenza A (H1N1) Pandemic in Japan organized by Japanese Circulation Society. A national survey on myocarditis associated with the 2009 influenza A (H1N1) pandemic in Japan. Circ J. 2010;74(10):2193-2199.

Spoto S, Valeriani E, Locorriere L, et al. Influenza B virus infection complicated by life-threatening pericarditis: a unique case-report and literature review. BMC Infect Dis. 2019;19:40.

Hayden FG, Sugaya N, Hirotsu N, et al. Baloxavir Marboxil for Uncomplicated Influenza in Adults and Adolescents. N Engl J Med. 2018;379:913-923.

Case 27. A 9-Year-Old Boy with Abdominal Pain, Vomiting, Lethargy, Headache, and Fever for 2 Days: Coxsackievirus Myocarditis

Yi-Jung Chang

Keywords

Coxsackievirus · Myocarditis · Abdominal pain

Key Points

- Coxsackievirus B is the most common etiology associated with viral myocarditis.
- Usually with a history of a recent respiratory or gastrointestinal illness (anorexia, abdominal pain, and vomiting) within the previous 2 weeks.
- Severe abdominal pain, often accompanied by gastrointestinal symptoms and fever, may be the first and most prominent symptom of myocarditis.
- Children with gastrointestinal symptoms may be a predictor poor prognosis.
- A high index of suspicion in children with nonspecific symptoms is mandatory for an early diagnosis and an adequate management for children with myocarditis.
- Timely use of ECMO can improve the survival rate in children with acute fulminant myocarditis when conventional treatment failed.

Case Report

A 9-year-old boy was taken to the emergency room with a 2-day history of abdominal pain, vomiting, lethargy, headache, fever, and loose stools. Abdominal pain, vomiting and lethargy worsened the day before admission. In the emergency room, the child is bedridden and crying with abdominal pain. His vital signs were as follows: a heart rate of 120 beats/min, respiratory rate 24 breaths/min, and a blood pressure of 72/30 mmHg. Due to the severity of abdominal pain, heart sounds and abdominal findings are difficult to be assessed. Laboratory tests showed white cell count 9900/μL, segmented 76%, lymphocytes 20%, monocytes 4%, platelet 293,000/μL, and hemoglobin 12.4 g/dL Blood biochemistry data showed sugar 182 mg/dL, blood urea nitrogen 37 mg/dL, creatinine 1.8 mg/dL, aspartate transaminase 481 U/L, alanine transaminase 471 U/L, sodium 144 mEq/L, potassium 4.0 mEq/L, chloride 108 mEq/L and C-reactive protein 18.0 mg/L (normal, < 5 mg/L). Arterial blood gas showed metabolic acidosis (PH 7.310, HCO_3 17.8 mm/L). Other significant laboratory

Y.-J. Chang (✉)
Department of Pediatrics, Chang Gung Memorial Hospital, and Chang Gung University College of Medicine, Taoyuan, Taiwan

Y.-C. Huang et al. (eds.), *Paediatric Infectious Diseases*,
https://doi.org/10.1007/978-981-19-7276-8_27

studies included the following: a troponin-I of 111.65 ng/mL, a Ca of 6.0 mg/dL, and an albumin of 2.4 g/dL. Chest X-ray showed a normal heart size, clear lung fields. Echocardiography showed poor ventricular function, with an ejection fraction of 19%. The patient's systolic blood pressure dropped below 70 mmHg, which was not responding to isotonic fluid and dopamine treatment. His consciousness level declined, with a Glasgow coma scale score of 12 points. The patient was transferred to the pediatric intensive care unit immediately. Two hours after admission, he developed ventricular tachycardia and coma. Cardiopulmonary resuscitation was performed immediately and extracorporeal membrane oxygenation (ECMO) was established and commenced. After 45 min of resuscitation, the vital signs returned and was able to be maintained. However, he passed away on the thirteenth hospitalization day due to cerebral hemorrhage, possibly a complication of ECMO treatment. Viral studies demonstrated elevated coxsackievirus B1 antibody titers and throat swab for virus isolation and identification revealed positive for coxsackievirus B1.

Discussion

Severe abdominal pain, often accompanied by gastrointestinal symptoms and fever, may be the first and most prominent symptom of myocarditis. The abdominal pain may be triggered by myocarditis-associated poor gastrointestinal perfusion. Craver et al. reported that children with acute myocarditis by influenza B initially manifested by vomiting and diarrhea. Hsiao et al. described gastrointestinal symptoms as primary presentation of the pediatric myocarditis in Taiwan. These non-specific symptoms are usually more suggestive of other diagnoses (such as respiratory infections, gastroenteritis, appendicitis), and may lead to incorrect initial diagnoses in children with myocarditis.

Myocarditis is defined as an inflammation of the muscular walls of the heart. The true incidence of myocarditis is likely underestimated because the disease can be sub-clinical or mild enough to go unrecognized in the context of a viral syndrome. Myocarditis is an uncommon diagnosis, accounting for 0.05% of pediatric admissions, and approximately 2 in 100,000 patient-years. The clinical features and course of myocarditis can be classified as fulminant, acute, or subacute; the more rapidly the disease develops, the higher is the case fatality rate. Myocarditis can be caused by a variety of infectious agents, including viruses, bacteria, fungi, rickettsiae, and protozoa, as well as non-infectious triggers such as toxins, and allergic (immunologic) reactions. Lately, the occurrence of myocarditis/pericarditis following mRNA vaccination against coronavirus disease-2019 (COVID-19) increased in a big number of cases deserving more observation. The most common causes of myocarditis in children are viruses, including enterovirus, parvovirus B19, adenovirus, influenza A virus, human herpes virus, Epstein-Barr virus, cytomegalovirus, hepatitis C virus, and human immunodeficiency virus. Enteroviruses, especially coxsackievirus B, account for 25% of viral myocarditis cases. Enteroviruses contact with human hosts via the respiratory or gastrointestinal tracts. The heart is the second goal. The process of enterovirus infection of the heart muscle is divided into three stages: Patients usually develop fever, myalgia, and discomfort a few days before the onset of symptoms of cardiac insufficiency. It may be clinically silent, or initially manifested as a systemic disease with viral symptoms. At a later point in time, as the rhythm develops, the peripheral pulse decreases, the liver enlarges, and the cardiac performance may become poor. None of these clinical findings can be considered pathognomonic for viral myocarditis. Early diagnosis of myocarditis depends on the level of clinical suspicion.

Evidence of myocardial involvement (such as electrocardiographic changes, records of left ventricular dysfunction, or evidence of myocardial inflammation through myocardial histological studies or imaging) can help make a diagnosis of myocarditis. Definite acute myocarditis should be based on the results of endocardial biopsy by Dallas standards. Probable acute myocarditis is defined as acute myocarditis that is determined clinically by a pediatric cardiologist based on the patient's medical history, physical examination, and laboratory examination results in the absence of an endocardial biopsy. Patients with virus myocarditis often have a history of a recent respiratory or, less commonly, gastrointestinal illness (anorexia, abdominal pain, and vomiting) within the previous 2 weeks. The classic electrocardiogram shows sinus tachycardia with low-pressure QRS complex and flat ST-T waves. A chest X-ray may show evidence of cardiac hypertrophy, increased pulmonary vascular markers, and pleural effusion in later stage. Initial chest film may appear normal as illustrated by the present case.

The most important aspect in the management of children with myocarditis is early and appropriate recognition before further clinical deterioration occurs. Atypical presentations of this uncommon disease are challenging to physicians. Children with gastrointestinal symptoms may be a predictor for poor prognosis. They are often given excessive intravenous fluids, which may aggravate heart failure. As shown by this patient, the condition may deteriorate within hours. Children with very high troponin levels (troponin I > 45 ng/mL) or reduced ejection fraction (left ventricle ejection fraction <42%) in the first 24 h were at high risk of mortality, which should be transferred to a center with intensive care unit, pediatric cardiology and cardiothoracic surgery capabilities. Conventional treatment includes inotropic drug support, afterload reduction and diuresis. When conventional measures fail, extracorporeal membrane oxygenation (ECMO) support can be used. Timely use of ECMO can improve the survival rate in children with acute fulminant myocarditis.

The case illustrates that coxsackievirus B is a common etiology of pediatric myocarditis that may present with gastrointestinal symptoms, including abdominal pain and vomiting. A high index of suspicion in such children with nonspecific symptoms is mandatory for an early diagnosis and an adequate management for children with myocarditis.

Further Reading

Chang YJ, Chao HC, Hsia SH, Yan DC. Myocarditis presenting as gastritis in children. Pediatr Emerg Care 2006;**22**:439-40.

Pollack A, Kontorovich AR, Fuster V, Dec GW. Viral myocarditis--diagnosis, treatment options, and current controversies. Nat Rev. Cardiol. 2015;**12:**670-80.

Aretz HT, Billingham ME, Edwards WD, Factor SM, Fallon JT, Fenoglio JJ Jr, Olsen EG, Schoen FJ. Myocarditis. A histopathologic definition and classification. Am J Cardiovasc Pathol. 1987;**1**:3-14.

Chang YJ, Hsiao HJ, Hsia SH, Lin JJ, Hwang MS, Chung HT, et al. Analysis of clinical parameters and echocardiography as predictors of fatal pediatric myocarditis. PLoS One. 2019;**14**:e0214087.

Lin KM, Li MH, Hsieh KS, Kuo HC, Cheng MC, Sheu JJ, et al. Impact of Extracorporeal Membrane Oxygenation on Acute Fulminant Myocarditis-related Hemodynamic Compromise Arrhythmia in Children. Pediatr Neonatol. 2016;**57**:480-87.

Hsiao HJ, Hsia SH, Wu CT, Lin JJ, Chung HT, Hwang MS, et al. Clinical presentation of pediatric myocarditis in Taiwan. Pediatr Neonatol. 2011;**52**:135-9.

Freedman SB, Haladyn JK, Floh A, Kirsh JA, Taylor G, Thull-Freedman J. Pediatric myocarditis: emergency department clinical findings and diagnostic evaluation. Pediatrics. 2007;**120**:1278-85.

Stefanski HE, Thibert KA, Pritchett J, Prusty BK, Wagner JE, Lund TC. Fatal Myocarditis Associated With HHV-6 Following Immunosuppression in Two Children. Pediatrics. 2016;137(1)

Abzug MJ. Nonpolio Enteroviruses. In Nelson's Textbook of Pediatrics. 20th ed. Philadelphia, PA: Elseiver. 2016:1561-8.e1.

Part V

Gastrointestinal Tract Infection

Case 28. A 14-Year-Old Male Adolescent with Progressive Lethargy, Nausea, Shortness of Breath, and Weight Loss: Liver Abscess

Pai-Jui Yeh and Hsun-Chin Chao

Keywords

Liver abscess · Children · *Klebsiella pneumonia* · Pyogenic

Key Points

- An uncommon yet important intra-abdominal infectious disease of children.
- Variable presentations, but mostly include fever and abdominal pain.
- *Klebsiella pneumoniae* remains the most prevalent pathogen in Taiwan.
- Higher clinical suspicion for children with history of hepatobiliary, hematological disease, malignancy, or other immunocompromised status.
- Proper antimicrobial therapy with timely drainage generally yields an adequate treatment response and improved outcome.

Case Report

A 14-year-old obese (body weight 79 kg (weight for age percentile >97)) boy without specific medical history was referred to our emergency department due to progressive lethargy and fever for 1 day. Accompanied symptoms included nausea, near-syncope discomfort, shortness of breath, and weight loss of 13 kg within 6 months. Chronic medication usage and surgical history were denied. Physical examination found injected throat, right upper abdominal tenderness, dehydration, and hypotension. Laboratory evaluation were notable for hyperglycemia (639 mg/dL), bandemia (25%), thrombocytopenia (71,000/μL), coagulopathy (international normalized ratio (INR) 1.8), acute kidney injury (creatinine 1.92 mg/dL), electrolyte imbalance (Na 123 mEq/L, Cl 89 mEq/L), elevated liver enzymes (aspartate aminotransferase (AST) 379 U/L, alanine aminotransferase (ALT) 299 U/L), elevated lactate level (50.4 mg/dL), high serum C- reactive protein (CRP) level (345.5 mg/L, normal <5 mg/L), and high procalcitonin level (25.37 ng/mL, normal <0.15 ng/mL). Due to suspected septic shock, he was admitted to intensive care unit for critical management.

Aggressive fluid replacement and inotropic agent were applied to stabilize the hemodynamic status. Empiric antimicrobial therapy comprising vancomycin, ceftriaxone, and amikacin was administered. Since blood culture soon reported the growth of *Klebsiella pneumonia*, ceftriaxone was continued accordingly. Abdominal computed tomography (CT) disclosed an ovoid, loculated hypodense lesion with internal air bubbles in the

P.-J. Yeh · H.-C. Chao (✉)
Division of Pediatric Gastroenterology, Department of Pediatrics, Chang Gung Memorial Hospital, and Chang Gung University College of Medicine, Taoyuan, Taiwan
e-mail: hero@cgmh.org.tw

Y.-C. Huang et al. (eds.), *Paediatric Infectious Diseases*,
https://doi.org/10.1007/978-981-19-7276-8_28

segment 8 of liver, measured 6.5 cm in longest length approximately, in favor of liver abscess (Fig. 1). The findings of abdominal sonography were also compatible with abscess formation (Fig. 2). CT-guided aspiration and pigtail drainage were performed on the fourth day of admission, and the pinkish abscess yielded *Klebsiella pneumonia* as well. With the improvement of fever and abdominal discomfort, he was transferred to ordinary ward for antimicrobial therapy and risk factor investigation.

As history reviewed in detail, he had relevant symptoms for diabetes mellitus (DM) (polydipsia and polyuria for a month) and positive familial history for DM. Laboratory examination revealed a high level of glycohemoglobin (HbA1c, 16%), hypertriglyceridemia (384 mg/dL), and a positive result of non-insulin dependent diabetes mellitus (NIDDM) via glucagon stimulation test. With dietary modification and insulin program suggested by endocrinologist, the sugar level was properly controlled. Secondly, immune function profile was checked and disproved a predisposing immunodeficiency.

As the pigtail drainage amount decreased, serial sonography also demonstrated the gradual resolution of abscess. Transient fever with bilateral pleural effusion was encountered, yet subsided with symptomatic management and empiric vancomycin regarding presumed catheter infection. Pigtail was removed 10 days later, and he was discharged smoothly after 3 weeks of hospitalization. Overall, he received a total of 40 days of antibiotics therapy, including intravenous and oral (cefixime) form for 21 and 19 days, respectively. The last abdominal sonography 6 weeks post diagnosis reported a complete resolution of intrahepatic lesion. Thereafter, he received outpatient follow up for T2DM management, without recurrence of liver abscess.

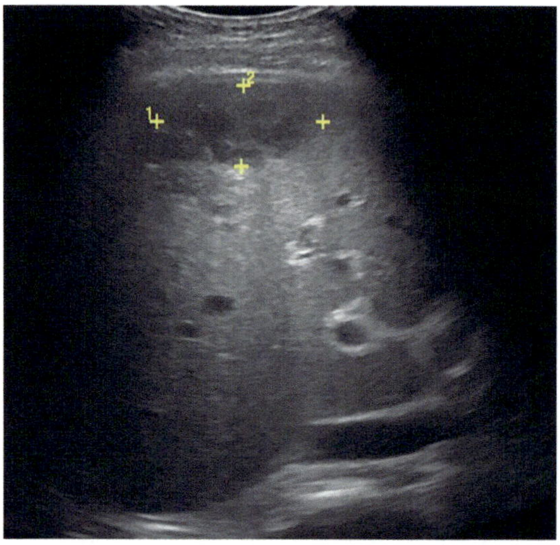

Fig. 2 Abdominal sonography: a heterogeneous, hypoechoic mass in the segment 8 of liver, without internal calcification

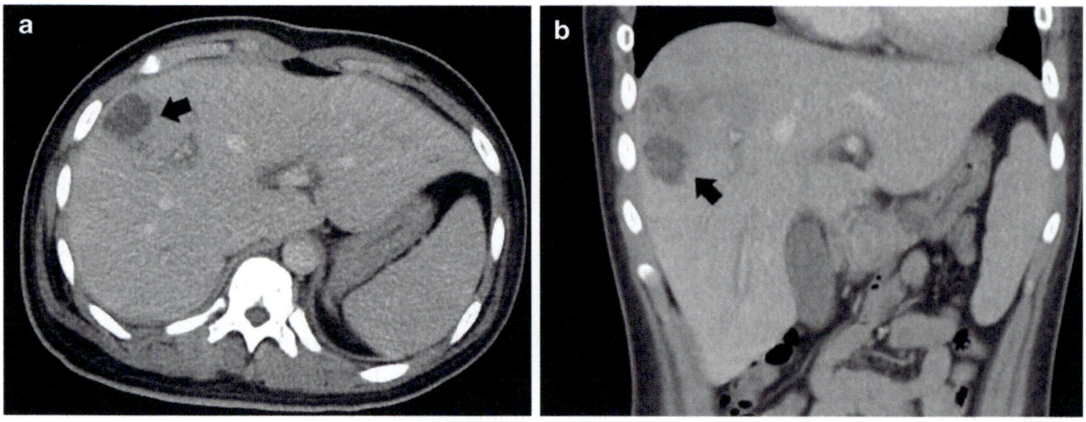

Fig. 1 Computer tomography images of the liver abscess: a loculated hypodense lesion in the segment 8 of the liver (arrows), (**a**) axial view; (**b**) coronal view

Discussion

Liver abscess is an important yet relatively uncommon disease in children. The incidence rates varied among studies from different countries, reflecting a possible association with sanitation, healthcare access, and nutritional condition. A declining trend of pediatric incidence was observed in three consecutive studies in Taiwan, evolving from 20 per 100,000 admissions in 1979–1992 to 8.3 in 1986–2001 and 5.39 in 2011–2018. The age at diagnosis is around 8–10 years old, while some reports from developing countries revealed a younger range. Gender preponderance appeared inconsistent among prior data. Underlying diseases and predisposing host factors that are possibly associated include diabetes mellitus, biliary tract anomalies, immunocompromised status (malignancy, chemotherapy, immunosuppressant user, or malnutrition), abdominal trauma, chronic granulomatous disease, sickle cell disease, certain parasitic infections, systemic sepsis, perforated appendicitis, umbilical infection, and incorrect umbilical venous catheterization. Nonetheless, the majority of pyogenic liver abscesses are cryptogenic.

Common presenting symptoms include fever and abdominal pain. Prolonged febrile period before the actual diagnosis is not uncommon. The pain pattern can also be diverse, although the right upper quadrant is mostly involved. Subdiaphragmatic irritation could cause pleural effusion and other nonspecific respiratory symptoms. Jaundice is less prevalent, with a low correlation to laboratory hyperbilirubinemia. The Fontan triad (fever, right hypochondrium pain, hepatomegaly) is proposed to describe the initial presentation, yet is not universally specific. Rarely, liver abscess may complicate with sepsis or acute abdomen due to rupture and peritonitis.

Abnormal laboratory parameters may include leukocytosis, anemia, and elevated acute phase reactants (procalcitonin, erythrocyte sedimentation rate, CRP) and altered liver enzyme levels. Hyperbilirubinemia is not usually observed. In addition, the correlation between these abnormalities and severity was less obvious and none of them was specific for the diagnosis. Among the reported series, positive rate of abscess culture and blood culture are around 19.2–73.3% and 13.3–28.9%, respectively. Although *Staphylococcus aureus* is the leading causal pathogen in the majority of pediatric reports, several studies from East Asia for both adults and children disclose a dominance of *Klebsiella pneumoniae*. Incidence of amebic abscess range from null to 50% among different regional studies, while most of these data were reported from Latin America and Africa. Culture-proved tubercular or fungal abscess are relatively scarce, which shall raise the suspicion of predisposing immunodeficiency.

Abdominal sonography is a valuable screening modality owing to its lower cost, lack of radiation, and non-invasive properties. Typical lesions present with acoustic enhancement, an abscess wall, a peripheral halo, septation, and internal debris. Computed tomography or magnetic resonance imaging assist in the differentiation from bilioma, cyst, hepatic metastases, or other mimicking masses. Commonly, abscesses develop in the right lobe, as a solitary lesion, with a diverse range of size, yet mostly exceed 5 cm at the time of diagnosis.

With a lack of treatment guideline, differences of therapeutic strategies are observed among reported series. Nevertheless, antibiotics therapy contributes to a crucial part of management. First-line parenteral antibiotics can be started from ampicillin or cephalosporin, plus an aminoglycoside and metronidazole. Second-line regimens include a third-generation cephalosporin or even carbapenem, depending on the culture result, clinical severity, responses to the treatment, and regional concern of antimicrobial resistance. Except for some individual circumstances, the duration of therapy generally comprises 2–4 weeks of parenteral antibiotics followed by oral antibiotics to complete a 4–6 week course. The effectiveness of exclusive antibiotics therapy to achieve a cure appears variable, ranging from 7 to 31.6%. Percutaneous drainage (PD) enhances therapeutic efficacy by evacuating abscess and providing microbial information. The reported success rate of PD can reach over 90%, while a failure could be related to the characteristics of lesion. The average duration of PD is around 1–2 weeks, adjusted by the response of lesion. The associated complications such as bacteremia, hemobilia, hemoperitoneum, or iatrogenic infection shall be monitored. Referring to the surgical approach, the optimal strategy is still debated. Firstly, the ileal cut-off size of an abscess to decide between percutaneous or surgical drainage remains controversial, even in adults. Secondly, the invasiveness and risks of intra-abdominal adhesion should be considered, especially for children. Despite the efficacy, most of the current series tend to preserve surgical intervention for patients with medical or PD failure, a ruptured or large lesion, or concurrent intra-abdominal pathology. More comprehensive studies are needed to evidence these concepts.

With the advance of diagnostic accuracy and therapeutic modalities, the mortality rate has been reduced from 42% to <15% or even null in recent studies. Prognostic determinants ever suggested in adult studies include certain clinical signs (abdominal pain and tachypnea), laboratory parameters (ALT >154 IU/L, hemoglobin <10 g/dL, high blood urea nitrogen), lesion characteristics (ruptured, gas-forming), microbial test (multi-drug-resistant isolates, anaerobic), major underlying disease (malignancy and severe organ dysfunction), and a high Acute Physiology and Chronic Health Evaluation II score at admission. For children, possible indicators for poor prognosis include jaundice, liver failure, acute abdomen with sepsis, bilirubin level >3.5 mg/dL, encephalopathy, large volume of abscess, multiple abscesses, and hypoalbuminemia (<2 mg/dL). Nevertheless, a pediatric stratification system is still lacking.

The diagnosis of pediatric liver abscess requires a high index of suspicion, particularly in susceptible children with a history of hepatobiliary, hematological disease, and malignancy. With timely diagnosis and proper management, the overall treatment response and outcome are generally improving.

Further Reading

Kong MS, Lin JN. Pyogenic liver abscess in children. J Formos Med Assoc 1994;93:45-50.

Tsai CC, Chung JH, Ko SF, et al. Liver abscess in children: a single institutional experience in southern Taiwan. Acta Paediatr Taiwan 2003;44:282-6.

Yeh P-J, Chen CC, Lai MW, Yeh HY, Chao HC. Pediatric Liver Abscess: Trends in the Incidence, Etiology, and Outcomes Based on 20-Years of Experience at a Tertiary Center. Front Pediatrs 2020;8:111.

Kouassi-Dria AS, Moh NE, Aké YL, et al. Liver abscess of children in Côte-d'Ivoire. Annals of Pediatric Surgery 2018;14:51-5.

Muorah M, Hinds R, Verma A, et al. Liver abscesses in children: a single center experience in the developed world. J Pediatr Gastroenterol Nutr 2006;42:201-6.

Chuang CC, Wu SF, Chen AC, Tsai MF, Lin CY, Chen W. Pitfalls in a sonographic diagnosis of liver abscess in children. Pediatrics and neonatology 2012;53:98-104.

Mishra K, Basu S, Roychoudhury S, Kumar P. Liver abscess in children: an overview. World J Pediatr 2010;6:210-6.

Waghmare M, Shah H, Tiwari C, Khedkar K, Gandhi S. Management of Liver Abscess in Children: Our Experience. Euroasian J Hepatogastroenterol 2017;7:23-6.

Roy Choudhury S, Khan NA, Saxena R, Yadav PS, Patel JN, Chadha R. Protocol-based management of 154 cases of pediatric liver abscess. Pediatric surgery international 2017;33:165-72.

Kleinman RE, Goulet O, Mieli-Vergani G, Sanderson IR, Sherman PM, Shneider BL. Walker's pediatric gastrointestinal disease: pathophysiology, diagnosis, management. 2018.

Tsai FC, Huang YT, Chang LY, Wang JT. Pyogenic liver abscess as endemic disease, Taiwan. Emerging infectious diseases 2008;14:1592-600.

Liu Y, Wang JY, Jiang W. An Increasing Prominent Disease of Klebsiella pneumoniae Liver Abscess: Etiology, Diagnosis, and Treatment. Gastroenterol Res Pract 2013;2013:258514.

Case 29. A 5-Month-Old Female Infant with Fever, Lethargy, Bulging Anterior Fontanelle Following Acute Gastroenteritis 2 Weeks Ago: Nontyphoidal *Salmonella* Enterocolitis with Invasive Diseases

Ming-Han Tsai and Yhu-Chering Huang

Keywords

Salmonella · Children · Bacteremia

Key Points

- There are significant geographic serotypes and serogroups variabilities in the occurrence of nontyphoidal *Salmonella* (NTS) bacteremia.
- Though antimicrobial therapy is not indicated for uncomplicated NTS enterocolitis, a short course (3–5 days) of intravenous ceftriaxone may be beneficial to a subset of patients with high CRP and longer duration of fever.
- Extremes of age and patients with immunosuppressing conditions are at risk for NTS bacteremia.
- Third generation cephalosporin (ceftriaxone) remains the drug of choice in the treatment of NTS bacteremia, though an increasing resistance was noted recently.
- A 10–14-day course of ceftriaxone therapy is likely adequate for previously healthy children with uncomplicated bacteremia.
- Longer duration of antimicrobial therapy (4–6 weeks) is warranted for children with immunosuppression for whom recurrence or extraintestinal foci may occur.

M.-H. Tsai (✉)
Department of Pediatrics, Chang Gung Memorial Hospital at Keelung, Keelung, Taiwan

Chang Gung University College of Medicine, Taoyuan, Taiwan
e-mail: a12270@cloud.cgmh.org.tw

Y.-C. Huang
Department of Pediatrics, Chang Gung Memorial Hospital, Chang Gung University, Taoyuan, Taiwan
e-mail: ychuang@cgmh.org.tw

Case 1

A 1-year-old, previously healthy boy was admitted to the hospital because of frequent diarrhea (mucus with blood-tinged content; 10–20 times/day) for 2 days. Associated symptoms included fever (39.1 °C) and postprandial vomiting (2–3 times/day). Decreased urine output with nearly no tears when crying was found. There was no specific contact or cluster history. On admission,

Y.-C. Huang et al. (eds.), *Paediatric Infectious Diseases*,
https://doi.org/10.1007/978-981-19-7276-8_29

the patient appeared a little lethargic and had a body temperature of 37.0 °C, a heart rate of 148 beats/min, and a respiratory rate of 28 breaths/min. The abdomen revealed soft, mildly distended, hyperactive bowel sound without tenderness.

Laboratory evaluation revealed the following: leukocyte count, 9400/mm^3 with 65% segmented neutrophils, 5% banded neutrophils, 24% lymphocytes, and 5% monocytes; hemoglobin, 13.3 g/dL; platelet count, 154,000/mm^3; C-reactive protein, 53.3 mg/L; and stool routine, trace occult blood without mucus or pus.

The abdominal radiograph revealed nonspecific bowel gas pattern. Abdominal sonography revealed bowel dilatation. Because of his lethargic appearance and suspected severe bacterial enterocolitis, intravenous ceftriaxone (50 mg/kg/day) was administered empirically. On the third day, fever subsided and the frequency of diarrhea decreased to four times per day. Both blood culture and stool culture yielded *Salmonella enterica* serogroup D, susceptible to ampicillin and ceftriaxone. The stool specimen for rotavirus and norovirus detection all showed negative. Repeated blood culture and stool culture for Salmonella on day 5 all showed negative. Ceftriaxone was discontinued on the eighth day of hospitalization, and he was discharged on day 9.

Case 2

A 5-month-old female infant had intermittent fever for 3 days and lethargic appearance, decreased appetite and intake for 1 day. She was brought to a local hospital, in where bulging fontanelle, a high fraction of band neutrophils (14%, WBC 4350/μL) and an elevated serum C-reactive protein (CRP) (268 mg/L) were noted. She was transferred to a medical center. Tracing back the history, she had fever with diarrhea 24 days prior to this admission and hospitalized at this medical center for 5 days with a final diagnosis of acute gastroenteritis due to norovirus infection. However, stool culture result reported positive for *Salmonella sp.* 1 day after discharge. On arrival at the medical center, the vital signs were body temperature 36.7 °C, heart rate 163/min, respiratory rate 32/min, and blood pressure 91/64 mmHg. The initial laboratory data showed white blood count (WBC) 3300/μL, lymphocytes 25.1%, monocytes 4.0%, neutrophils 30%, band form 45%, meta-myelocyte 5%, platelet 285,000/μL, hemoglobin 9.8 g/dL, and C-reactive protein 301 mg/L. The initial impression was bacterial meningitis and empiric antibiotics with vancomycin and ceftriaxone were administered.

On day 2 of admission, lumbar puncture was done, cerebrospinal fluid (CSF) showing WBC 290/μL, neutrophil 72%, lymphocyte 22%, monocyte 5%, sugar <5 mg/dL (blood sugar 283 mg/dL), protein 236 mg/dL, and positive for *Streptococcus pneumoniae* antigen test. CSF culture subsequently yielded *Salmonella* sp. Empiric vancomycin, levofloxacin, and ceftriaxone were administered. On the second day of admission, brain ultrasound examination revealed bilateral subdural effusion. Fever persisted under antibiotic treatment. Magnetic resonance image (MRI) of brain was performed on the 11th day of admission and revealed that complicated meningitis with bilateral subdural empyema and secondary acute infarcts at the right frontal and left corona radiate. An operation for external drainage was performed by the neurosurgeon on Day 13 of admission. The analysis of subdural fluid obtained on surgery revealed no pleocytosis, low sugar level (9 mg/dL), high protein level (1233 mg/dL), but negative for bacteria culture. On Day 21, fever subsided and both vancomycin and levofloxacin were discontinued, while ceftriaxone was continued. Serial brain ultrasound examinations showed improving ventriculomegaly and resolving subdural effusion gradually. The patient was finally discharged without significant neurologic deficits after a total of ceftriaxone therapy for 6 weeks. The patient continued to develop well with milestones and had no significant neurologic deficits till aged 6 years at follow-up.

Both the bacterial isolates identified from stool and CSF specimens were subsequently characterized as *Salmonella* Poona and shared the same pulsed-field gel electrophoresis pattern. A case of acute gastroenteritis with subsequent meningitis due to *Salmonella* Poona in an infant was molecularly documented.

Discussion

Acute gastroenteritis (AGE) causes substantial complications and is the second leading cause of death worldwide in children younger than 5 years of age. Though rarely lethal in the developed countries, the disease's burden of AGE in children younger than 5 years of age is still huge. Among the etiologies responsible for childhood AGE, rotavirus is the most common pathogen worldwide before the introduction of the rotavirus vaccine. As expected, AGE due to rotavirus decreased markedly after the introduction of rotavirus vaccines. However, currently, rotavirus vaccine is not included in national immunization program (NIP), but used in the private sector in most Asian countries. In Taiwan, though not included in NIP, the uptake rate of rotavirus vaccine was approximately 60% among the eligible infants since 2013. The positive rate of rotavirus among pediatric inpatients <5 years of age with AGE decreased significantly from 43% in 2001–2003, to 21.2% in 2009–2011 and less than 10% in 2014–2017. In a prospective study conducted in ten major hospitals across Taiwan from 2014 to 2017, enteric pathogen was detected in 1983 (42.19%) of 4700 children aged <5 years hospitalized with AGE, and the three most common etiologies were *Salmonella* spp. (12.5%), norovirus (11.2%), and rotavirus (8.7%).

Nontyphoidal *Salmonella* (NTS) infection, caused by *Salmonella enterica* subspecies *enterica* other than *Salmonella* Typhi and *Salmonella* Paratyphi, is a foodborne illness with a global heavy burden. The main manifestation of NTS infection is diarrheal enteritis, resulting from the ingestion of contaminated food; however, it may also cause invasive NTS infections beyond the gastrointestinal tract, such as bacteremia, meningitis, endovascular infections, or other focal infections, including osteomyelitis and abscess. A report of the Global Burden of Diseases, Injuries, and Risk Factors Study (GBD) 2017 estimated that there were 535,000 cases of invasive NTS diseases and 77,500 related deaths worldwide in 2017.

NTS infection usually results from ingestion of contaminated food and water. It can also be acquired via the fecal–oral route, either from other humans or farm or pet animals. Recent studies from Taiwan revealed that consumption of purchased groundwater within 1 week was an independent risk factor associated with increased risk of salmonellosis. Additionally, 41.8% of 67 food samples collected from either supermarkets or traditional markets were contaminated by *Salmonella* and *Salmonella* was detected in 94.1%, 66.7%, and 8.6% of examined pork, chicken, and vegetables, respectively.

The common presentation of NTS infection is gastroenteritis. The incubation period may range from 4 h to 72 h after the ingestion of contaminated food or water. Symptoms may include fever and chills, nausea and vomiting, abdominal cramping, and diarrhea. If fever is present, it generally subsides within 72 h. Diarrhea is usually self-limiting, which may last for 3–7 days, and may be grossly bloody. *Salmonella* is excreted in feces after infection, a process lasting for a median of 5 weeks. In young children, the excretion may be prolonged; however, in older children, the excretion lasting for longer than 8 weeks after infection is uncommon (Tsai et al. 2007). Bacteremia may occur in 5% of individuals with gastrointestinal illness caused by NTS, especially in the elderly, immunocompromised patients, or younger children. Several studies from Taiwan all revealed that bacteremia occurred in 6–8% of pediatric patients hospitalized with AGE caused by NTS. Adult patients with NTS bacteremia are more likely to have underlying conditions such as immunocompromise, predisposing them to primary bacteremia, extra-intestinal organ involvement, and higher mortality rate. However, among children with NTS bacteremia in resource-rich settings, most have associated gastroenteritis, have no underlying comorbid illness, and recover uneventfully. In a study of NTS bacteremia in pediatric patients (2010–2018) in Taiwan, there was no significant difference in terms of the proportion of patients with underlying diseases or immunocompromised diseases between patients with bacteremia and without bacteremia.

More than 2500 known serotypes of NTS can cause human disease. *S.* Enteritidis and *S.* Typhimurium are the most commonly isolated pathogenic serotypes and, therefore, are most frequently isolated from the blood. Some less frequently isolated serotypes can be more invasive than others and are more likely to cause bacteremia, including *S. enterica* serotypes Dublin, Choleraesuis, Virchow, Infantis, Newport, and Heidelberg. In Taiwan, by O-antigen grouping, serogroup B was found to be the predominant group in children with gastrointestinal illness as well as in those with bacteremia during 1996–2006, while *Salmonella* serogroup D, though a less frequently identified serogroup, had a higher proportion for the development of NTS bacteremia. Since 2007, especially in the 2010s, there was a significant decline in the proportion of serogroup B with a concomitant rise in serogroup D, and serogroup D became the most common serogroup of NTS bacteremia in children.

For uncomplicated gastroenteritis caused by NTS, antimicrobial therapy is not indicated because it does not shorten the duration of illness and may prolong the duration of fecal excretion. However, certain patients, such as young infants <3 months old, patients with toxic appearance and suspected extraintestinal infection, immunocompromised patients, and patients with severe colitis, would benefit from empirical antibiotic treatment. In a previous observational study, we found that a short course (3–5 days) of intravenous ceftriaxone may be beneficial to a subset of patients with high CRP (>100 mg/L) and longer duration of fever (>2 days prior to admission) among children with NTS AGE, but without bacteremia.

Antimicrobial resistance is a global problem with NTS in the past decades, and overall resistance increased from 20 to 30% in the early 1990s to 70% in some countries in the 2000s. High resistance rates of ampicillin and trimethoprim/sulfamethoxazole, especially among the prevalent serotypes *S.* Enteritidis and *S.* Typhimurium, were found globally. Third generation cephalosporin was usually the drug of choice for treatment of NTS bacteremia in children. Fluoroquinolones are frequently avoided in children because of cartilage abnormalities observed in developing animals. Possibly owing to the increasing use of third generation cephalosporin, increasing resistance of NTS isolates to ceftriaxone has been reported, more frequently in Asia and the United States. In the United States, the number of ceftriaxone-resistant blood isolates has approximately doubled, from 2.5% (1996–2007) to 5% (2003–2013). In northern Taiwan, resistance of non-bacteremic NTS isolates to ceftriaxone increased significantly from 3 to 4% in 2010–2012 to 11–14% in 2018–2019. Continuous surveillance on the antimicrobial resistance of NTS in the future is necessary.

The optimal duration of antimicrobial treatment for NTS bacteremia depends upon the immune status of the host. A 10–14-day course of antimicrobial therapy for otherwise healthy individuals is likely appropriate. We previously analyzed 199 episodes of NTS bacteremia in previously healthy children. Approximately one-third of the patients who had no focal infection received a treatment course of appropriate antibiotics therapy <7 days and recovered uneventfully. We speculated that a shorter duration, less than 10 days, of appropriate antibiotic therapy may be adequate for NTS bacteremia in otherwise healthy children. However, a prospective, randomized study is needed. A longer duration of antimicrobial therapy (4–6 weeks) is warranted for immunocompromised patients and those with focal infections such as osteomyelitis and meningitis.

In summary, bacteremia due to NTS infection is a serious complication that may not be suspected in the setting of mild primary infection. Factors affecting the incidence of NTS bacteremia include *Salmonella* serotype, geographic location, and host factors, including extremes of age and immunosuppressing conditions. Third generation cephalosporin (eq. ceftriaxone) remains the drug of choice in the treatment of NTS bacteremia. A 10–14-day course of antimicrobial therapy is likely adequate for previously healthy children with uncomplicated bacteremia. Longer duration of antimicrobial therapy (4–6 weeks) is warranted for children with immunosuppression for whom recurrence or extraintestinal foci may occur.

Further Reading

Roth GA, Abate D, Abate KH, Abay SM, Abbafati C, Abbasi N, et al. Global, regional, and national age-sex-specific mortality for 282 causes of death in 195 countries and territories, 1980-2017: a systematic analysis for the Global Burden of Disease Study 2017. Lancet 2018;392: 1736-88.

Lin FJ, Huang YC, Huang YC, et al., Clinical and epidemiological features in hospitalized young children with acute gastroenteritis in Taiwan: A multicentered surveillance through 2014e2017, J Formos Med Asso, https://doi.org/10.1016/j.jfma.2021.06.001.

Chen HM, Wang Y, Su LH, Chiu CH. Nontyphoidal *Salmonella* infection: microbiology, clinical features, and antimicrobial therapy. Pediatr Neonatol 2013;54: 147-52.

GBD 2017 Non-Typhoidal *Salmonella* Invasive Disease Collaborators. The global burden of non-typhoidal salmonella invasive disease: a systemic analysis for the Global Burden of Disease Study 2017. Lancet Infect Dis 2019;19: 1312-24.

Lee CM, Lee MS, Yang TL, Lee KL, Yen TY, Lu CY, et al. Clinical features and risk factors associated with bacteremia of nontyphoidal salmonellosis in pediatric patients, 2010-2018. J Formos Med Assoc 2021;120: 196-203.

Tsai MH, Huang YC, Chiu CH, Yen MH, Chang LY, Lin PY, et al. Nontyphoidal *Salmonella* bacteremia in previously healthy children: analysis of 199 episodes. Pediatr Infect Dis J 2007;26: 909-13.

Shen H, Chen H, Ou Y, Huang T, Chen S, Zhou L, et al. Prevalence, serotypes, and antimicrobial resistance of *Salmonella* isolates from patients with diarrhea in Shenzhen, China. BMC Microbiol 2020;20: 197.

Lo HY, Lai FP, Yang YJ. Changes in epidemiology and antimicrobial susceptibility of nontyphoid Salmonella in children in southern Taiwan, 1997-2016. J Microbiol Immunol Infect. 2020;53: 585-591.

Su LH, Teng WS, Chen CL, Lee HY, Li HC, Wu TL, et al. Increasing ceftriaxone resistance in Salmonellae, Taiwan. Emerg Infect Dis 2011;17: 1086-1890.

Angelo KM, Reynolds J, Karp BE, Hoekstra RM, Scheel CM, Friedman C. Antimicrobial resistance among nontyphoidal *Salmonella* isolated from blood in the United States, 2003-2013. J Infect Dis 2016;214: 1565-70.

Chen CY, Hsieh PH, Chang CY, Yang ST, Chen YH, Chang K, et al. Molecular epidemiology of the emerging ceftriaxone resistant non-typhoidal *Salmonella* in southern Taiwan. J Microbiol Immunol Infect 2019;52: 289-96.

Chang YJ, Chen YC, Chen NW, Hsu YJ, Chu HH, Chen CL, Chiu CH. Changing Antimicrobial Resistance and Epidemiology of Non-Typhoidal *Salmonella* infection in Taiwanese children. Front Microbiol. 2021;12:648008

Chen CJ, Wu FT, Hsiung CA, Chang WC, Wu HS, Wu CY, Lin JS, Huang FC, Huang YC. Risk factors for salmonella gastroenteritis in children less than five years of age in Taiwan. Pediatr Infect Dis J. 2012 Dec;31(12):e239-43.

Case 30. A 6-Year-Old Boy with Fever, Abdominal Pain, and Diarrhea Followed by Progressive Abdominal Distention: Salmonella Enterocolitis Complicated with Toxic Megacolon

Wei-Hsuan Lin and Yhu-Chering Huang

Keywords

Salmonella · Enterocolitis · Toxic megacolon

Key Points

- Nontyphoidal *Salmonella* (NTS) gastroenteritis is usually self-limited.
- For uncomplicated gastroenteritis caused by NTS, there is no evidence of any clinical benefit of antibiotic therapy in otherwise healthy children and adults.
- Certain patients, such as young infants <3 months old, patients with toxic appearance and suspected extraintestinal infection, immunocompromised patients, and patients with severe colitis, would benefit from empirical antibiotic treatment.
- Toxic megacolon (TM) is one of the complications of NTS gastroenteritis, and should be suspected if a patient with an acute colitis develops worsening abdominal pain, distension, reduced bowel sounds, and persistent fever.
- Toxic megacolon must be managed aggressively, and failure of medical management or clinical worsening is an indication for early surgical intervention.

Case Report

A 6-year-old previously healthy boy suffered from fever, diffuse abdominal pain, and diarrhea without bloody stool. He was admitted to a local hospital initially on the third day of illness. Physical examination disclosed abdominal distention, but no rebounding tenderness. Initial lab data showed WBC 5290/μL, segmented 74%, platelet 196,000/μL, hemoglobin (Hb) 11.7 g/dL, and the biochemistry data revealed elevated C-reactive protein (CRP) 241 mg/L (normal, <5 mg/L), hyponatremia (127 mmol/L), and hypokalemia (3.4 mmol/L). His brother and mother also had diarrhea recently. An abdominal sonography examination indicated

W.-H. Lin (✉)
Division of Pediatric Infectious Diseases, Department of Pediatrics, Chang Gung Memorial Hospital, and Chang Gung University College of Medicine, Taoyuan, Taiwan

Y.-C. Huang
Pediatrics, Chang Gung Memorial Hospital, Chang Gung University, Taoyuan, Taiwan
e-mail: ychuang@cgmh.org.tw

Y.-C. Huang et al. (eds.), *Paediatric Infectious Diseases*,
https://doi.org/10.1007/978-981-19-7276-8_30

that he had enterocolitis. The stool routine analysis showed WBC 0–5/HPF with negative occult blood. Antibiotics with ceftriaxone 100 mg/kg/day was applied to him since the first day of admission. Stool culture obtained on the first day yielded *Salmonella* serogroup D1, which was susceptible to ampicillin, ceftriaxone, and fluoroquinolones. During the hospitalization, the patient had progressive abdominal distention. An abdominal plain film was taken, showing distended bowel loops without subdiaphragmatic free air. Second stool culture was obtained on the third day of hospitalization which still yielded *Salmonella* serogroup D1 with the same susceptibility testing results. On the seventh day of hospitalization, fever and abdominal pain persisted. Follow-up lab data showed leukocytosis (WBC 15,980/μL, segmented 58%), platelet 435,000/μL, and Hb 11.1 g/dL. The CRP level was ever decreased to 148 mg/L on hospital day 4, but raised again on hospital day 7 (232 mg/L). Hyponatremia and hypokalemia were both returned to normal range after intravenous fluid supplement. Blood culture obtained on hospitalization day 1 and day 3 were both negative of bacterial growth. Since distended abdomen and abdominal pain didn't improve, an abdominal CT examination was performed on hospital day 7, showing distended colon, but no pneumoperitoneum or intra-abdominal abscess. Physical examination at this point still revealed no muscle guarding, no tenderness, or rebounding tenderness.

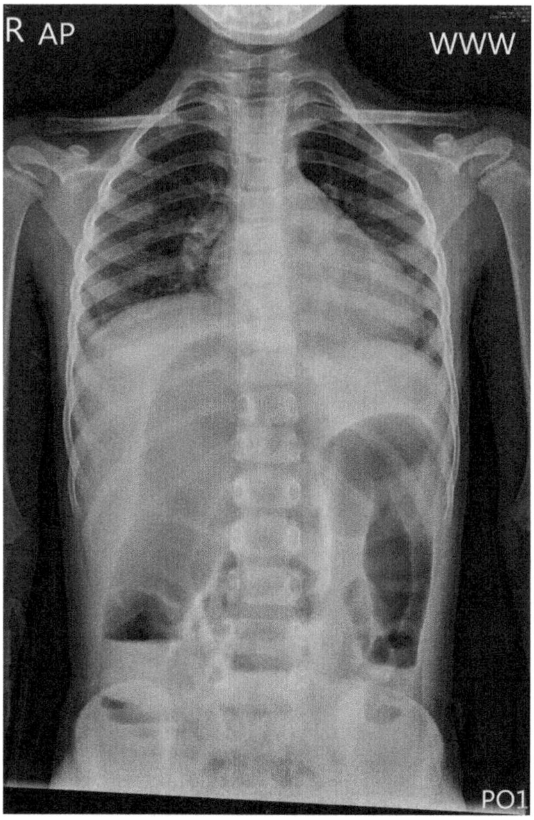

Fig. 1 On arrival at the medical center, the plain abdominal film showed distended colon, the diameter of colon was 4.4 cm, 1.4 times the width of first lumbar vertebra

On the same day, since fever persisted and abdominal distention was noted, he was transferred to a medical center. On arrival at the medical center, the plain abdominal X-ray showed distended colon, the diameter of colon was 4.4 cm, 1.4 times the width of first lumbar vertebra (Fig. 1). Three hours later, follow-up plain abdominal film showed the diameter of colon was 6 cm, which was 1.6 times the width of first lumbar vertebra (Fig. 2). Rectal tube was inserted later on the same day. Few hours after insertion of rectal tube, the distended colon on plain abdominal film improved a lot (Fig. 3). Blood culture was obtained again on arrival at the medical center which still showed negative. After ceftriaxone usage for 10 days, it was switched to Ertapenem due to persistent fever. Fever lasted for a total of 10 days and subsided on the day when ceftriaxone was substituted by Ertapenem. Follow-up laboratory data 3 days after admission showed CRP level had decreased to 53 mg/L and 12.5 mg/L on hospital day 6, respectively. Stool culture obtained on the day of admission didn't yield *Salmonella sp.* again. His symptoms improved on the fifth day after insertion of rectal tube, and it was removed afterwards. One day after removal of rectal tube, follow-up X-ray showed fair distributed bowel gas (Fig. 4). The total duration of antibiotics usage was 2 weeks (Ceftriaxone+Ertapenem). He was ultimately discharged on hospital day 9 with a final diagnosis of salmonella enterocolitis complicated with toxic megacolon.

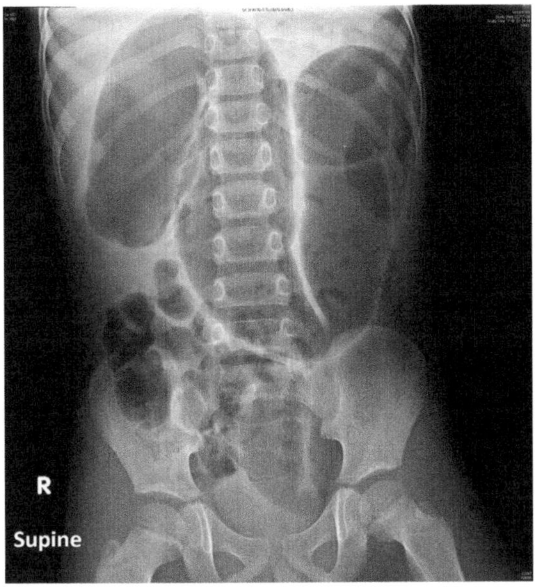

Fig. 2 Three hours after arrival at the medical center, follow-up plain abdominal film showed the diameter of colon was 6 cm, which was 1.6 times the width of first lumbar vertebra

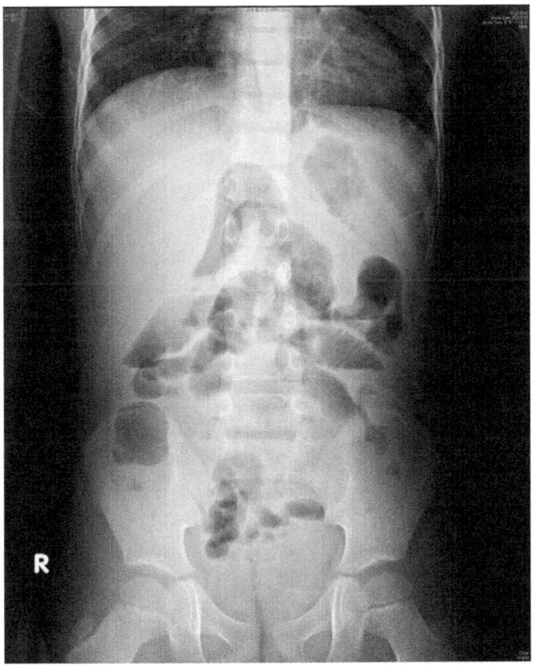

Fig. 3 Few hours after insertion of rectal tube on the same day of arrival at the medical center, the distended colon on X-ray improved a lot

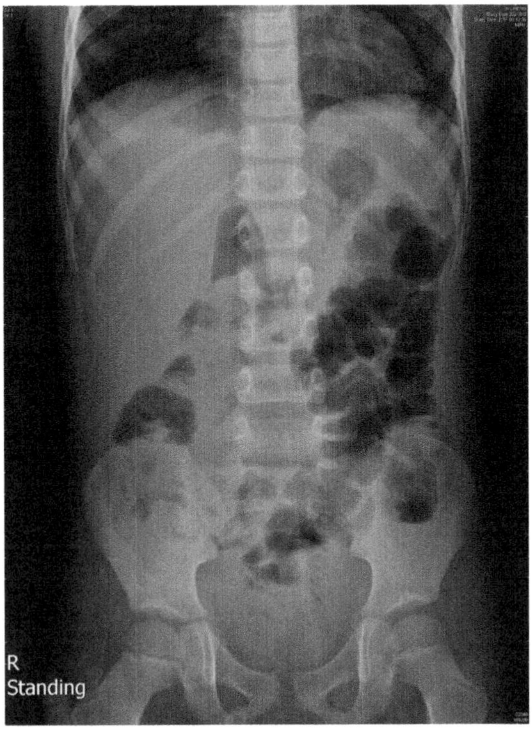

Fig. 4 One day after removal of rectal tube (Hospital day 6 in the medical center), follow-up X-ray showed fair distributed bowel gas

Discussion

Enteric fever is caused by *Salmonella typhi* and *Salmonella paratyphi.* Other *Salmonella* serotypes are known as nontyphoidal salmonellae (NTS). NTS are frequently isolated from the stool of patients with gastroenteritis, which can range from mild to severe; invasive infections can be severe and potentially life-threatening. NTS causes an estimated 1.35 million infections, 26,500 hospitalizations, and 420 deaths each year in the Unites States, resulting in enormous medical cost. Most NTS infection is a self-limited, uncomplicated gastroenteritis that does not require antimicrobial treatment. Nevertheless, it may develop to invasive infections, such as bacteremia, osteomyelitis, and meningitis, which may require antimicrobial therapy. In a study from Taiwan, young children aged 1–4 years (76% of

453 cases) accounted for most NTS cases <18 years old, followed by infants (14.3%). Among the 453 isolates, 6.8% (31/453) of the *Salmonella* isolates were from blood and 90.9% (412/453) from stools. Bacteremia often develops in children younger than 5 years old. It was also reported that fever greater than 5 days was associated with the presence of invasive *Salmonella* infection.

The incubation period of *Salmonella* is approximately 4 h–72 h from the ingestion of contaminated food or water. Symptoms include acute onset of fever and chills, nausea and vomiting, abdominal cramping, and diarrhea. If a fever is present, it usually subsides within 72 h. Diarrhea, usually lasting 3–7 days, is self-limiting and may be grossly bloody. *Salmonella* is excreted in feces after infection, the duration of fecal shedding may last for a median of 5 weeks or even longer in young children.

To date, more than 2500 NTS serotypes have been identified. In a study from Taiwan during 2001 to 2011, children younger than 5 years old were more likely to have serogroup B infection than older children. However, although serogroup B has accounted for largest proportion of nontyphoid *Salmonella* infections, serogroup D *Salmonella* surpasses that of serogroup B for patients older than 5 years.

Nontyphoidal salmonellosis is one of the major causes of foodborne disease, which is most associated with consumption of contaminated poultry, eggs, and milk products. In a study from Taiwan, 67 food samples collected from two supermarkets and five traditional markets were examined for *Salmonella*. A total of 28 (41.8%) samples were contaminated by *Salmonella*. *Salmonella* was detected in 94.1% of examined pork, 66.7% of chicken, and 8.6% of vegetables. *S.* Anatum (6, 21.4%), *S.* Albany (6, 21.4%), and *S.* Derby (5, 17.9%) were the top three isolated serotypes.

Antibiotics such as ciprofloxacin, azithromycin, and ceftriaxone are sometimes needed to treat patients with severe *Salmonella* infections. A previous meta-analysis showed that antibiotic therapy in immunocompetent children and adults with non-severe *Salmonella* gastroenteritis is not beneficial. However, in certain circumstances, such as young infants younger than 3 months, patients with toxic appearance and suspected extraintestinal infection, immunocompromised patients, and patients with prolonged duration of symptoms, empirical antibiotic treatment is beneficial to these patients. Antimicrobial-resistant *Salmonella* infections can be more severe and have higher hospitalization rates. According to US Centers for Disease Control and Prevention, antibiotic-resistant nontyphoidal Salmonella infections are rising. It reached 16% for at least one resistant antibiotic in 2017, 10% for ciprofloxacin, and 3% for ceftriaxone. This resistant strain spread rapidly. In 2018, it accounted for 25% of *Salmonella* Infantis infections in people. However, the resistance rate differs in different serotypes and different antibiotics. *S.* Enteritidis, one of the most frequently isolated *Salmonella* serotypes, is relatively more susceptible to antimicrobial agents than are other common serotypes. Another prevalent serotype, *S.* Typhimurium, was found having much higher rate of antimicrobial resistance. Among 453 pediatric patients in Taiwan in 2017, the antimicrobial resistance rates among the isolates were: ampicillin (47.6%), chloramphenicol (34.9%), trimethoprim-sulfamethoxazole (30.7%), ceftriaxone (5.9%), ciprofloxacin (22.1%), and imipenem (0.2%). Among the 453 isolates, 122 (26.9%) were resistant to ciprofloxacin or ceftriaxone or both, indicating these were highly resistant strains. *S.* Anatum was the most common (54.1%, $n = 66$), ceftriaxone- or ciprofloxacin-resistant strains, followed by *S.* Typhimurium (15.5%, $n = 19$), and *S.* Enteritidis (9.8%, $n = 12$). For patients with invasive *Salmonella* infections that are resistant to both ciprofloxacin and ceftriaxone, carbapenems may be the final option.

Toxic megacolon (TM) is one of the complications of *salmonella* infection. Clinical suspicion of TM should be raised if a patient with an acute colitis develops worsening abdominal pain, distension, reduced bowel sounds, fever, dehydration, lethargy, and increasing white cell count. Signs and symptoms of acute colitis that are frequently resistant to therapy are often present for at least 1 week prior to the onset of acute dilatation. TM caused by *S.* Enteritidis has been described in adults, but it can also affect young children. This species is more commonly involved in both intestinal and extraintestinal salmonellosis than others. A previous study reported that 3% of TM are associated with NTS infection.

Toxic megacolon must be managed aggressively. Narcotic and anticholinergic drugs must be avoided. Antibiotic therapy should ideally be based on the cultured organism. Failure of medical management or clinical worsening is an indication for early surgical intervention. During an 11-year period reviewing 75 hospitalized children diagnosed with NTS gastroenteritis and toxic megacolon in Taiwan, 36% of these children developed intestinal perforation. Among these patients, age >1 year old; serum CRP >200 mg/L; colon diameter >2.5 times the width of L1 vertebral body; inadequate early hydration (urine amount of first 8 h collected on admission <16 mL/kg/8 h); and delay in rectal tube insertion (effective rectal tube insertion beyond 24 h after admission) were found to be the risk factors associated with intestinal perforation.

In summary, NTS-infected pediatric inpatients with a higher risk of invasive diseases may require antimicrobial therapy. However, antibiotic-resistant NTS infections are on the rise in recent years worldwide. Toxic megacolon is one of the severe complications of NTS enterocolitis, and early recognition and administering adequate treatment can avoid developing intestinal perforation.

Further Reading

US CDC https://www.cdc.gov/drugresistance/pdf/threats-report/nt-salmonella-508.

Chang YJ, Chen MC, Feng Y, et al. Highly antimicrobial-resistant Nontyphoidal Salmonella from retail meats and clinical impact in children, Taiwan. Pediatr Neonatol 2020;61:432-438.

Su LH, Chiu CH, Chu C, Ou JT. Antimicrobial resistance in nontyphoid Salmonella serotypes: a global challenge. Clin Infect Dis 2004;39:546-551.

Chen HM, Wang Y, Su LH, Chiu CH. Nontyphoid salmonella infection: microbiology, clinical features, and antimicrobial therapy. Pediatr Neonatol 2013;54:147-152.

Feng Y, Chang YJ, Fang SH, Su LH, Li HC, Yang HP, et al. Emergence and Evolution of High-Level Cephalosporin-Resistant *Salmonella* Goldcoast in Northern Taiwan. Open Forum Infect Dis 2019;6: ofz447.

Chaudhuri A, Bekdash BA. Toxic megacolon due to Salmonella: a case report and review of the literature. Int J Colorectal Dis 2002;17:275-279.

Chao HC, Chiu CH, Kong MS, et al. Factors associated with intestinal perforation in children's non-typhi Salmonella toxic megacolon. Pediatr Infect Dis J 2000;19:1158-1162.

Tsai MH, Huang YC, Lin TY, Huang YL, Kuo CC, Chiu CH. Reappraisal of parenteral antimicrobial therapy for nontyphoidal Salmonella enteric infection in children. Clin Microbiol Infect 2011; 17: 300-305.

Chiou CS, Hong YP, Liao YS, Wang YW, Tu YH, Chen BH, et al. New Multidrug-resistant Salmonella enterica serovar Anatum clone, Taiwan, 2015-2017. Emerg Infect Dis 2019;25 144-147.

Case 31. A 14-Year-Old Girl with Prolonged Fever: Typhoid Fever

Hao-Ting Hsu and Po-Yen Chen

Keywords

Adolescent · Prolonged fever · *Salmonella* typhi

Key Points

- Typhoid fever was an uncommon transmissible disease in the developed countries.
- Sporadic cases or clusters could occur following environmental contamination by imported cases.
- Prolonged fever was among the common manifestations. Laboratory studies were largely non-specific.
- Diagnosis relied on the isolation of the bacteria from blood, bone marrow, or bile specimen.
- Widal test was of low sensitivity, but useful in endemic areas without available culturing facilities.

H.-T. Hsu
Department of Pediatrics, Taichung Veterans General Hospital, Taichung, Taiwan

P.-Y. Chen (✉)
Pediatrics, Taichung Veterans General Hospital, National Chung Hsing University, Taichung City, Taiwan
e-mail: pychen@vghtc.gov.tw

Case Report

A previously healthy 14-year-old girl had intermittent symptoms of fever, abdominal pain, and mild diarrhea for 1 month. She lived in a rural area in central Taiwan. She received treatment in the local clinics. Because of poor response to the treatment, she was admitted to a local hospital where the blood culture upon admission yielded *Escherichia coli*. She was on parenteral antibiotic treatment and the symptoms resolved 4 days later. She discharged and received sequential oral amoxicillin/clavulanate therapy. Unfortunately, she developed fever up to 39 °C 8 days after discharge, which was accompanied by vomiting and diarrhea. The fever persisted for 8 days again, and she was brought back to the same hospital. The workup for the febrile episode disclosed leukopenia with a white blood cell count (WBC) of 4050/μL, thrombocytopenia with a platelet count of 109,000/μL and an elevated C-reactive protein (CRP) level of 5.4 mg/dL. She was referred to a medical center for the prolonged fever.

She was febrile but alert and with stable vital signs upon arrival at the medical center. Physical examination was unremarkable. Laboratory studies showed a WBC count of 4350/μL, platelet count of 123,000/μL, CRP level of 5.169 mg/dL, ESR level of 40 mm/h. The tests for renal and liver functions, urine analysis, and blood gas were all within normal limits. The roentgenography for the chest and abdomen were both negative findings. Hepatomegaly was identified on the abdominal sonography.

Y.-C. Huang et al. (eds.), *Paediatric Infectious Diseases*,
https://doi.org/10.1007/978-981-19-7276-8_31

Table 1 The proposed four-stage investigation procedure of fever of unknown origin

Stage	Investigation procedure
I	*General history, physical examination, screening test:* Laboratory studies showed mild leucopenia, thrombocytopenia, elevated CRP level. Blood and urine cultures were repeated
II	*Detailed history, repeat physical examination and specific screening test:* She was a high school student and lived near a factory and farmland. She had two domestic dogs and a hamster, and she did not get any bite from them. She did not take any special food or exotic dishes. The abdominal sonogram did not find any lesion except mild hepatomegaly. The Widal test was non-reactive
III	*Specific diagnostic test and invasive test:* Ga-67Inflammatory scan with SPECT/CT was arranged and no definite evidence of gallium-avid lesion was identified
IV	*Therapeutic try:* empiric antibiotic

For the unusual clinical course of this teenager, a comprehensive survey of the prolonged fever was conducted in accordance with the proposed four-stage investigation procedure of fever of unknown origin (FUO) (Table 1).

On the second day of admission, a gram-negative bacillus was identified from the blood culture which was subsequently recognized as *Salmonella* Typhi. She received ceftriaxone treatment and became afebrile on the third day of hospitalization. The whole-body inflammatory scan identified no infectious foci. She was discharged on the seventh day and continued an additional 5-day course of oral cefixime treatment. In the follow-up outpatient clinic, three consecutive sets of stool every 24 h were collected for the culture of *S.* Typhi and all showed negative findings.

Discussion

This previously healthy girl had prolonged fever and intermittent abdominal discomfort for a long period. The initial identification of *E. coli* bacteremia was unusual, but appeared to respond well to the parenteral antimicrobial therapy. The S. typhi might have been incorrectly identified as *E. coli* and the duration of the antimicrobial therapy was not sufficient in this patient. Without the typical presentations, including the rose spot rash and relative bradycardia, it was difficult to suspect typhoid fever simply on the clinical ground in this case in clinical settings where the disease was extremely uncommon. Fortunately, *S.* Typhi was soon identified from her blood culture, and she responded well to the adequate parenteral ceftriaxone.

Although the global burden of enteric fever has decreased over the past two decades, the prevalence remains high in Southeast Asia, India, and Africa. Typhoid fever is a notifiable infectious disease in Taiwan and must be reported to the Taiwan Centers for Disease Control (CDC) within 24 h after diagnosis. There are an average of 10–20 cases each year in Taiwan, including indigenous and imported cases. Most of the imported cases were from Indonesia, India, Myanmar, and the Philippines.

There is no known animal reservoir of *S.* Typhi in nature and human is the only known host. The pathogen replicates within the reticuloendothelial system, a hallmark of enteric fever, and is responsible for the clinical findings of prostration, generalized sepsis, and hepatosplenomegaly. Typhoid fever is a febrile illness, which usually develops 5–21 days after ingestion of the causative microorganism in contaminated food or water. The classic presentation in the first week of illness is rising fever and bacteremia. The fluctuated and worsening fever, headache, weakness and fatigue, muscle aches, dry cough, poor appetite and weight loss, abdominal pain, diarrhea, constipation, and rose spots on the trunk and abdomen can occur in the second week of infection. Patients in their third-week of illness may develop hepatosplenomegaly and gastrointestinal complications, including secondary bacteremia and peritonitis. As a result of bacteremic seeding, focal extra-intestinal complications can occur in the central nervous system, hepatobiliary, cardiovascular, respiratory, genitourinary, and musculoskeletal systems.

The laboratory evaluation is non-specific, but commonly presents with anemia, either leucopenia or leukocytosis, elevated liver enzymes, and thrombocytopenia. Widal Test is an agglutination test that detects serum agglutinins (H and O) in patients' serum. *Salmonella* antibody starts appearing in serum at the end of the first week and rises sharply during the third week of fever. It is preferable to test two specimens of sera at an interval of 7–10 days to demonstrate a rising antibody titer. A single Widal test is of little clinical relevance, especially in endemic areas. This is due to recurrent exposure to typhoid-causing bacteria, immunization, and high chances of cross-reaction from other infections such as malaria and non-typhoid salmonella. In acute typhoid fever, O agglutinins can usually be detected 6–8 days after the onset of fever and H agglutinins after 10–12 days. When facilities for culturing are not available, the Widal test remains useful in the diagnosis of typhoid fever in the endemic areas.

The definitive diagnosis of typhoid fever depends on the isolation of *S.* Typhi from the culture of blood or bone marrow aspirate (while stools are useful for the diagnosis of typhoid carriers). Bone marrow is a sanctuary for *S.* Typhi and provides an important source of diagnostic culture material even after the initiation of antimicrobial therapy. The positive yield rate of blood culture is 40–80% and stool culture is a fast and simple test providing a positive yield rate of up to 30–40% However, stool culture was often negative by the time when systemic symptoms bring individuals to medical attention.

Successful treatment usually results in clinical improvement within 3–5 days in uncomplicated cases. In children, beta-lactam antibiotics (ceftriaxone, cefotaxime, or cefixime), azithromycin, ciprofloxacin, and ofloxacin can be used. The widespread and increasing antimicrobial resistance has increased especially in Southeast Asia and thus narrowed the treatment options for travel-related enteric fever.

Further Reading

Chien YL, Huang FL, Huang CM, Chen PY. Clinical approach to fever of unknown origin in children. J Microbiol Immunol Infect 2017;50(6):893-898.

Su CP, Chen YC, Chang SC. Changing characteristics of typhoid fever in Taiwan. J Microbiol Immunol Infect. 2004;37(2):109-14.

Liu PY, Wang KC, Hong YP, Chen BH, Shi ZY, Chiou CS. The first imported case of extensively drug-resistant Salmonella enterica serotype Typhi infection in Taiwan and the antimicrobial therapy. J Microbiol Immunol Infect. 2021 Aug;54(4):740-744.

Wang KY, Lee DJ, Shie SS, et al. Population structure and transmission modes of indigenous typhoid in Taiwan. *BMC Med Genomics* 2019;12: 126.

Manesh A, Meltzer E, Jin C, Britto C, Deodhar D, Radha S, Schwartz E, Rupali P. Typhoid and paratyphoid fever: a clinical seminar. J Travel Med 2021;28(3):taab012.

Masuet-Aumatell C, Atouguia J. Typhoid fever infection - Antibiotic resistance and vaccination strategies: A narrative review. Travel Med Infect Dis 2021;40:101946.

Crump JA. Progress in Typhoid Fever Epidemiology. Clin Infect Dis 2019;68(Suppl 1):S4-S9.

Kumar P, Kumar R. Enteric Fever. Indian J Pediatr 2017;84(3):227-230.

Stephens I, Levine MM. Management of typhoid fever in children. Pediatr Infect Dis J 2002;21(2):157-8.

Case 32. A 10-Year-Old Girl with Progressive Abdominal Distension and Intermittent Fever for 2 Months: Abdominal Tuberculosis

Wah-Tin Tiew and Yhu-Chering Huang

Keywords

Tuberculosis · Abdominal · Peritonitis

Key Points:

- Abdominal tuberculosis (TB) accounts for approximately 5% of all cases of tuberculosis and can present as TB lymphadenopathy, peritoneal TB, gastrointestinal TB, and visceral TB.
- In TB endemic areas, abdominal TB should be considered in patients with non-specific constitutional symptoms and long-lasting abdominal symptoms.
- In addition to confirmatory tests of TB, chest radiography and abdominal image studies should be performed for the diagnosis of abdominal TB to avoid delay in treatment.
- Once suspected of abdominal TB, anti-tuberculous therapy should be initiated as soon as possible and a response to therapeutic anti-TB medication may indirectly confirm the diagnosis.
- Surgery is reserved for tissue diagnosis and the management of complications.

Case Report

A 10-year-old female child was admitted due to progressive abdominal distension and intermittent fever for 2 months. She had loss of weight and her appetite was poor with no episodes of vomiting or altered bowel habit. There was no contact with anyone having tuberculosis disease, and she denied night sweats, chronic cough, or skin discoloration. Physical examination revealed a thin girl with poor muscle bulk and fair hydration status. Her body temperature was 37.8 °C, pulse rate 98/min, blood pressure 104/54 mmHg. BCG scar was present. There were multiple sub-centimeter cervical lymph nodes palpable. Her abdomen was grossly distended with visible bowel loops and presence of hepatomegaly of 3 cm. Examination of respiratory, cardiovascular, and central nervous system was unremarkable. She was initially treated for bacterial peritonitis with broad spectrum antibiotics and given intravenous fluid for adequate hydration.

W.-T. Tiew (✉)
Ministry of Health, Putrajaya, Malaysia

Y.-C. Huang
Pediatrics, Chang Gung Memorial Hospital, Chang Gung University, Taoyuan, Taiwan
e-mail: ychuang@cgmh.org.tw

Y.-C. Huang et al. (eds.), *Paediatric Infectious Diseases*,
https://doi.org/10.1007/978-981-19-7276-8_32

Initial laboratory data showed leukocytosis (WBC 10,300/μL, segmented 47.7%, lymphocytes 44.2%), thrombocytosis (platelet 567,000/μL), and hemoglobin (Hb) 11.1 g/dL. Her serum albumin was 31 g/L, blood urea nitrogen (BUN) 4.6 mmol/L, sodium 136 mEq/L, potassium 4.6 mEq/L, creatinine 35 mmol/L.

Tuberculin skin test (TST) done on her left forearm and measured 20 mm after 72 h of inoculation. Urgent contrast enhanced computed tomography of abdomen showed presence of focal irregular enhancing bowel wall thickening at caecum, ileocecal valve, and terminal ileum. Multiple enlarged mesenteric, paracortic, and aortocaval nodes were seen. Small complex ascites was seen at pelvis area. There was also presence of minimal right pleural effusion with adjacent atelectatic changes.

In view of positive Tuberculin skin test and findings in CT abdomen highly suggestive of Tuberculosis, chest radiograph was ordered to look for primary focus. And it was reported as prominent mediastinum with air space opacities at right middle lobe and blunted right costophrenic angle. Acid-fast bacilli was not seen on sputum stained with auramine-rhodamine. Sputum for Xpert MTB/rif (GeneXpert®) assay was reported as *Mycobacterium tuberculosis complex* detected and rifampicin resistance not detected.

Diagnosis of disseminated tuberculosis disease involving abdomen, lungs, and lymph nodes was made. Anti-tuberculosis therapy with four drugs regimen, including isoniazid (H), rifampicin (R), pyrazinamide (Z) and ethambutol (E) was initiated according to recommended dosing by World Health Organization (WHO). She was able to tolerate the medication well without much side effects. Nutrition support wise, total parenteral nutrition was initiated via peripherally inserted central catheter. Her condition improved tremendously with anti-tuberculous therapy, i.e., her abdominal distension resolved, hence surgical intervention was not indicated. She gained weight during her stay in ward. Follow-up ultrasonography of abdomen showed improving bowel wall thickening and resolved complex ascites. Prior to discharge after 2 weeks of hospital stay, education on importance of compliance to anti-tuberculosis therapy and relevant side effects was given to her parents. Case was notified to nearest district health office for screening of close contact.

She completed 9 months of anti-tuberculous therapy, i.e., 2 months of HRZE, plus 7 months of HR successfully without complications. There was no relapse of disease found after 1 year of outpatient follow-up.

Discussion

Abdominal tuberculosis accounts for around 5% of all cases of tuberculosis worldwide and about 11–12% of extrapulmonary tuberculosis. There are four forms of abdominal tuberculosis, i.e., tuberculous lymphadenopathy, peritoneal tuberculosis, gastrointestinal (GI) tuberculosis, and visceral tuberculosis involving intra-abdominal solid organs. The involvement of the peritoneum, GI tract, and/or liver are the most common forms of abdominal tuberculosis. In clinical practice, different forms may coexist.

The pathogenesis of abdominal tuberculosis is rather complex. Abdominal tuberculosis may occur via ingestion of infected sputum (infrequently with ingestion of unpasteurized milk or undercooked meat, check this fact), or hematogenous spread in cases of pulmonary tuberculosis or miliary tuberculosis or via lymphatic drainage, or even direct spread from adjacent organs. After the ingestion of infected sputum or milk, approximately after 2–4 weeks, infected mucosal layer of the GI tract may develop caseous necrosis that leads to ulceration of the overlying mucosa, which can later spread into the deeper layers and into the adjacent lymph nodes and into the peritoneum. In cases of active pulmonary tuberculosis or miliary tuberculosis, tubercle bacilli spread hematogenously and seeded in abdominal solid organs, kidneys, lymph nodes, and peritoneum. Direct spread into the peritoneum from infected adjacent foci, including the fallopian tubes or adnexa, or psoas abscess or tuberculous spondylitis could also occur. Lastly, it can spread through lymphatic channels from infected nodes.

As shown in the illustrated case, fever, abdominal pain/discomfort, weight loss, abdominal distention/mass, and ascites are the common presenting symptoms. These symptoms usually persist for weeks to months before the patients seek medical help and the diagnosis of abdominal TB is made. Abdominal tuberculosis is often challenging to diagnose due to its variable clinical manifestations depending upon the form of disease and difficulty in obtaining tissue for diagnosis. Besides, abdominal tuberculosis can also mimic certain conditions such as Crohn's disease and malignancy. The diagnosis of abdominal tuberculosis should be suspected in patients who present with symptoms such as fever, abdominal pain, abdominal distension, weight loss, vomiting, and abdominal mass, plus had significant exposure history such as history of prior TB infection or disease, known or possible TB exposure or history of travelling to area or countries endemic.

Tuberculin skin test (TST) or blood for Interferon-Gamma Release Assays (IGRAs) are useful screening tests for tuberculosis infection. Adequate radiological (such as computed tomography, CT) and histopathological studies are needed to make the diagnosis, hence, efforts should be made to collect clinical specimens such as tissue or lymph nodes biopsy and peritoneal fluids for tissue diagnosis, as well as for culture and drug susceptibility test.

The histopathological changes suggestive of Mycobacterium tuberculosis-infected tissue is presence of necrotizing granulomatous inflammation, composed of epithelioid histiocytes surrounding a central necrotic zone, and can be accompanied by a variable number of multinucleated giant cells and lymphocytes. Non-necrotizing granulomas can be present as well.

Acid-fast bacilli (AFB) positivity in ascitic fluid smear is low. While the use of nucleic acid test (NAAT) is also limited in the diagnosis of abdominal TB due to its low sensitivity though high specificity. The sensitivity of Xpert MTB/Rif on ascitic fluid, peritoneal and intestinal tissue were reported as 70%, 19%, and 8.1%, respectively, while specificity was 100% for all types of specimen samples.

Approximately 15–25% of cases with abdominal tuberculosis have concomitant pulmonary TB. Therefore, obtaining chest radiograph, and subsequent sputum collection would be helpful to diagnose pulmonary tuberculosis or military TB.

Computed Tomography of abdomen is very helpful in evaluation of abdominal tuberculosis. Findings on CT are dependent on areas involved. In intestinal tuberculosis, CT can demonstrate concentric mural thickening, especially at the ileocecal region with or without proximal intestinal dilatation, though other parts of intestine can be affected as well. Presence of thickening of the peritoneal, ascites, lymph nodes, and thickening of the mesentery and omentum can be seen in peritoneal TB.

In words, diagnosis of abdominal TB is a challenge to clinicians. The clinical manifestations are non-specific, for weeks to months and have varied pictures, which may mimic a variety of other abdominal disorders. Abdominal images, performed subsequently in most cases, usually reveal abnormal findings, but the findings are also non-specific. Unless a high index of suspicion is maintained, the diagnosis can easily be missed or delayed, resulting in increased morbidity and mortality.

Antituberculous therapy should be initiated for abdominal tuberculosis. However, the direct evidence for the optimal duration of treatment is lacking. Most international guidelines, including World Health Organization recommended four drugs, i.e., isoniazid (H), Rifampicin (R), pyrazinamide (Z) and ethambutol (E) for 2 months during the intensive phase and two drugs, Isoniazid and rifampicin for 6 months for maintenance phase, for all types of abdominal TB. Surgical intervention may be considered after adequate duration of antituberculous therapy depending on patient's treatment response. Nutritional rehabilitation via total parenteral nutrition may be considered as part of supportive therapy.

In TB endemic areas, abdominal TB should be considered in patients with non-specific constitutional symptoms and long-lasting abdominal symptoms. In addition to confirmatory tests of

TB, including PPD test, TB interferon-diagnostic tests, and mycobacterial tests, chest radiography and abdominal image studies should be performed for the diagnosis of abdominal TB to avoid delay in treatment. Response to therapeutic anti-TB medication may indirectly confirm the diagnosis. Surgery is reserved for tissue diagnosis and the management of complications.

Further Reading

Saluja SS, Ray S, Pal S, et al. Hepatobiliary and pancreatic tuberculosis: a two decade experience. BMC Surg. 2007;7:10.

Limsrivilai J, Shreiner AB, Pongpaibul A, et al. Meta-analytic Bayesian model for differentiating intestinal tuberculosis from Crohn's disease. Am J Gastroenterol 2017; 112: 415–27.

Sharma V, Bhatia A, Malik S, Singh N, Rana SS. Visceral scalloping on abdominal computed tomography due to abdominal tuberculosis. Ther Adv Infect Dis 2017; 4: 3–9.

Debi U, Ravisankar V, Prasad KK, Sinha SK, Sharma AK. Abdominal tuberculosis of the gastrointestinal tract: revisited. World J Gastroenterol 2014;20:14831-14840.

Sinan T, Sheikh M, Ramadan S, Sahwney S, Behbehani A. CT features in abdominal tuberculosis: 20 years' experience. BMC Med Imaging 2002;2:3.

Rufai SB, Singh S, Singh A, Kumar P, Singh J, Vishal A. Performance of Xpert MTB/RIF on Ascitic Fluid Samples for Detection of Abdominal Tuberculosis. J Lab Physicians 2017; 9: 47-52.

Bera C, Michael JS, Burad D, et al. Tissue Xpert™ MTB/Rif assay is of limited use in diagnosing peritoneal tuberculosis in patients with exudative ascites. Indian J Gastroenterol 2015; 34: 395–398.

Kumar S, Bopanna S, Kedia S, et al. Evaluation of Xpert MTB/RIF assay performance in the diagnosis of abdominal tuberculosis. Intest Res 2017;15:187-194.

Horvath KD, Whelan RL. Intestinal tuberculosis: return of an old disease. Am J Gastroenterol 1998;**93**:692–696.

World Health Organization. Treatment of drug-susceptible tuberculosis: rapid communication. Geneva, 2021.

World Health Organization. Rapid communication on updated guidance on the management of tuberculosis in children and adolescents. Geneva, 2021.

World Health Organization. WHO operational handbook on tuberculosis. Module 3: Diagnosis – rapid diagnostics for tuberculosis detection 2021 update. Geneva, 2021.

Lin YS, Huang YC, Lin TY. Abdominal tuberculosis in children: a diagnostic challenge. J Microbiol Immunol Infect 2010;43:188-93.

Part VI

Urinary Tract Infection

Case 33. An 8-Month-Old Female Infant with Fever and Pyuria: Acute Lobar Nephronia

Chi-Hui Cheng

Keywords

Acute lobar nephronia · Urinary tract infections · Image diagnosis scheme Antibiotic treatment duration · Uropathogen

Key Points

- Acute lobar nephronia (ALN) is a severe renal parenchymal infection and may represent an early stage of renal abscess formation.
- ALN cases present similar clinical symptoms as patients with acute pyelonephritis and renal abscesses.
- A systemic imaging work-up scheme using ultrasound screening followed by computed tomography (CT) examination could enhance the efficacy of CT performance and the sensitivity of overall diagnosing of ALN.
- *Escherichia coli* is the most common pathogen identified from ALN cases.
- A 3-week antibiotic therapy is recommended for the treatment of ALN.
- ALN likely progresses to renal scarring, if not properly treated.

Case Report

An 8-month-old female patient was brought to the emergency department of a medical center due to intermittent fever without any symptoms. Blood tests revealed serum C-reactive protein level (CRP): 126 mg/L (normal, <5 mg/L), WBC: 21,000/μL, Hb: 9 g/dL, and platelet count: 320,000/μL. A urine analysis showed pyuria (urine WBC > 500/mL). With the impression of urinary tract infection, empirical antibiotics with cefazolin + gentamicin were administered. She was then admitted for further care.

After admission, renal echo revealed bilateral nephromegaly without a focal mass: left kidney sized 6.8 cm, and right kidney sized 7.2 cm. Thus, an abdominal computed tomography (CT) was arranged and decreased nephrogenic density after contrast medium administration was noted on both kidneys (Fig. 1). A diagnosis of bilateral acute lobar nephronia (ALN) was made. Urine culture subsequently yielded *E. coli* with a colony count $>10^5$ CFU/mL which was sensitive to both cefazolin and gentamicin.

C.-H. Cheng (✉)
Division of Pediatric Nephrology, Department of Pediatrics, Chang Gung Memorial Hospital, Taoyuan, Taiwan

Department of Pediatrics, College of Medicine, Chang Gung University, Taoyuan, Taiwan

Y.-C. Huang et al. (eds.), *Paediatric Infectious Diseases*,
https://doi.org/10.1007/978-981-19-7276-8_33

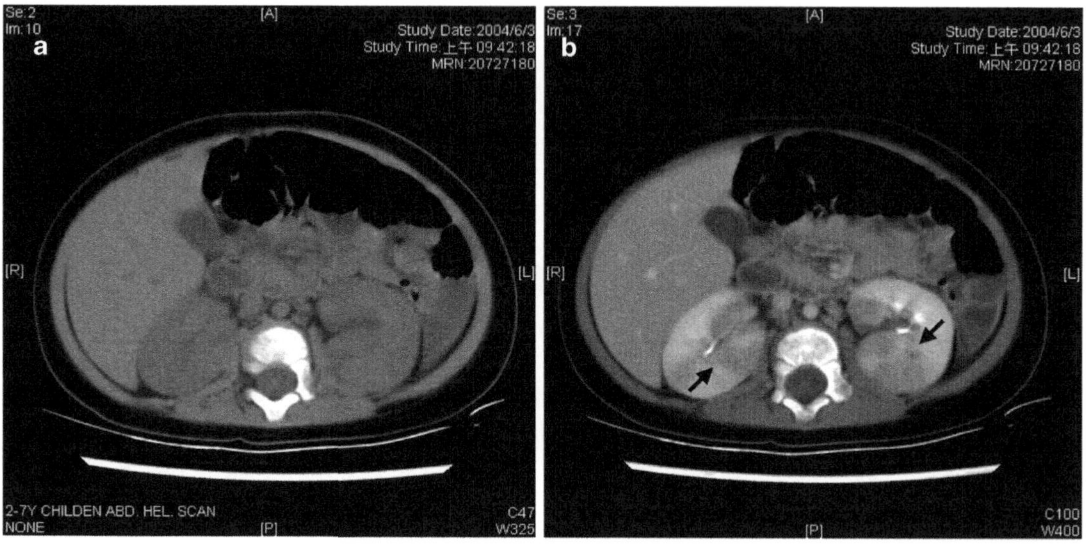

Fig. 1 Characteristic pre-contrast (**a**) and contrast-enhanced (**b**) CT scans for an 8-month-old patient with acute lobar nephronia who presented with severe bilateral nephromegaly, but without a focal mass sonographically. No attenuation area was seen in the kidney before enhancement. (Reproduced with permission from (Cheng et al. 2006))

Four days after the intravenous antibiotic treatment, her fever subsided. Under the stable condition, she was discharged with oral antibiotics for continued therapy.

Discussion

Studies have indicated that approximately 3% of prepubertal girls and 1% of prepubertal boys have been diagnosed with urinary tract infections (UTIs). The clinical severity of acute renal bacterial infection spans continuously from an uncomplicated lower UTI (i.e., cystitis) to frank abscess formation. Among these UTIs, renal parenchymal infections, including uncomplicated acute pyelonephritis (APN), acute lobar nephronia (ALN), and intrarenal abscess, are considered to be the more serious forms of UTI.

Acute lobar nephronia (ALN), also known as acute focal bacterial nephritis (AFBN), has been diagnosed with ever-increasing frequency in patients, due to the advancement of non-invasive imaging-technique modalities. ALN presents as a localized non-liquefactive inflammatory renal bacterial infection, which typically involves one or more lobes. It has previously been indicated as a complicated form of acute renal infection, representing the progression of the inflammatory process of acute pyelonephritis (APN). ALN may also represent a relatively early stage of the development of the renal abscess. The typical clinical presentations of ALN include fever, flank pain, leukocytosis, pyuria, and bacteriuria, which are quite similar to those with renal abscess or APN.

Sonographically, ALN generally presents as severe nephromegaly or a poorly defined, irregularly margined focal mass with hyper-, iso-, or hypoechogenicity, depending on the temporal sequence of the lesions and the resolution of the disease. Although renal ultrasonography (US) has been considered as the best and most effective screening method, various false positive and false negative findings have been reported previously. Computed tomography (CT), instead, has been currently recognized as the most sensitive and specific imaging modality for diagnosing ALN. CT images of the ALN-infected areas typically appear as wedge-shaped, poorly defined regions of decreased nephrogenic density after contrast medium administration, as shown in the illustrated case, and mass-like hypodense lesions in the more severe form. CT, however, is costly and requires the sedation of a young patient. We have recently developed a systemic imaging work-up scheme using US screening followed by CT. In this imaging scheme, all patients with UTI underwent the renal US during the 1st—second day following their hospital admission. The CT assessment followed immediately when the initial US findings met either one of these two criteria, evidence of (1) unilateral or bilateral nephromegaly; and (2) a focal renal mass. For children who presented with borderline nephromegaly ultrasonographically, CT was performed when the patient remained febrile for 72 h after antibiotic-treatment commencement. With this scheme, not only the efficacy of CT performance but also the sensitivity of overall diagnosing of ALN appears to be improving.

With the application of renal ultrasonography and CT, ALN has been diagnosed with increased frequency, even at early stages. Thus, we can observe more details of the clinical characteristics and clinical course of ALN in pediatric patients. The incidence rate of ALN is 8–10% among Taiwanese children with febrile UTIs.

Escherichia coli has been recognized as the most frequent cause of gram-negative bacterial extraintestinal infections in humans, including neonatal meningitis and various UTIs such as cystitis, prostatitis, pyelonephritis, acute lobar nephronia, and bacteremia. Our early studies showed that *E. coli* was the most common pathogen identified from the patients with ALN, having a higher percentage of pathogens than the first-time UTIs. Complex pathogen-host interactions determine the patient's susceptibility to bacterial infections. Through the urovirulence factor analyses, we have noted that the *pap*G class II gene (gene associated with P-fimbriae of uropathogenic *E. coli*) was the most strongly associated pathogenic determinant for the pediatric ALN patients who have no underlying diseases except vesicoureteral reflux. However, pulsed-field gel electrophoresis analysis indicated that no major genotype was associated with the disease category. Thus, the major pathogenic determinants of *E. coli* may be associated with the specific uropathogenic genes, but not the bacterial lineage itself.

ALN is a severe disease entity, with extensive renal parenchymal involvement. Thus, it makes ALN likely progress to be a renal scar. Indeed, through a prospective randomized clinical trial study, we have noted that ALN is associated with a very high incidence of renal scarring in children, in comparison to APN, irrespective of the duration of antibiotic treatment.

Treatment for patients with ALN generally requires sequential intravenous/oral antibiotic therapy as does the treatment regimen for uncomplicated APN. Surgical intervention is rarely needed for ALN patients, except for those with concomitant urological abnormalities which may increase the risk of occurrence of acute bacterial infection. Although it has been suggested that the treatment duration for ALN needs to be at least the same as that for uncomplicated APN, recommendations for the duration of antibiotic treatment remain somewhat inconclusive. With the assistance of the ALN diagnosis scheme developed, we found that all ALN patients receiving a 3-week antibiotic course were successfully treated, whereas treatment failures (17.1% of treated patients) were noted in the 2-week treatment group. This observation suggests that the 2-week antibiotic treatment, usually scheduled for APN, may not be adequate for the treatment of ALN. Rather, a 3-week antibiotic treatment scheme was recommended for ALN.

Further Reading

Mattoo TK, Shaikh N, Nelson C. Contemporary management of urinary tract infection in children. Pediatrics 2021:147:e2020012138

Zaontz MR, Pahira JJ, Wolfman M, Gargurevich AJ, Zeman RK. Acute focal bacterial nephritis: a systematic approach to diagnosis and treatment. J Urol 1985;133:752-7.

Shimizu M, Katayama K, Kato E, Miyayama S, Sugata T, Ohta K. Evolution of acute focal bacterial nephritis into a renal abscess. Pediatr Nephrol 2005;20:93-5.

Rathore MH, Barton LL, Luisiri A. Acute lobar nephronia: a review. Pediatrics 1991;87:728-34.

Klar A, Hurvitz H, Berkun Y, et al. Focal bacterial nephritis (lobar nephronia) in children. J Pediatr 1996;128:850-3.

Cheng CH, Tsau YK, Hsu SY, Lee TL. Effective ultrasonographic predictor for the diagnosis of acute lobar nephronia. Pediatr Infect Dis J 2004;23:11-4.

Cheng CH, Tsau YK, Su LH, Lin CL, Lin TY. Comparison of urovirulence factors and genotypes for bacteria causing acute lobar nephronia and acute pyelonephritis. Pediatr Infect Dis J 2007;26:228-32

Cheng CH, Tsau YK, Lin TY. Effective duration of antimicrobial therapy for the treatment of acute lobar nephronia. Pediatrics 2006;117:e84-9.

Cheng CH, Tsau YK, Chen SY, Lin TY. Clinical courses of children with acute lobar nephronia correlated with computed tomographic patterns. Pediatr Infect Dis J 2009;28:300-3.

Cheng CH, Tsau YK, Chang CJ, et al. Acute lobar nephronia is associated with a high incidence of renal scarring in childhood urinary tract infections. Pediatr Infecti Dis J 2010;29:624-8.

Case 34. A 2-Year-Old Girl with Fever for 2 Weeks despite Oral Antibiotic Therapy: Renal Abscess in Children

Chi-Hui Cheng

Keywords

Renal abscess · Urinary tract infections
Combinatory image diagnosis scheme
CT diagnosis · Antibiotic treatment duration

Key Points

- Renal abscesses have been considered a very rare but severe form of renal infection.
- Renal abscesses can result from hematogenous spread or as a complication of infection from the lower urinary tract.
- Patients with renal abscess manifest similar clinical symptoms to those with acute pyelonephritis or acute lobar nephronia.
- Ultrasonography plus subsequent computed tomography confirmation has become the main diagnostic scheme for renal abscesses.
- A prolonged antibiotic course (3–6 weeks) plus pus drainage, if needed, is usually recommended for renal abscess treatment. For unresponsive cases, a surgical manipulation is recommended.

C.-H. Cheng (✉)
Division of Pediatric Nephrology, Department of Pediatrics, Chang Gung Memorial Hospital, Taoyuan, Taiwan

Department of Pediatrics, College of Medicine, Chang Gung University, Taoyuan, Taiwan

Case Report

A 2-year-old female suffered from intermittent high fever up to 39 ~ 41 °C for 2 weeks. Mild cough but no rhinorrhea was noted. Pharyngitis and acute otitis media (AOM) were told initially, but fever persisted despite empiric antibiotic therapy. Her appetite and activity were rather well during these 2 weeks. No dysuria but frequent urination was noted in the recent 1 month. There was also mild diarrhea since 3 days ago. The characteristic of the stool was loose, not watery or blood-tinged. Furthermore, multiple maculopapular skin rashes appeared over her bilateral lower limbs 2 days ago. She was brought to our outpatient department. A chest X-ray showed increased infiltration over bilateral lung fields, and atypical pneumonia was suspected. Due to her prolonged fever, she was admitted for further evaluation and treatment.

Intermittent high fever up to 40 °C was still noted after admission. Zithromax for 5 days was given under the impression of Mycoplasma pneumonia (Mycoplasma pneumoniae IgM Ab positive 1:32). Urine routine on admission revealed

Y.-C. Huang et al. (eds.), *Paediatric Infectious Diseases*,
https://doi.org/10.1007/978-981-19-7276-8_34

hematuria (urine OB 4+) and pyuria (urine WBC >100/high power field). With suspected urinary tract infection, we gave her empirical antibiotics with cefazolin plus netromycin initially.

A Renal echo examination was performed on hospital day 2 and showed enlarged left kidney sized 9.56 cm × 3.86 cm, and a normal right kidney sized 7.28 cm × 3.53 cm, suspected left side lobar nephronia, with abscess formation (Fig. 1). An abdominal computed tomography (CT) was arranged and showed multilobulated abscess formation over the left kidney (Fig. 2). The possible pathogens included *Staphylococcus aureus* according to the opinions of the Infectious Disease specialist, the nephrologist, and the urologist. Due to her persistent spiking fever and the finding of abdominal CT, we shifted antibiotics to prostaphlin plus cefotaxime on hospital day 3 for better *Staphylococcus aureus* and Gram-negative pathogen coverage.

Furthermore, the urologist was consulted and a percutaneous tube was inserted for abscess drainage on hospital day 4. A urine culture on admission reported *E. coli* and *K. pneumoniae*

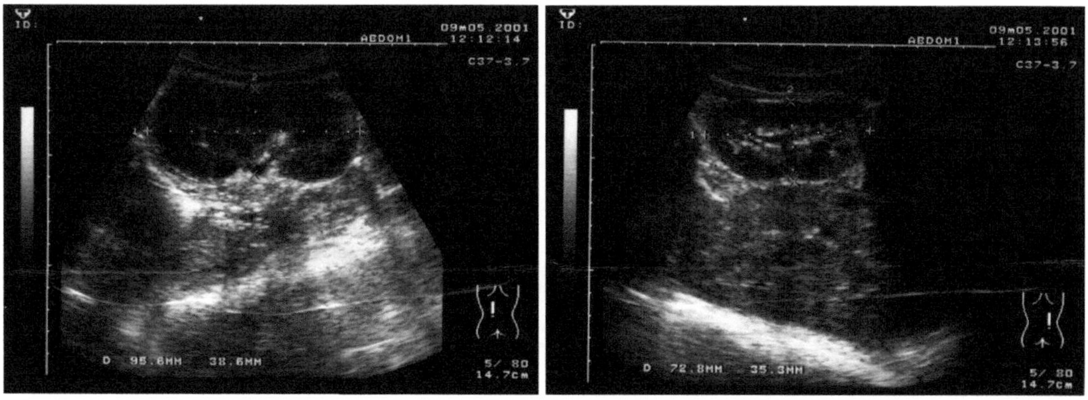

Fig. 1 The renal ultrasonography images showed an enlarged left kidney (9.56 cm × 3.86 cm) and a normal-sized right kidney (7.28 cm × 3.53 cm)

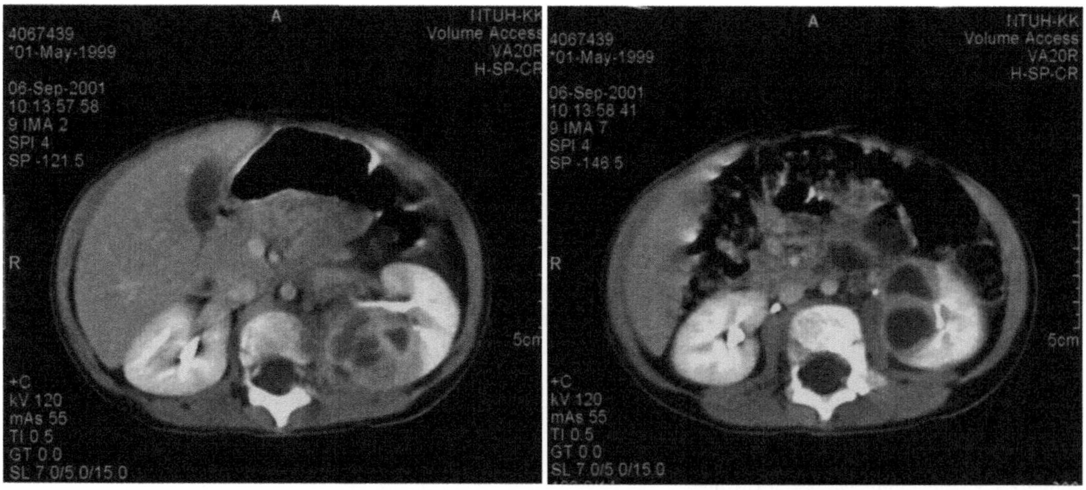

Fig. 2 The contrast-enhanced CT scan showed a puffy appearance of the left kidney, more in the superior and medial aspect, with multilobulated abscesses formation and involvement of the Gerota's fascia and left psoas muscle. Swelling of the left paraspinal muscle is also noted. Renal abscess is compatible with multilobulated abscess formation

with a colony count of 30,000 CFU/mL. Initial acid-fast stain and Gram's stain of the renal pus specimen were negative, but the specimen subsequently yielded *E. coli* which was resistant to first generation cephalosporin but sensitive to second and third generation of cephalosporins. We continued cefotaxime treatment and discontinued prostaphlin later according to the culture results. Her appetite and activity were better gradually and the skin rash also much decreased. However, spiking high fever persisted.

The drainage tube was removed on hospital day 11 and her fever subsided on the same day. Under the stable condition, she was discharged on hospital day 18 with sequential oral antibiotic therapy for a total of 4-week treatment course.

Discussion

Renal abscesses which are suppurative processes localized in the renal parenchyma are considered as a very rare but severe form of renal infection in children. Renal abscesses can result from hematogenous spread or as a complication of lower urinary tract infection. *S. aureus* and *E. coli* are reported to be the most common pathogens isolated. Other anaerobic bacteria were also reported to cause pediatric renal abscesses related to malignancy, pyelonephritis, or orodental infections. In our previous study, *E. coli* was the most common bacteria isolated, implicating that most of the renal abscesses resulted from the complications of ascending infections. Besides, vesicoureteral reflux (VUR) may not be a prerequisite factor for the development of renal abscess because the proportion of VUR (43%) is quite close to that in children with uncomplicated UTIs as well as those with acute pyelonephritis (APN), or acute lobar nephronia (ALN).

Patients with renal abscess usually manifest fever, lumbar pain, abdominal pain, raised erythrocyte sedimentation rates, leukocytosis, and less often have positive results for blood and urine cultures. This vague characteristic symptomatology has posed a great challenge for clinicians to differential diagnosis this disease from other severe renal infections, such as APN and ALN.

Ultrasonography (US) and computed tomography (CT) have been frequently employed for the imaging diagnosis of various renal infections. However, due to low specificity associated with sonographic images for renal lesions, additional computed tomography is usually required for renal abscess detection as well as defining the disease extension. Rote et al. attributed this scenario to the rare observation of a unique picture of sonolucency. When the infection has not progressed to a distinct mass of sufficient size, echography may just show an enlarged kidney.

Ultrasonography plus subsequent CT confirmation has become the main diagnostic scheme for the detection of renal abscesses. A feature of ultrasonographic-marked nephromegaly indicated that the patient might be in the early stage of renal abscess formation or as an ALN. We have included marked nephromegaly as the ultrasonographic indication for the subsequent CT diagnosis in our early study. With this imaging modality, a relatively shorter period for CT-diagnosed renal abscess after the onset of symptoms and signs and a shorter fever continuation after antibiotic treatment were noted. Henceforth, including sonographic marked nephromegaly as one of the admission indications for the subsequent CT diagnosis should be of great benefit in preventing renal abscesses from progressing into a more extended or advanced state due to late diagnosis, and thus in turn, leading to a shorter fever duration after the initiation of antibiotic treatment.

Pus drainage, if needed, and a prolonged antibiotic treatment course (3–6 weeks) are commonly recommended for renal abscess treatment if the abscess size is small or no perirenal involvement is noted. Nevertheless, for protracted and poor responsive cases, expeditious surgical manipulation is recommended.

Further Reading

Cheng CH, Tsau YK, Hsu SY, Lee TL. Effective ultrasonographic predictor for the diagnosis of acute lobar nephronia. *Pediatr Infect Dis J*. 2004;23(1):11-14.

Wang YT, Lin KY, Chen MJ, Chiou YY. Renal abscess in children: a clinical retrospective study. *Acta Paediatr Taiwan*. 2003;44(4):197-201.

Angel C, Shu T, Green J, Orihuela E, Rodriquez G, Hendrick E. Renal and peri-renal abscesses in children: proposed physio-pathologic mechanisms and treatment algorithm. *Pediatr Surg Int*. 2003;19(1-2):35-39.

Cachat F, Gehri M, Guignard JP. The role of uroradiological studies in children with renal abscess. *Pediatrics*. 2002;109(1):165-166.

Chen CY, Kuo HT, Chang YJ, Wu KH, Yang WC, Wu HP. Clinical assessment of children with renal abscesses presenting to the pediatric emergency department. *BMC Pediatr*. 2016;16:189.

Brook I. The role of anaerobic bacteria in perinephric and renal abscesses in children. *Pediatrics*. 1994;93(2):261-264.

Cheng CH, Tsai MH, Su LH, Wang CR, Lo WC, Tsau YK, et al. Renal abscess in children: a 10-year clinical and radiologic experience in a tertiary medical center. *Pediatr Infect Dis J*. 2008;27(11):1025-1027.

Ilyas M, Mastin ST, Richard GA. Age-related radiological imaging in children with acute pyelonephritis. *Pediatr Nephrol*. 2002;17(1):30-34.

Cheng CH, Tsau YK, Lin TY. Effective duration of antimicrobial therapy for the treatment of acute lobar nephronia. *Pediatrics*. 2006;117(1):e84-89.

Dougherty FE, Gottlieb RP, Gross GW, Denison MR. Neonatal renal abscess caused by Staphylococcus aureus. *Pediatr Infect Dis J*. 1991;10(6):463-466.

Part VII

Bone and Joint Infection

Case 35. An 11-Month-Old Infant with Limping Gait for 1 Week: Osteomyelitis Caused by Bacillus Calmette–Guérin (BCG) Vaccine

Chih-Jung Chen

Keywords

Osteomyelitis · Bacillus Calmette–Guérin (BCG) vaccine

Key Points

- Rare but severe complication after BCG vaccination.
- Mostly occur in immunocompetent individuals in approximately 1 year (range, 3–36 months) after BCG vaccination.
- Long bones of lower extremity are the most commonly involved skeletons.
- Prognosis is generally good except for those with vertebrate osteomyelitis and multifocal infections.
- Delayed vaccination at later infancy is associated with reduction of BCG osteomyelitis, but local reactions and regional lymphadenopathy are inversely increased.

C.-J. Chen (✉)
Division of Pediatric Infectious Diseases, Department of Pediatrics, Chang Gung Memorial Hospital, Taoyuan, Taiwan

College of Medicine, Chang Gung University, Taoyuan, Taiwan

Molecular Infectious Diseases Research Center, Chang Gung Memorial Hospital, Taoyuan, Taiwan
e-mail: chinjung@cgmh.org.tw

Case Report

An 11-month-old previously healthy girl presented to a local hospital with limping gait for 1 week. She had received the vaccines in the extended program of immunization, which included the Tokyo-172 strain of Bacillus Calmette–Guérin (BCG) vaccine administration at the age of 1 month. The initial physical examination of the lower limbs revealed limitations of abduction and adduction of the right hip joint. Sonography and roentgenography revealed widening of the right hip joint with accumulated synovial fluid. Under the impression of synovitis, she was on conservative treatment for 1 month. However, the limping gait did not improve, and fever was occasionally observed by her family during the period of conservative treatment. The arthrocentesis and arthrotomy of the right hip joint were finally arranged, which disclosed pus-like material in the joint space. The pathology study revealed chronic inflammation of the synovial membrane without acid-fast bacilli. The culture of synovial fluid yielded no organism. With the diagnosis of right septic hip, she started oral dicloxacillin treatment and was subsequently admitted to the hospital for systemic intravenous antibiotic therapy with a regimen of ceftriaxone and teicoplanin. She failed antimicrobial treatment and became unable to walk after the surgery.

Follow-up roentgenography and magnetic resonance imaging (MRI) revealed defects and

Y.-C. Huang et al. (eds.), *Paediatric Infectious Diseases*,
https://doi.org/10.1007/978-981-19-7276-8_35

osteolytic lesions of the proximal right femoral bone. She was febrile and immobile. Hemogram and biochemistry studies revealed leukocytosis with a peripheral white blood cell count of 14,300/μL, elevated C-reactive protein of 12.3 mg/L, and elevated erythrocyte sedimentation rate of 53 mm/h. She received another arthrotomy of the right hip joint along with a debridement and sequestration operation of the right femoral bone. The PCR test targeting *Mycobacterium tuberculosis* on the debridement samples of right femoral osteomyelitis was positive. The anti-tuberculosis regimen with isoniazid, rifampin, and pyrazinamide was administered. Unfortunately, the antimycobacterial therapy was complicated with hepatotoxicity 1 week after treatment. The regimen was replaced with streptomycin and ethambutol due to the substantial elevation of AST (577 U/L) and ALT (633 U/L) levels.

The liver enzyme returned to the normal range 10 days after stopping isoniazid, rifampin, and pyrazinamide. Readministration of the antimycobacterial regimen with isoniazid, rifampin, and moxifloxacin was successful, and no additional elevation of liver enzymes was observed. However, she experienced an episode of dislocation of the right hip joint. MRI further revealed the progression of right femoral osteomyelitis with surrounding myositis, which required the third surgery for debridement. The PCR test remained positive for *M. tuberculosis* and turned out to be BCG strain later by the central laboratory of Taiwan Centers for Diseases Control. Moxifloxacin was discontinued 2 months later, and the anti-tuberculosis regimen with isoniazid and rifampin was continued. She was unable to walk for a period of time, but improved gradually. She continued the anti-tuberculosis regimen for a total of 14 months, achieved a complete recovery, and continued well for 10-year follow-up.

Discussion

BCG is a live vaccine that contains an attenuated strain of *Mycobacterium bovis* and is currently produced by more than 40 manufacturers worldwide. The common seed strains used in BCG vaccines include Pasteur-1173 P2, Copenhagen-1331, Glaxo-1077, Tokyo-172, Russian and Moreau substrains. Although the immunogenicity was different for each substrain, the clinical efficacy favoring certain seed strains was not consistently demonstrated, and no recommendation was made on one strain over the other. BCG has been used in humans for 100 years since 1921 and is generally considered a vaccine with an acceptable safety profile and appreciable effectiveness in preventing severe tuberculosis diseases, including meningitis and disseminated diseases. However, BCG was also among the currently used vaccines with the most common reactogenicity. Mild local adverse reactions, such as papule in 2–4 weeks, ulceration in 1–2 months, and scar formation in 2–5 months, occurred in almost all BCG vaccinees after immunization. Cutaneous abscess and regional lymphadenopathy could be identified in 1–2% of individuals after BCG vaccination. It appeared that the incidences of adverse reactions were largely dependent on the seed strains used for BCG vaccination. For instance, the more immunogenic substrains of Pasteur and Copenhagen were reported to be associated with greater incidences of reactogenicity compared to the Tokyo, Glaxo, and Moreau strains. The above-mentioned mild adverse reactions were usually self-limited. No aggressive surgical or medical treatment was needed.

Osteomyelitis/osteitis is a rare but severe adverse reaction of BCG with a wide variation of incidences from 1 case per 3000 to 10^8 doses in different reports using different seed strains of *M. bovis* from distinct countries. The disease might be overlooked, and misdiagnosis could occur, especially in settings where the incidence was low, laboratory identification of *M. bovis* was not established or healthcare personnel was less experienced with this illness. Furthermore, given the nature of the long incubation time and insidious onset, the clinical suspicion of BCG osteomyelitis can be difficult, and the time to achieve a correct diagnosis is usually prolonged. Familiarity with the clinical characteristics of BCG-related osteomyelitis was essential for early suspicion and timely diagnosis.

The commonly involved bones in BCG-related osteitis were long bones of lower extremities, foot, ribs/sternum, long bones of upper extremities, and hands. The spine was less commonly affected. In a Taiwanese study characterizing BCG osteomyelitis between 1999 and 2014, only 2.8% of cases had spondylitis. The intervals between vaccination and symptom onset were approximately 7–18 months in most of the cases receiving vaccination in early infancy, although a wider range from 3 to 36 months was reported. It has been noted that the lower extremity long bone was usually associated with a longer interval. The common initial manifestations included local redness and/or swelling of the affected bone, palpable mass, limping or inability to walk. Fever can also be identified in 20% of cases. Hemogram and biochemistry studies of peripheral blood are usually unremarkable, with slight elevation of white blood cell counts and inflammation markers. Etiology diagnosis depends on acid-fast staining, culture or PCR targeting *M. bovis* on the biopsy or surgical specimen. Sometimes the microbiological diagnosis cannot be achieved, and the histology study was strongly suggestive if caseous necrosis or granulation tissue was revealed. With effective antimycobacterial therapy, most of the patients recovered completely. A wide operation to remove the infected bone tissue would cause destruction of the affected skeleton and was not necessary. Poor prognosis can sometimes be encountered, especially in children with vertebrate involvement or multifocal infections. An average duration of half a year is usually required for functional recovery of BCG osteomyelitis.

The postponement of BCG vaccination in elderly patients during infancy was reported to be associated with a lower incidence of osteomyelitis in vaccinees. In Taiwan, where the Tokyo-172 strain was used for BCG vaccination, delayed vaccination from neonates to after 5 months of age was associated with a 68% reduction in the risk of osteomyelitis. However, the policy change of immunization at an older age was also inversely associated with an 8.82-fold increase in injection site reactions, a 2.24-fold increase in regional lymphadenopathy and a shorter onset duration for both complications.

Further Reading

Huang CY, Chiu NC, Chi H, Huang FY, Chang PH. Clinical Manifestations, Management, and Outcomes of Osteitis/Osteomyelitis Caused by Mycobacterium bovis Bacillus Calmette-Guérin in Children: Comparison by Site(s) of Affected Bones. J Pediatrics 2019; 207: 97–102.

Huang W, Chiu NC, Chi H, Huang FY, Huang CY. Inoculation Age of Bacillus Calmette-Guérin Tokyo-172 Strain and Vaccine-related Adverse Reactions in Taiwan Birth Cohort of 2012–2017. Clin Infect Dis 2021;**73**: e1554–e1559.

Dara M, Acosta CD, Rusovich V, Zellweger JP, Centis R, Migliori GB. Bacille Calmette-Guerin vaccination: the current situation in Europe. Eur Respir J 2014; 43: 24-35.

Case 36. A 12-Year-Old Adolescent with Fever, Vomiting, General Skin Rash Following a Preceding Minor Trauma Over Left Hip: Disseminated Community-Associated Methicillin-Resistant Staphylococcus Aureus Infection

Yhu-Chering Huang

Keywords

Community-associated · Methicillin-resistant Staphylococcus aureus · Pyomyositis Arthritis · Pulmonary septic emboli

Key Points

- *S. aureus* is a common pathogen in humans throughout the life.
- Colonization of *S. aureus* in human is common, and infection of *S. aureus* is usually preceded by colonization.
- Purulent formation is the key element, and erythematous skin rash and dissemination of diseases are common manifestations and also diagnostic clues of the infections caused by *S. aureus.*
- A local soft tissue swelling without overlying erythematous skin manifestation but with a discrepantly severe pain sensation usually suggests a deep soft tissue infection and requires a rapid management.
- Treatment of *S. aureus* infection depends on the disease severity, sites of infection, and local antibiogram.
- The rate of MRSA among community-associated *S. aureus* infection in Asian countries ranged from 2.5% to >50%.

Case Report

A 12-year-old previously healthy female adolescent had minor trauma over left hip area 1 week ago. She developed fever, vomiting, and dizziness 5 days ago, and cough and rhinorrhea 2 days ago. She sought medical care at a clinic. She developed general erythematous skin rash with itching and wheal formation after medication and then was sent to a regional hospital. General weakness and respiratory distress were noted there. Blood pressure (BP) showed 74/44 mmHg, pulse rate (PR) 138/min, and respiratory rate (RR) 15/min. Laboratory inves-

Y.-C. Huang (✉)
Pediatrics, Chang Gung Memorial Hospital, Chang Gung University, Taoyuan, Taiwan
e-mail: ychuang@cgmh.org.tw

Y.-C. Huang et al. (eds.), *Paediatric Infectious Diseases*,
https://doi.org/10.1007/978-981-19-7276-8_36

tigations showed a white blood cell (WBC) count of 22,200/mm^3 with 92% segmented neutrophils and 7% lymphocytes. Serum C-reactive protein (CRP) concentration was 120 mg/L (normal, <5 mg/L), serum blood urea nitrogen (BUN) 30 mg/dL (normal, <20 mg/dL), serum creatinine 2.1 mg/dL, serum creatine phosphokinase (CPK) 729 U/L (with CK-MB 18 U/L). Under the impression of anaphylactic shock, sepsis, and rhabdomyolysis, she was referred to a medical center. Rechecked laboratory data at the medical center showed a WBC count of 4000/mm^3 with 73% segmented neutrophils and 4% band neutrophils, serum CRP 485 mg/L, BUN 19 mg/dL, and serum creatinine 1.1 mg/dL. Physical examination showed limited range of motion and tenderness over left hip (no local erythema and swelling). Left hip arthritis was highly suspected, empiric oxacillin plus ceftriaxone were administered intravenously and a consultation of orthopedic specialist was arranged immediately. Bedsides, echo-guided aspiration of left hip joint was performed, revealing turbid fluid. Emergent operation for left hip arthritis with arthrotomy, debridement, and drainage was conducted.

On the second day of hospitalization, fever was still noted; dyspnea, subcostal retraction, and wheezing breathing sound were noted. A chest radiography (Fig. 1) showed probably septic emboli and right side pleural effusion/empyema, which were confirmed by the subsequent chest computed tomography (CT) (Fig. 2). Blood culture yielded Staphylococcus-like and was subsequently identified as methicillin-resistant *S. aureus* (MRSA) on hospital day 3. Synovial fluid also yielded MRSA. Antibiotics were shifted to vancomycin. The patient continued to experience fever. Follow-up laboratory tests still revealed leukocytosis (WBC 22,400/mm^3) and high CRP level up to 358 mg/L. On day 9, a chest surgery was performed, which included right lower lobe (RLL) lobectomy and bronchoplasty for gangrene change with purulent discharge of RLL, closure of bronchial fistula for multiple bronchopleural fistulas of right middle lobe, and decortication of pleura of right side empyema. Pus cultures from the lung specimen again yielded MRSA.

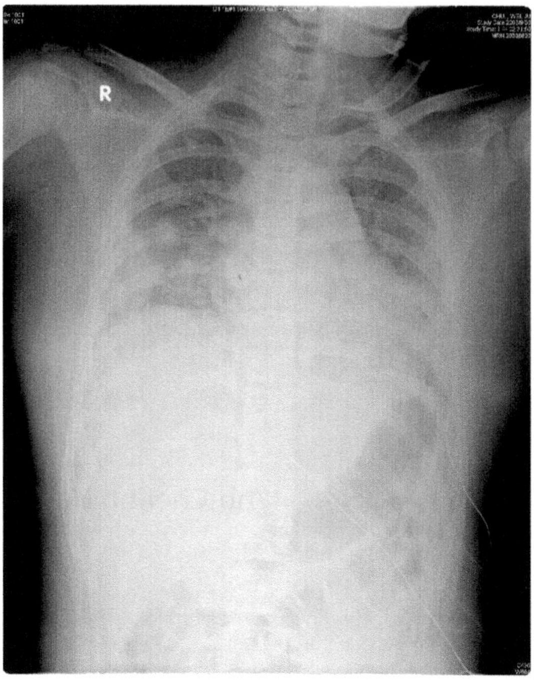

Fig. 1 A chest radiography on Hospital day 2 showed probably septic emboli and right side pleural effusion/empyema

Fever still noted, with stationary respiratory condition and left thigh pain. On Day 15, chest CT showed improving lung condition, whereas lower extremities CT demonstrated pyomyositis of left adductor magnus (Fig. 3). A third operation was performed, revealing grayish red pus accumulation of 400 mL in the muscle belly at the proximal thigh level and extending to proximal pelvic cavity through obturator foramen, and debridement and drainage were done. Pus culture again yielded MRSA. Antibiotics were shifted to teicoplanin plus meropenem on Day 16. Fever subsided on Day 21. Meropenem was discontinued on Day 23. Fever developed again on Day 25. Considering drug fever, we changed antibiotics to linezolid on Day 30. Fever was gone on Day 33 and she was discharged on Day 45 after admission.

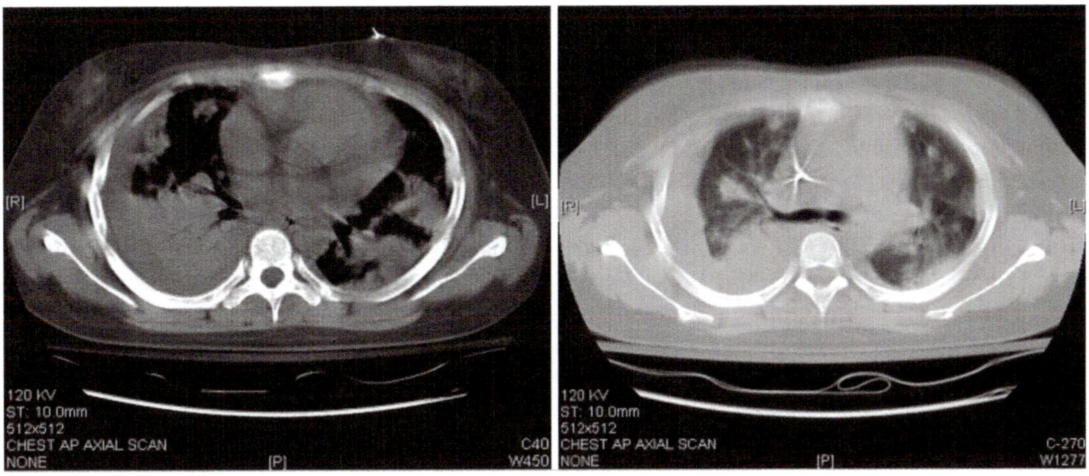

Fig. 2 A chest computed tomography demonstrated septic emboli of both lung fields and right side pleural effusion/empyema

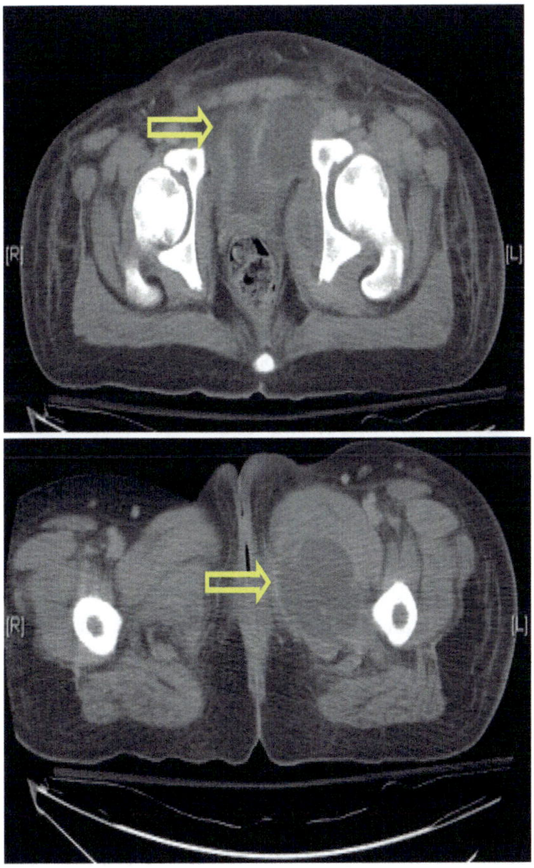

Fig. 3 A computed tomography of thighs demonstrated pyomyositis of left adductor magnus (arrow)

All the three MRSA isolates shared same molecular characteristics, which were sequence type 59/pulsotype D/Staphylococcal chromosomal cassette type V_T/Panton-Valentine leukocidin-positive, a local endemic community-associated MRSA (CA-MRSA) clone in Taiwan. The final diagnosis is disseminated MRSA infection with left hip arthritis, pneumonia complicated with empyema and bronchopleural fistulas, and pyomyositis of left adductor magnus, in post-operation status.

Discussion

S. aureus is a common pathogen in humans throughout their life. It can cause a broad spectrum of diseases, from skin and soft tissue infection (SSTI), fasciitis, pyomyositis, bone and joint infection, pneumonia, bacteremia, endocarditis, to septicemia with shock and toxic shock syndrome (TSS), etc.

Colonization of *S. aureus* in human is common, particularly in infants and young children, and can be identified in 20–40% of general population, mostly in nares, oropharynx, and skin surface of body. A longitudinal study conducted between 2009 and 2011 in northern Taiwan revealed that more than 90% of the babies ever had *S. aureus* colonization during the first 2 years of life. Forty percent of the babies were ever colonized with MRSA. Both the acquisition and the colonization rate of *S. aureus*, including MRSA, peaked in the first 4 months of life, and then declined gradually.

Infection is usually preceded by colonization. Minor injury with or without gross disruption of skin integrity may introduce colonizing *S. aureus* into the inner tissue, even bloodstream, and result in infection and disease. The lesion site of infection is not infrequently seen in a distant site other than the site of injury. Clinically, purulent formation is key element of *S. aureus* infection. Erythematous skin rash and dissemination of diseases are common manifestations and are also the diagnostic clues of the infections caused by *S. aureus*, as shown in the illustrated case.

Purulent change of the lesion site with pus/abscess formation is a typical presentation of *S. aureus* infection and can be frequently seen clinically, from superficial infection of skin and appendages (manifested as impetigo, furuncle, carbuncle, cutaneous abscess, wound infection), subcutaneous tissue infection (cellulitis), deep tissue infection (such as fasciitis, myositis, pyomyositis), bone and joint infection to internal organ involvement (renal or liver abscess). Over the lesion site, local erythematous change, swelling, warm sensation and pain, tender sensation are commonly seen in these conditions. However, the more superficial the lesion site (such as carbuncle, cutaneous abscess) is involved, the more prominent the local erythema on the overlying skin can be observed. In contrast, the deeper the (infection) lesion site (such as fasciitis, pyomyositis) is involved, the less prominent the overlying skin change can be identified initially, but may present profoundly several hours or even 1–2 days later. However, local swelling and a discrepantly severe pain sensation is usually complained under this condition. In this illustrated case, in addition to hip arthritis and pneumonia with empyema, pyomyositis of left adductor magnus was not identified and not diagnosed until a CT scan examination was performed for lower extremities due to persistent fever and left thigh pain, but without local findings. Pyomyositis is a bacterial infection of skeletal muscle with resultant abscess formation, usually seen in tropical areas and occasionally seen in temperate areas, and almost always due to *Staphylococcus aureus*. It usually involves large muscles such as quadriceps femoris muscle, as the illustrated case, abdominal muscles, psoas muscle, etc. Risk factors include immunosuppression, concurrent *S. aureus* infection, malnutrition, trauma, and injection drug use. Clinically, the lesion may manifest swelling, severe muscle pain and tenderness and "woody" sensation when palpation is perfomed, while no overlying skin change can be observed.

With toxin release, erythematous skin rash is an important and common presenting sign of *S. aureus* infection, accompanying with either SSTI (previously named as surgical scarlet fever in this condition), scalded skin syndrome, deep tissue infection, or toxic shock syndrome. Rash manifestations may present as scarlatiniform rash, general red sea-like rash, or nonspecific general erythematous macular rash and subsequent skin desquamation may occur in certain cases several days later.

Dissemination of *S. aureus* following SSTIs to distant bone and joints or internal organs such as kidney, liver, or endocardium, etc. with resultant "metastatic" infections could be occasionally seen, as shown in the illustrated case, and should be kept in mind clinically.

The prevalence of community-associated (CA)-MRSA varied markedly from country to country. The rate of MRSA among CA *S. aureus* infection can range from <1% to >50% in different countries and is usually higher in children than in adults. The rate of MRSA among CA *S. aureus* infection in Asian countries ranged from 2.5% to >50%. As the clonality, molecular epidemiology of CA-MRSA in Asia showed a clonal heterogeneity, with different clones in different countries. However, a few clones were shared by several countries. Currently in Taiwan, MRSA accounted for 60–70% of community-onset *S. aureus* clinical isolates from pediatric patients and Taiwan clone (ST59/SCCmec VT/PVL-positive, clindamycin non-susceptible) and USA300 (ST8/SCCmec IV/PVL-positive, clindamycin susceptible) are two major clones.

Treatment of *S. aureus* infection depends on the severity of disease entities as well as the local epidemiology of antibiotic resistance pattern. For superficial SSTI with cutaneous abscess, incision and drainage is usually adequate when the lesion size is small (less than 5 cm). Otherwise, antibiotics may be needed. Oral agents such as clindamycin, trimethoprim-sulfamethoxazole (TMP-SMX), and minocycline are used for empiric outpatient therapy of skin and soft tissue infections (SSTIs) associated with CA-MRSA, depending on the local antibiotic resistogram. For severe and/or invasive MRSA infections, most clinicians use vancomycin (IV) or teicoplanin for the empiric and definitive therapy. Linezolid, PO or IV, is recommended for treatment of severe SSSIs and pneumonia caused by MRSA. Daptomycin (IV) should be considered in patients with MRSA bacteremia and right-sided endocarditis as well as in complicated SSSIs, but should not be used to treat MRSA pneumonia. Tigecycline and telavancin are alternative (IV) treatments for SSSIs caused by MRSA Ceftaroline, a parenteral agent, is approved for SSSIs and community-acquired pneumonia caused by MRSA. Several agents for MRSA, including tedizolid, dalbavancin, and oritavancin, are newly licensed or are in ongoing trials.

Further Reading

Chuang YY, Huang YC. Molecular epidemiology of community-associated methicillin-resistant *Staphylococcus aureus* in Asia. Lancet Infect Dis 2013;13:698-708.

Chen CJ, Huang YC. New epidemiology of *Staphylococcus aureus* in Asia. Clin Microbiol Infect 2014; 20: 605–623.

Huang YC, Chen CJ. USA 300 (sequence type 8) became a major clone of methicillin-resistant Staphylococcus aureus in northern Taiwan. Int J Antimicrob Agents. 2022 Jan 25:106534. https://doi.org/10.1016/j.ijantimicag.2022.106534.

Turner NA, Sharma-Kuinkel BK, Maskarinec SA, Eichenberger EM, Shah PP, Carugati M, Holland TL, Fowler VG Jr. Methicillin-resistant Staphylococcus aureus: an overview of basic and clinical research. Nat Rev Microbiol 2019; 17:203-218.

Huang YC, Su LH, Lin TY. Nasal carriage of methicillin-resistant Staphylococcus aureus in contacts of an adolescent with community-acquired disseminated disease. Pediatr Infect Dis J 2004; 23: 919–922.

Liu C, Bayer A, Cosgrove SE, Daum RS, Fridkin SK, Gorwitz RJ, et al. Clinical Practice Guidelines by the Infectious Diseases Society of America for the Treatment of Methicillin-Resistant Staphylococcus Aureus Infections in Adults and Children. Clin Infect Dis 2011;52: e18-55.

Part VIII

Skin and Soft Tissue Infection

Case 37. A 4-Year-Old Boy with Left Leg Pain and Limping Gait Following Mucoid Diarrhea 2 Weeks Ago: Salmonella Pyomyositis

Ping-Ing Lee

Keywords

Pyomyositis · Salmonellosis · Magnetic resonance imaging · *Staphylococcus aureus*

Key Points

- Pyomyositis is a hematogenous infection of the skeletal muscles and is more prevalent in tropical areas.
- *Staphylococcus aureus* is the most common causative organism.
- Symptoms and signs of pyomyositis are usually scanty and unapparent except for local pain and tenderness. It may be difficult to differentiate with other possible diagnoses including septic arthritis, and osteomyelitis, because the infection is contained by the overlying fascia.
- Serum muscle enzyme levels may be normal or elevated in cases with pyomyositis.
- Magnetic resonance imaging is the preferred imaging technique for diagnosis.
- Salmonellosis is a foodborne infection that is more prevalent in areas with traditional wet markets and close contacts between humans and animals. The infection is more prevalent in young children.

P.-I. Lee (✉)
Department of Pediatrics, National Taiwan University Children's Hospital, National Taiwan University, Taipei, Taiwan
e-mail: pinging@ntu.edu.tw

Case Report

A previously healthy 4-year-old boy had diarrhea with mucoid/watery stool 14 days ago. Blood streaked stool was noted once. The symptom of diarrhea improved gradually in following days. Left leg pain with limping gait and fever up to 40 °C was noted 2 days ago. On arrival at the hospital, tenderness over left hip was noted. There was no apparent swelling and redness over the legs and the joints. He was admitted to our hospital.

At admission, the white blood cell count was 10,390/μL with 38.2% segmented neutrophil. C-reactive protein level as 6.5 mg/L. Radiography of both hips was unremarkable except for soft tissue swelling at left upper thigh. Magnetic resonance imaging (MRI) showed diffuse soft tissue swelling near the left pelvic sidewall, extending to the left ischiorectal fossa, left perineum, left femoral adductors and obturator muscles. A rim enhancing lesion, about 2.7 cm in diameter, was noted near the left femoral adductors (Figs. 1 and 2).

Y.-C. Huang et al. (eds.), *Paediatric Infectious Diseases*,
https://doi.org/10.1007/978-981-19-7276-8_37

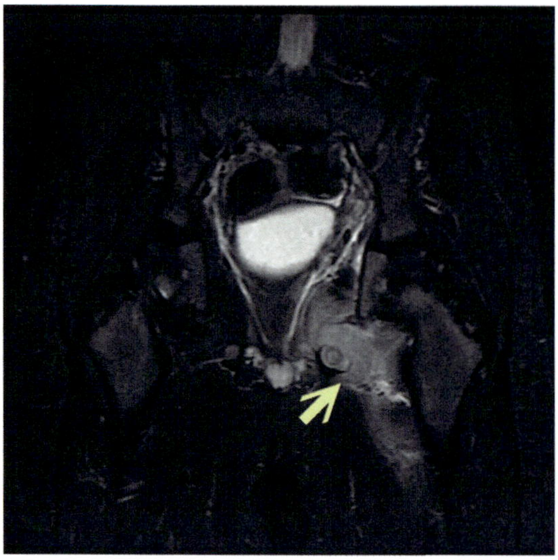

Fig. 1 Magnetic resonance imaging showed diffuse soft tissue swelling (arrow) near the left pelvic sidewall

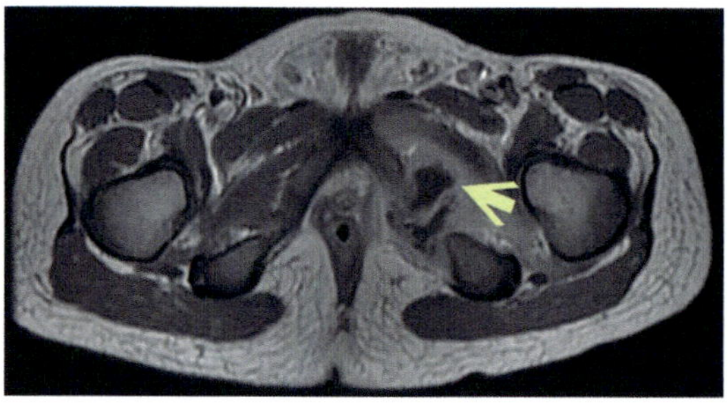

Fig. 2 Magnetic resonance imaging showed a rim-enhancing lesion near the left femoral adductors (arrow), about 2.7 cm in diameter

Debridement and fasciotomy were performed on left femoral adductors. Pus culture grew Salmonella O9 (group D1) that was susceptible to cefotaxime, ceftazidime, trimethoprim/sulfamethoxazole, and ciprofloxacin. Stool culture did not show significant bacteria pathogen. Intravenous cefotaxime was given for 2 weeks followed by 1 week of oral cefixime with complete recovery.

Discussion

Pyomyositis is a bacterial infection of muscle that occurs usually in the absence of a predisposing site of infection. The offending pathogen usually arise from hematogenous spread, rather that extension of infection from adjacent tissues. The presumed pathogenesis is thought to reflect initial bacteremia. Local trauma of muscles may predispose to produce pyomyositis.

Pyomyositis is also known as tropical pyomyositis because it is more prevalent in tropical areas. However, it distributes all over the world. It is possible that a higher incidence of bacterial infections, and hence a higher chance of hematogenous bacterial spread, in tropical areas may account for a higher incidence of pyomyositis in tropical areas. The isolated *Salmonella* species in present case is indeed a more common pathogen in tropical areas with traditional wet markets and close contacts between humans and animals.

Clinically, pyomyositis is characterized by fever, localized muscle pain, swelling, and tenderness. The most frequent sites of involvement are the large muscles of the lower extremities and the trunk muscles. However, a variety of other muscles' involvements have been reported. Leukocytosis and elevated C-reactive protein level are common. Serum muscle enzyme levels may be normal or elevated. This is quite different from the case of viral myositis that is usually accompanied by an obvious increase of serum muscle enzymes.

For the present case, it is difficult to differentiate among possible diagnoses of pyomyositis, septic arthritis, and osteomyelitis because the lesion is located deep in left thigh. Because the infection is contained by the overlying fascia, there is usually no apparent redness and swelling over the lesion of pyomyositis. The only abnormal physical finding in the present case was local tenderness. Normal appearance of plain X-ray cannot exclude the possibility of osteomyelitis and septic arthritis. Typical changes of osteomyelitis, including thickened periosteum and osteolytic lesion, may appear on plain film several days after the disease onset. Mild septic arthritis may also appear normal in joint X-ray examination.

Prompt image diagnosis is essential for the evaluation of patients with focal limb pain because the possible need for surgical exploration must be assessed immediately. Ultrasonography may be helpful in detecting soft tissue swelling, abscess, and joint effusion, but it cannot evaluate the possibility of osteomyelitis. MRI is the most useful study in assessment of such patients. It can demonstrate and differentiate clearly the involvement of joint, bone, and muscle. For cases with pyomyositis, T1-weighted MRI image may show a slight increase in signal intensity with a surrounding enhanced rim. The T2-weighted image will show a diffuse increase in signal intensity of the lesion. Although computed tomography is more readily available, it cannot demonstrate details of myositis and it is poor to demonstrated bone and joint lesions that may be associated with pyomyositis.

Staphylococcus aureus is the most common cause of pyomyositis. *S. aureus* is responsible for 95% of pyomyositis in tropical areas. Whereas in temperate areas, *S. aureus* is the cause of 60–70% of cases. Blood cultures are positive in only 5–35% of the cases, and metastatic infections in other tissues are rare. Other possible pathogens include salmonella, streptococcus, *Streptococcus pneumoniae*, enterococcus, gram-negative bacilli, nontuberculous mycobacteria, and fungus.

Drainage of formed abscesses is necessary, not only for treatment but also for identification of offending pathogen. Initial antibiotic therapy should be active against methicillin-resistant *S. aureus* (MRSA) because of the increasing incidence of community-acquired MRSA infections. For young children living in areas prevalent for salmonella infection, appropriate coverage of this gram-negative organism may be necessary. The prognosis after appropriate treatment of pyomyositis is excellent.

Salmonellosis is a foodborne infection that is more prevalent in Taiwan because many people in Taiwan are more willing to purchase meat from traditional wet markets rather than supermarkets. Fresh poultry products are frequently contaminated by salmonella. Salmonella gastroenteritis is more prevalent in hot seasons. The incidence increases with decreasing age. Infants had the highest annual incidence of 525 cases/100,000 person-years in Taiwan.

The most common manifestation of salmonella infection is enterocolitis that may be complicated by septicemia, pneumonia, arthritis, and osteomyelitis. Pyomyositis is not a frequent complication. The antibiotic resistance rate of salmonella has been increasing in recent years, including the resistance rate to fluoroquinolone and the third-generation cephalosporins. At present, the drug of choice for empiric treatment of salmonellosis is the third-generation cephalosporins in children.

Further Reading

Pasternack MS. Myositis and myonecrosis. In: Mandell GL, Bennett JE, Dolin R, eds. Mandell, Douglas, and Bennett's Principles and Practices of Infectious Diseases, 9th edition. Philadelphia: Churchill Livingstone, 2020.

Chiu NC, Hsieh MC, Chi H, Huang FY. Clinical characteristics of pyomyositis in children: 20-year experience in a medical center in Taiwan. J Microbiol Immunol Infect 2009;42:494-9.

Lovejoy JF 3rd, Alexander K, Dinan D, Drehner D, Khan-Assad N, Lacerda IRA. Team approach: pyomyositis. JBJS Reviews 2017;5:e4.

Chou H, Teo HE, Dubey N, Peh WC. Tropical pyomyositis and necrotizing fasciitis. Semin Musculoskelet Radiol 2011;15:489-505.

Agarwal V, Chauhan S, Gupta RK. Pyomyositis. Neuroimaging Clin N Am 2011;21:975-83.

Phadke PS, Gandhi AR, More SA, Joshirao RP. Salmonella pyomyositis with concurrent sacroiliac osteomyelitis presenting as piriformis syndrome: a rare case. J Postgrad Med 2017;63:44-6.

Hwang JH, Shin GW, Lee CS. Community-onset pyomyositis caused by a *Salmonella enterica* serovar enteritidis sequence type 11 strain producing CTX-M-15 extended-spectrum beta-lactamase. J Clin Microbiol 2015;53:1439–41.

Lee CM, Lee MS, Yang TL, et al. Clinical features and risk factors associated with bacteremia of nontyphoidal salmonellosis in pediatric patients, 2010-2018. J Formos Med Assoc 2021;120(1 Pt 1):196-203.

Lo HY, Lai FP, Yang YJ et al. Changes in epidemiology and antimicrobial susceptibility of nontyphoid salmonella in children in southern Taiwan, 1997-2016. J Microbiol Immunol Infect 2020;53:585-91.

Feng Y, Chang YJ, Pan SC, et al. Characterization and source investigation of multidrug-resistant *Salmonella Anatum* from a sustained outbreak, Taiwan. Emerg Infect Dis 2020;26:2951-5.

Tseng CF, Chiu NC, Huang CY, et al. The epidemiology of non-typhoidal salmonella gastroenteritis and campylobacter gastroenteritis in pediatric inpatients in northern Taiwan. J Microbiol Immunol Infect 2019;52:449-55.

Hung YT, Lay CJ, Wang CL, Koo M. Characteristics of nontyphoidal salmonella gastroenteritis in Taiwanese children: A 9-year period retrospective medical record review. J Infect Public Health 2017;10:518-21.

Chen CJ, Wu FT, Hsiung CA, et al. Risk factors for salmonella gastroenteritis in children less than five years of age in Taiwan. Pediatr Infecti Dis J 2012;31:e239-43.

Huang IF, Kao CH, Lee WY, et al. Clinical manifestations of nontyphoid salmonellosis in children younger than 2 years old--experiences of a tertiary hospital in southern Taiwan. Pediatr Neonatol 2012; 53:193-8.

Chen PL, Li CY, Hsieh TH, et al. Epidemiology, disease spectrum and economic burden of non-typhoidal salmonella infections in Taiwan, 2006-2008. Epidemiol Infect 2012;140:2256-63.

Part IX

Other Specific Infection/Syndrome

Case 38. A 6-Year-Old Boy with Fever, Sore Throat, and a Crusted Wound on the Left Flank: Scrub Typhus

Hsin Chi

Keywords

Zoonotic disease · *Orientia tsutsugamushi* Doxycycline · Painless eschar · Vasculitis

Key Points

- A Zoonotic disease, due to infection of *Orientia tsutsugamushi*
- Transmitted via the bite of chiggers, larval stage of *Leptotrombidium delicense*
- Infection causes vasculitis, can be mild or severe in children and can affect almost every organ system
- Drug of choice is doxycycline 4 mg/kg/day
- No vaccines are currently available.

Case Report

A 6-year-old previously healthy boy had a spiking high fever up to 39 °C, sore throat and one crusted wound (about 0.5 cm × 0.5 cm) on the left flank 4 days prior to this admission. The symptoms did not improve despite of medications from a local clinic. He was brought to our ER. Rapid tests for influenza, adenovirus, group A *Streptococcus* were done. Oral antibiotic cephalexin was prescribed due to a positive group A Streptococcus rapid test. One day before admission, he vomited after eating food and showed decreased activity and appetite, so he was brought to our ER again. Then he was admitted to our ward for further management under the impression of acute pharyngitis, group A *Streptococcus* infection related.

On admission, an eschar-like wound was found on his left flank (Fig. 1a). Laboratory examinations revealed leukopenia (3.2×10^9 cells/L) with a neutrophil count of 62% and lymphocyte 33%, thrombocytopenia (112×10^9 cells/L) and elevated C-reactive protein (17.74 mg/L).

On the second day of hospitalization, epigastric pain with vomiting episodes developed. His abdomen was distended with hypoactive bowel sound. NPO with intravenous fluid hydration was done. Reddish maculopapular rashes over trunk and face were noted on hospital day 3 (Fig. 1b).

Tracing back his travel history, he had visited Taitung and Lanyu (in eastern part of Taiwan) for 1 week (13 days prior to fever onset) and climbed Xiangshan (a hill in Taipei city) 4 days prior to fever onset. Scrub typhus is endemic in both areas. Subsequently, scrub typhus was suspected, and doxycycline was immediately administered on hospital day 3. The abdominal

H. Chi (✉)
Division of Pediatric Infectious Diseases, Department of Pediatrics, MacKay Children's Hospital, Taipei, Taiwan

MacKay College of Medicine, Taipei, Taiwan
e-mail: chi.4531@mmh.org.tw

Y.-C. Huang et al. (eds.), *Paediatric Infectious Diseases*,
https://doi.org/10.1007/978-981-19-7276-8_38

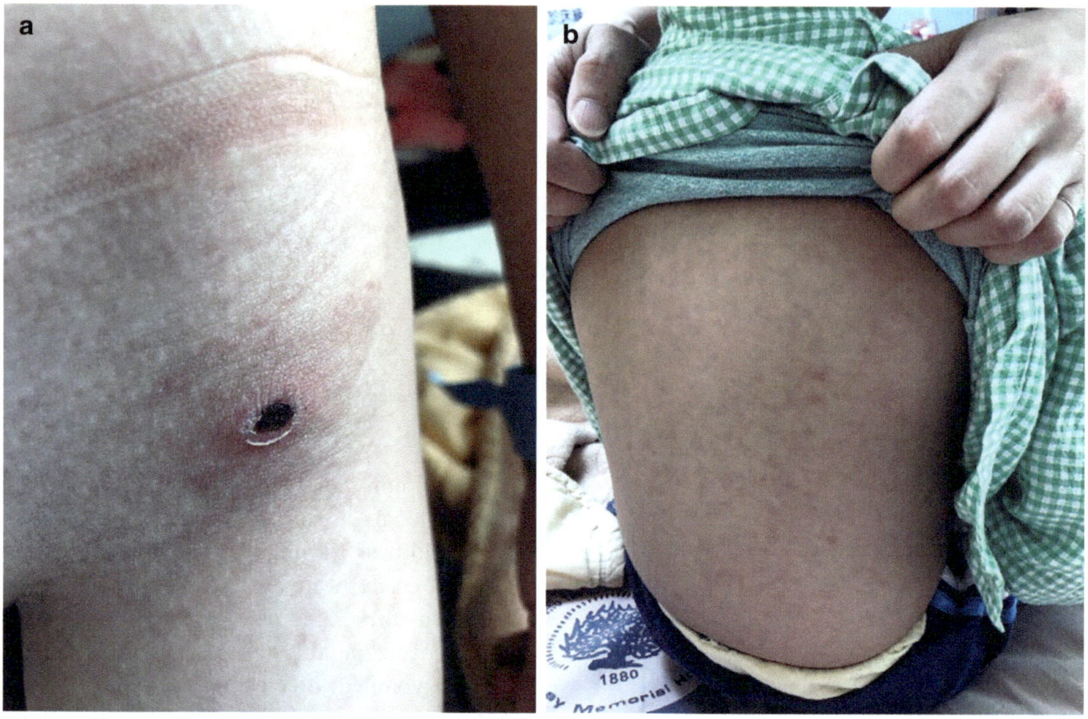

Fig. 1 (**a**) Eschar-like lesion over left flank area. (**b**) Maculopapular rashes over chest and abdomen

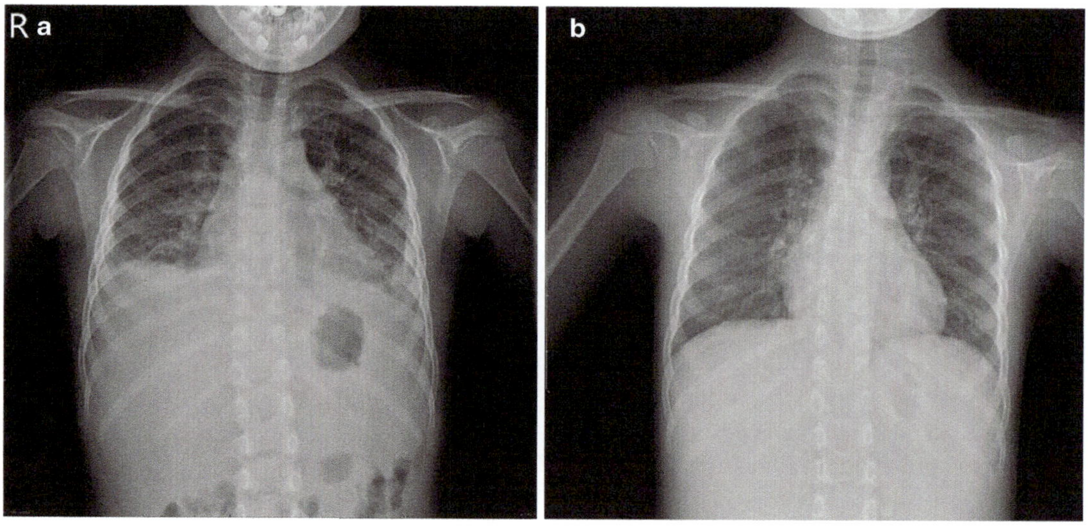

Fig. 2 (**a**) Bilateral pleural effusions on CXR. (**b**) Resolution of pleural effusions on CXR

echo revealed moderate ascites, mild bilateral pleural effusion, and acute cholecystitis. The CXR revealed bilateral pleural effusions (Fig. 2a). The laboratory examination revealed leukopenia (2.3×10^9 cells/L) with a neutrophil count of 71% and band 13%, thrombocytopenia (50×10^9 cells/L), anemia (Hb 109 g/L), elevated transaminase values (aspartate transaminase 153 IU/L, alanine transaminase 124 IU/L), hypokalemia (2.8 mmol/L), elevated C-reactive protein (55.29 mg/L), hypoalbuminemia (29 g/L), elevated lactate dehydrogenase (482 IU/L), and elevated γ-glutamyltransferase (46 IU/L). Tests for EBV serology, CMV serology and anti-streptolysin O titer were negative. We also immediately sent a blood specimen to the central laboratory of Taiwan Centers for Diseases Control for scrub typhus real-time PCR test and Immunofluorescence assay (IFA). Follow-up laboratory examination on hospital day 5 revealed normal WBC count (6.7 × 10^9 cells/L) with neutrophil 55%, Band 2%, improving thrombocytopenia (72 × 10^9 cells/L), hemoglobin (122 g/L), elevated transaminase values (aspartate transaminase 144 IU/L, alanine transaminase 132 IU/L), hypokalemia (3.1 mmol/L), hypoalbuminemia (29 g/L), and decreasing C-reactive protein (39.95 mg/L). Fever subsided 48 h after the start of doxycycline. The diagnosis of scrub typhus was confirmed by qPCR of *O. tsutsugamushi* and positivity of IFA-IgM, IFA-IgG. He was discharged with oral antibiotics and was followed up at outpatient department. The laboratory examination and CXR all revealed resolving results (Fig. 2b).

Discussion

Scrub typhus, a rickettsial exanthematous febrile disease, is endemic in Southeast Asia. It has been designated as a reportable communicable disease in Taiwan since 1955. It is a zoonotic disease caused by the infection of *Orientia tsutsugamushi*, which consists of many antigenically diverse strains. Scrub typhus is widely distributed in the western Pacific area and Asia, from Japan and South Korea to northern Australia, and the western border can reach Afghanistan and Pakistan. In Taiwan, both Taitung and Hualien counties, in eastern part of Taiwan, are endemic areas with the highest annual incidence rate of scrub typhus [1, 2].

Classical scrub typhus transmitted via the bite of the larvae of *Leptotrombidium delicense* (also called "chiggers" or "red bugs") is prevalent during early summer and autumn in Taiwan [3]. The larvae of such mites are approximately 0.2–0.4 mm in length. The larval stage is the only parasitic stage when the pathogen is transmitted to people and other vertebrates. In regions where scrub typhus is a constant threat, a natural cycle occurs through transovarial transfer from mite larvae to small mammals, such as field mice or rats, and people are incidental hosts. It seems that rodents are more commonly infested with the vectors during these seasons. Meanwhile, children, who are incidental hosts, have an increased risk of exposure because of higher numbers of field trips and outdoor activities in those periods.

O. tsutsugamushi infects endothelial cells and causes vasculitis, the predominant clinicopathologic feature of the disease. Scrub typhus can range from mild to severe in children and affect almost every organ system. It is characterized by fever, headache, myalgia, and vomiting. Half of the patients with scrub typhus show an eschar and a spotted rash [4]. Severe manifestations include pneumonitis, meningitis, encephalitis, disseminated intravascular coagulation, and multiorgan failure. Regional or generalized lymphadenopathy, hepatomegaly, and splenomegaly are noted in children with scrub typhus. Gastrointestinal symptoms, including abdominal pain, vomiting, and diarrhea, also occur in children. A single painless eschar with an erythematous rim at the site of the chigger bite and a maculopapular rash are present in less than half of the cases. Laboratory findings such as elevation of C-reactive protein (CRP), aspartate aminotransferase (AST) alanine aminotransferase (ALT) level are seen in most children. Hypoalbuminemia and proteinuria are also found [5, 6].

Positive laboratory diagnosis for scrub typhus is based on a positive real-time polymerase chain reaction test, or a fourfold increase in OT-specific immunoglobulin M or immunoglobulin G antibody in paired sera by using an indirect immunofluorescence assay technique.

Currently, the drug of choice is doxycycline (4 mg/kg/day PO or IV divided every 12 h; maximum: 200 mg/day), a member of the tetracycline family, and several studies have proved its effectiveness. Several alternative antimicrobials including tetracyclines, chloramphenicol, azithromycin, and quinolones can be used. Azithromycin is as effective as other anti-rickettsial drugs with higher treatment success rates, lower frequency of adverse effects, and longer time to defervescence [7]. Clinical trials showed that azithromycin is as effective, and that rifampicin is superior to doxycycline and can have a role as an alternative therapy, especially for pregnant women. Therapy should be continued for a minimum of 5 days and until the patient has been afebrile for at least 3 days to avoid relapse.

Serious complications include pneumonitis in 20–35% and meningoencephalitis in approximately 10–25% of children [8]. Prevention is based on avoidance of the chiggers that transmit *O. tsutsugamushi*. Protective clothing is the next most useful mode of prevention. No vaccines are currently available.

References

1. Chen HL, Chen HY, Horng CB. [Surveillance of scrub typhus in Taiwan]. J Microbiol Immunol Infect 1993;26:166-70.
2. Lee YS, Wang PH, Tseng SJ, Ko CF, Teng HJ. Epidemiology of scrub typhus in eastern Taiwan, 2000-2004. Jpn J Infect Dis 2006;59:235-8.
3. Lien JC, Lin SY, Lin HM. Field observation on the bionomics of Leptotrombidium deliensis, the vector of scrub typhus in the Pescadores. Acta Med Biol (Niigata) 1967;15:27-31.
4. Weng SC, Lee HC, Chen JJ, Cheng YJ, Chi H, Lin CY. Eschar: A Stepping Stone to Scrub Typhus. J Pediatr 2017;181:320- e1.
5. Huang CT, Chi H, Lee HC, Chiu NC, Huang FY. Scrub typhus in children in a teaching hospital in eastern Taiwan, 2000-2005. Southeast Asian J Trop Med Public Health 2009;40:789-94.
6. Jim WT, Chiu NC, Chan WT, Ho CS, Chang JH, Huang SY, et al. Clinical manifestations, laboratory findings and complications of pediatric scrub typhus in eastern Taiwan. Pediatr Neonatol 2009;50:96-101.
7. Lee SC, Cheng YJ, Lin CH, Lei WT, Chang HY, Lee MD, et al. Comparative effectiveness of azithromycin for treating scrub typhus: A PRISMA-compliant systematic review and meta-analysis. Medicine (Baltimore) 2017;96:e7992.
8. Lee HC, Ko WC, Lee HL, Chen HY. Clinical manifestations and complications of rickettsiosis in southern Taiwan. J Formos Med Assoc 2002;101:385-92.

Case 39. A 5-Month-Old Infant with Repeated Community-Acquired Pneumonia and Failure to Thrive: Pediatric Human Immunodeficiency Virus Infection

Wah Tin Tiew and Yhu-Chering Huang

Keywords

Human immunodeficiency virus · Vertical transmission · PCR

Key Points

- Prevention of mother-to-child transmission is important to reduce the number of new HIV infections. These strategies include universal opt-out screening for all pregnant women, combination antiretroviral therapy for HIV-infected pregnant women, elective cesarean delivery before labor onset, postnatal antiretroviral drugs, and complete avoidance of breastfeeding.
- For young children less than 18 months of age, the gold standard diagnostic test is HIV nucleic acid amplification tests.
- All HIV-infected children should receive antiretroviral drugs therapy while the treatment regimens should be individualized.
- Good adherence is important to ensure viral suppression and recovery of CD4 cells, as well as to prevent development of resistance and treatment failure.

Case 1

A 5-month-old female infant was born full term via spontaneous vaginal delivery with good Apgar score and had a birth weight of 2.88 kg. Maternal human immunodeficiency virus (HIV) rapid screening test during pregnancy was negative. The infant had a previous history of hospital admission at 3 months of age with severe community-acquired pneumonia due to adenovirus and parainfluenza-1 virus with superimposed bacterial infection, requiring mechanical ventilation and non-invasive ventilation for 12 days.

This admission, she presented to emergency department (ED) with fever, rapid breathing, and poor feeding. Physical examination revealed a cachexic infant who was tachypneic with chest wall retraction and nasal flaring. Lung auscultation showed reduced breath sounds bilaterally with crackles and rhonchi. She had extensive oral thrush, multiple cervical lymphadenopathy and

W. T. Tiew (✉)
Ministry of Health, Putrajaya, Malaysia

Y.-C. Huang
Pediatrics, Chang Gung Memorial Hospital, Chang Gung University, Taoyuan, Taiwan

Y.-C. Huang et al. (eds.), *Paediatric Infectious Diseases*,
https://doi.org/10.1007/978-981-19-7276-8_39

generalized dry unhealthy skin. Abdominal palpation revealed presence of hepatosplenomegaly. Neurologic examination was unremarkable.

Her initial laboratory data showed WBC 9980/μL, absolute neutrophils count 5040/μL, absolute lymphocyte count 2150/μL, thrombocytosis (platelet 347,000/μL), and hemoglobin (Hb) 7.4 g/dL. Her serum albumin was 25 g/L, blood urea nitrogen (BUN) 4.6 mmol/L, sodium 136 mEq/L, potassium 4.6 mEq/L, and creatinine 35 mmol/L. Parainfluenza-1 was detected from nasopharyngeal specimen. Blood culture was negative for bacteria.

She was treated as community-acquired pneumonia with intravenous amoxicillin-clavulanate and oral oseltamivir. Non-invasive respiratory support was applied for 4 days followed by oxygen supplementation via nasal cannula. While in the ward for nutritional rehabilitation, she developed new onset of fever with respiratory distress. RSV antigen was detected and her blood culture grew pan-susceptible nontyphoidal Salmonella. The infant's HIV Ag/Ab serology was tested reactive. Later, her mother's HIV Ag/Ab serology test was also reactive. Blood for HIV RNA viral load and CD4/CD8 was sent. Non-invasive ventilation (BiPAP) was applied and her chest X-ray showed collapsed-consolidation over right upper lobe (RUL) with patchy alveolar infiltration of both lungs. She was treated for opportunistic infections, presumed CMV pneumonitis as her blood for CMV viral load was 60,496 copies/mL with intravenous ganciclovir, presumed *Pneumocystis jiroveci* pneumonia (PJP) with intravenous sulfamethoxazole/trimethoprim (SXT/TMP) plus methylprednisolone. Her condition showed a little improvement; however, she still had respiratory distress and needed oxygen supplementation. Sputum for PJP PCR was negative. Sputum for acid fast bacilli smear was negative for 3 consecutive days. Repeated blood culture showed clearance of bacteria and blood for Mycobacterium culture did not grow nontuberculous Mycobacterium. Echocardiography done in 2D revealed dilated cardiomyopathy. Due to persistent respiratory distress and chest X-ray changes of RUL consolidation, she was started treatment for presumed Mycobacterium avium-intracellulare complex (MAC) infection empirically with clarithromycin, rifampicin, and ethambutol. Her condition slowly improved over a few weeks.

Her HIV RNA viral load was 5.2×10^6 copies/mL (6.76 log), while her CD4 was 105 cells/mm^3 (5%). Final diagnosis of newly diagnosed perinatally acquired HIV infection (US CDC clinical stage 3, immunological stage 3) with multiple opportunistic infections was made. She was started on combination anti-retroviral therapy (ART) with lamivudine (3TC), zidovudine (AZT), and nevirapine (NVP) after discussion with her parents, including assessment of readiness and compliance to treatment. Parents were given extensive education on HIV infection, treatment regimens and its side effects, as well as follow-up plan. Her father tested positive for HIV as well; both parents were also initiated on ARV treatment and followed up by a family medicine specialist. She was discharged after 3 months of hospital stay. Her HIV RNA viral load was decreasing in trend, and viral suppression (HIV viral load <20 copies/mL) was achieved after almost 1 year of ARV. Her CD4 cells recovery was good, 1898 cells/mm^3 (29%). She regained her growth potential and is currently doing well. It was a case of perinatally acquired HIV infection.

Case 2

A 3-year-old boy presented to emergency department (ED) of a medical center with fever, vesicular rash all over his body for 7 days, and an episode of seizure. Prior to this admission, he had four admissions for enterocolitis, two admissions for bronchopneumonia, and one admission for prolonged fever in a regional hospital. Physical examination revealed a thin child with body weight of 11 kg, with generalized vesicular rash and multiple cervical lymphadenopathy.

His initial laboratory data showed WBC 10,700/mm^3 (segmented neutrophils 38%, band 2%, monocytes 12%, lymphocytes 48%), raised C-reactive protein (67 mg/L), and positive varicella zoster serology (IgM+, IgG+). Diagnosis of varicella-zoster infection was made; however, this infection that he had was rather prolonged with extensive vesicular rash present even at day 7 of illness. He received intravenous acyclovir therapy and immunological assessment. His serum immunoglobulin levels are as follows: IgG: 4220 mg/dL (Normal range: 680–1530 mg/dL), IgA: 477 mg/dL (74.4–373.5 mg/dL), IgM: 104 mg/dL (40.2–167 mg/dL), IgE: 1940 IU/mL (<90 IU/mL). Lymphocytes subsets are as follows: B cell (CD19): 61.3% (7.8–22.8%); T cell (CD13): 25.8% (49.9–84.7%), Ts (CD8): 19.3% (24–33%); Th (CD4): 3.9% (41–53%); reversed CD4/CD8 ratio of 0.2 (1.4–1.9) and low absolute CD4 counts (196 cells/mm^3).

His HIV studies showed positive by ELISA serology and subsequently, by Western blot test. HIV RNA PCR was positive with RNA viral load of 2.8×10^5 copies/mL. Extensive investigations were carried out to determine the route of transmission. Vertical transmission was ruled out as both parents were negative for HIV ELISA and HIV PCR test. He had a blood transfusion (2 units PRBC and 10 units Platelets) 3 months prior to this admission; however, all ten donors tested negative for HIV ELISA, Western blot, and HIV PCR. There was no invasive medical procedure done in local medical clinics. Birth records at Obstetric clinic including other births were traced and reviewed, and found no possibility of switching. Investigations were also carried out on infants admitted to the same unit after he was born, as well as health care workers, but nothing of significance was found. Hence, it was concluded that HIV transmission route for this case was unknown, while the possibility of vertical transmission and blood products transmission was excluded.

Discussion

Pediatric HIV infection is largely preventable, through prevention of maternal to child transmission (PMTCT) program. The rate of transmission of HIV from a mother living with HIV to her child during antepartum, intrapartum, and postpartum period ranges from 15% to 45% without active prevention measures [1].

In Taiwan, a cumulative of 41,033 persons were diagnosed with HIV infection from 1984 till end of 2020. Among which, children aged less than 14 years, adolescents/young adults aged 15–24 years accounted for 0.15% and 23.8% of total cases, respectively, at the time of diagnosis. Perinatally acquired HIV infections were found mainly in HIV-infected children less than 14 year-old, while behaviorally acquired HIV infections mainly through unprotected sexual activity were common among youth aged 15–24 years. Other modes of transmissions include blood products transfusion, sharing needle while using injectable drugs and victim of sexual abuse.

Prevention of maternal-to-child transmission (PMTCT) program in Taiwan has been very successful in preventing new HIV infections among children, and only five cases of vertically transmitted HIV infections were diagnosed from 2011 to 2020 [2]. These preventive strategies include universal opt-out HIV screening for all pregnant women, provision of combination antiretroviral therapy (ART) for HIV-infected pregnant women, elective cesarean delivery before onset of labor and before rupture of membranes, and complete avoidance of breastfeeding [3].

About 20% of children with perinatally acquired HIV infections presented with severe clinical symptoms within first few months of life and may progress rapidly and lead to death [4]. Some children may manifest the disease later with mean age of diagnosis between 3 and 5 years, and may survive till 9–10 years old [5, 6]. Clinical presentations include unexplained wasting syndrome, recurrent and/or infections, generalized lymphadenopathy, hepatosplenomegaly, etc. [7, 8].

HIV diagnostic testing for infants younger than 18 months of age differs from that for older children, adolescents, and adults. Presence of passively transferred maternal HIV antibodies may be detectable in an exposed but uninfected infant's blood until approximately 18 months of age. Therefore, a negative serological testing of infants exposed to HIV and children before the age of 18 months is very informative. The gold standard for diagnostic testing of infants less than 18 months is HIV nucleic acid amplification tests [NAATs] by means of polymerase chain reaction (PCR) assays detecting HIV DNA or RNA [9].

For infants with known perinatal exposure, an HIV NAAT should be performed on infant's peripheral blood sample at birth or in the first few days of life for infants at highest risk of infection. Infants with a positive NAAT result at or before 48 h of age are considered to have in utero infection with HIV, whereas infants who have a negative NAAT result during first week of life and a subsequent positive test result are considered to have intrapartum infections [9]. If HIV NAAT is negative shortly after birth or at 14–21 days, they should be repeated at 1–2 months of age and again at 4–6 months of age [9, 10].

Infants with known perinatal exposure should receive postnatal antiretroviral drugs to reduce the risk of perinatal HIV transmission, either prophylaxis (one or more antiretroviral drugs) or presumptive HIV therapy (combination of three antiretroviral drugs), depending on risk of HIV acquisition [11].

For infants above 18 months old, older children, and adolescents, HIV serological testing is adequate for diagnosis confirmation. For infants and children with confirmed HIV infection, HIV DNA/RNA viral load and CD4 cells counts should be measured prior to starting treatment. There are two disease classification systems developed by WHO and US CDC, both involve clinical and immunological staging [7, 12, 13]. Careful and thorough physical examination and evaluation should be done to look for presence of opportunistic infections and treat it accordingly. Extensive education and counselling should be given to parents or caretakers or child (if older children and adolescent) regarding diseases, antiretroviral drugs and side effects, importance of treatment adherence to prevent development of resistance, and treatment failure.

All children or adolescents should receive combination antiretroviral therapy (cART) once their diagnosis is confirmed. Preferred regimens for initial therapy should include two nucleoside reverse transcriptase inhibitors (NRTI) plus an active drug from either non-nucleoside reverse transcriptase inhibitor (NNRTI), an integrase strand transfer inhibitor (INSTI), or a boosted protease inhibitor (PI). Choice of a regimen should be individualized based on patient's age, potential adverse effects, pill size, dosing frequency and result of drug resistance testing (if available), and preferences of the patient and caregivers [8, 14].

References

1. WHO. Global HIV Programme. Maternal-to-child transmission of HIV. Available at: https://www.who.int/teams/global-hiv-hepatitis-and-stis-programmes/hiv/prevention/mother-to-child-transmission-of-hiv
2. Taiwan Centers for Disease Control. HIV statistics. Available at: https://www.cdc.gov.tw/Category/Page/rCV9N1rGUz9wNr8lggsh2Q
3. American Academy of Pediatrics Committee on Pediatric AIDS. HIV testing and prophylaxis to prevent mother-to-child transmission in the United States. Pediatrics. 2008;122(5):1127-1134
4. Kovacs A, Scott GB. Advances in the Management and Care of HIV-Positive Newborns and Infants. In: Pizzo PA, Wilfert CM, eds. Pediatric AIDS. Philadelphia, Pa: Lippincott Williams & Wilkins; 2001:567-92
5. Vancouver, Canada, June, 1996. 7. Tovo PA, de Martino M, Gabiano C, et al. Prognostic factors and survival in children with perinatal HIV-1 infection. Lancet 1992;339:1249-53.
6. Bamhart HX, Caldwell MB, Thomas P, Nascola L, Ortiz I, Hsu H, Schulte J, Parrott R, Maldonado Y, Byers R, and the Pediatric Spectrum of Disease Clinical Consortium. Natural history of human immunodeficiency virus disease in perinatally infected children: an analysis from the Pediatric Spectrum of Disease Project. Pediatrics 1996;97:710-6.
7. Centers for Disease Control and Prevention (CDC). Revised surveillance case definition for HIV infection--United States, 2014. *MMWR Recomm Rep.* 2014;63(RR-03):1-10
8. Taiwan AIDS Society. Guidelines for diagnosis and treatment of HIV/AIDS, 5th edition 2018. Chapter 8. Available at http://www.aids-care.org.tw/journal/treatment.asp. Accessed at 26 October 2021.
9. Chadwick EG, Ezeanolue EE; COMMITTEE ON PEDIATRIC AIDS. Evaluation and Management of the Infant Exposed to HIV in the United States. *Pediatrics*. 2020;146(5):e2020029058. https://doi.org/10.1542/peds.2020-029058
10. Taiwan AIDS Society. Guidelines for diagnosis and treatment of HIV/AIDS, 6th edition 2020. Chapter 7. Page 1-6. Available at http://www.aids-care.org.tw/journal/treatment.asp. Accessed at October 26, 2021.

11. Panel on treatment of pregnant women with HIV infection and prevention of perinatal transmission. Recommendations for the use of antiretroviral drugs in pregnant women with HIV infection and interventions to reduce perinatal HIV transmission in the United States. Available at: https://clinicalinfo.hiv.gov/en/guidelines/perinatal/antiretroviral-management-newborns-perinatal-hiv-exposure-or-hiv-infection?view=full. *Accessed October 26, 2021.*
12. Centers for Disease Control and Prevention. 1994 revised classification system for human immunodeficiency virus infection in children less than 13 years of age. MMWR. 1994;43(No. RR-12)
13. World Health Organization. (2007). WHO case definitions of HIV for surveillance and revised clinical staging and immunological classification of HIV-related disease in adults and children. World Health Organization. https://apps.who.int/iris/handle/10665/43699
14. Panel on Antiretroviral Therapy and Medical Management of Children Living with HIV. Guidelines for the use of antiretroviral agents in Pediatric HIV infection. Available at: https://clinicalinfo.hiv.gov/en/guidelines/pediatric-arv/regimens-recommended-initial-therapy-antiretroviral-naive-children?view=full. Accessed on October 26, 2021

Case 40. A 6-Year-Old Girl with Fever and Neck Lymph Nodes Enlargement: Kikuchi-Fujimoto Disease

Chih-Hsien Chuang

Keywords

Kikuchi-Fujimoto disease · Fever Lymphadenopathy · Children · Systemic lupus erythematous

Key Points

- Kikuchi-Fujimoto disease is a benign, self-limiting disease of unknown etiology characterized by fever and cervical lymphadenopathy.
- Leukopenia is one characteristic finding. Abnormal liver function profiles and skin rashes may occasionally be observed.
- Kikuchi-Fujimoto disease is a disease by exclusion. The diagnosis of Kikuchi-Fujimoto disease may be suggested by histopathological findings.
- Male predominance was observed in pediatric population.
- Treatment options include non-steroidal anti-inflammatory drugs and steroid. Steroid is reserved for those with pathological verification of the diagnosis and with severe inflammation unresponsive to other treatments

C.-H. Chuang (✉)
Department of Pediatrics, Saint Paul's Hospital, Taoyuan, Taiwan
e-mail: doc1860@mail.sph.org.tw

Case Report

A 6-year-11-month-old girl was well until 3 weeks before admission when she had intermittent fever. Right neck swelling developed 1 week later. Other associated symptom was mild diarrhea without blood or mucus three times a day. One week before admission, she was evaluated in the outpatient clinic. She was a well-nourished and well-developed girl with scheduled vaccination including Bacillus Calmette–Guérin vaccine. Her body weight was 24.5 kg (50–85th percentile) and body height was 131.5 cm (>97th percentile). On physical examination, she had multiple enlarged lymph nodes in bilateral neck, which were tender on palpation. The largest one was 2 cm in diameter. The white cell count (WBC) was 2200/μL (segmented neutrophil 51%, lymphocyte 42%, eosinophil 1%, and atypical lymphocyte 6%), the hemoglobin level was 12 g/dL, and the platelet count was 134,000/μL. Blood biochemistry data included creatinine of 0.6 mg/dL, alanine transaminase of 38 U/L, and C-reactive protein of <0.3 mg/dL. Echocardiography showed negative findings. She was treated with cephalexin.

On the day of admission, she had fever for 3 weeks with multiple enlarged neck lymph nodes bilaterally, generalized myalgia, and body-weight loss of 2 kg. Blood tests showed erythrocyte sedimentation rate of 27 mm/h, lactate dehydrogenase of 1083 U/L, triglyceride of 276 mg/dL, ferritin of 819 mg/dL, negative

Y.-C. Huang et al. (eds.), *Paediatric Infectious Diseases*,
https://doi.org/10.1007/978-981-19-7276-8_40

antinuclear antibody, C3 of 98.5 mg/dL, and C4 of 34.3 mg/dL. Other laboratory tests were similar to the results 1 week ago. Screenings for Epstein-Barr virus, cytomegalovirus, and antistreptolysin O were negative. Examination of peripheral blood smear showed normocytic, normochromic red blood cells, decreased WBC, and slightly decreased platelet count. Ultrasonography of abdomen revealed negative finding. Bone marrow aspiration was performed to exclude hematological malignancy or hemophagocytic lymphohistiocytosis. The finding was reactive marrow. No increased percentage of blasts or malignant cells infiltration and no increased histiocytes or obvious hemophagocytosis were seen. She still had fever 1 week after admission. Excisional biopsy of right neck lymph nodes was performed. Pathological examination of the biopsy specimen revealed paracortical hyperplasia and patchy infiltrates, which are composed of a mixture of plasmacytoid dendritic cells, crescentic histiocytes, activated lymphoid cells, foamy macrophages, abundant apoptotic bodies, and areas of necrosis. The pathological diagnosis was histiocytic necrotizing lymphadenitis (Kikuchi-Fujimoto disease). Fever subsided 2 days after biopsy without any medications. Follow-up was uneventful for this patient.

Discussion

Enlargement of lymph node is common in children. The cause of abnormal enlargement of lymph node can result from benign to malignancy and the clinical features range from indolent to aggressive. Normal lymph nodes in children are usually less than 1 cm in diameter and less than 1.5 cm in diameter in inguinal area. The evaluation of lymphadenopathy is determined by clinical characteristics of children. Early excisional biopsy is indicated for children with warning signs. Warning signs included children with systemic symptoms (fever, weight loss, and night sweat, etc.), abnormal chest radiography, abnormal blood tests (complete blood counts, differential counts, or elevated lactate dehydrogenase), lymph nodes more than 2 cm in diameter with increased size from baseline, generalized lymphadenopathy, or lymph nodes in supraclavicular area.

Kikuchi-Fujimoto disease (KFD) or histiocytic necrotizing lymphadenitis is a distinctive clinicopathological entity first described independently by Kikuchi and Fujimoto in Japan in 1972. KFD is generally a benign, self-limiting disease of unknown etiology characterized by fever and cervical lymphadenopathy. KFD usually occurs in young Asian female adults under 30 years old. The female–male ratio is about 3–4:1 in adults. However, a male predominance was observed in pediatric population. The younger the patient was, the more male predominance was observed. Lymphadenopathy is the most common presentation of KFD. More than 90% of pediatric patients had cervical lymphadenopathy. More than half of the patients had tender or painful lymphadenopathy. Most of lymphadenopathy was multiple. Unilateral lymphadenopathy accounts for 70–80%. Typical lymph node size is 2–3 cm, most lymph nodes are less than 5 cm. Generalized lymphadenopathy is uncommon, accounting for less than 5% of cases. Fever is the second common presentation of KFD. The percentage of fever in adult is 30–50%. Fever is more prominent in children than adults. In patients with fever, the duration of fever ranged from one to several weeks. Hepatomegaly and splenomegaly are present in 5–8% of patients. Skin rashes developed in 16–40% of patients with male predominance and the presence is predisposed to a protracted clinical course.

There is no specific laboratory test for KFD. Leukopenia was one of the characteristic findings of KFD. In pediatric population, approximately 50% of KFD cases had leukopenia. Patients with prolonged fever had higher proportion of leukopenia than patients without. Inflammatory markers (such as erythrocyte sedimentation rate and C-reactive protein) and liver function tests (aspartate aminotransferase, alanine aminotransferase) may be mildly elevated. Lactate dehydrogenase was elevated in most patients. Anti-nuclear antibody (ANA) was positive in 10–20% patients. However, initial ANA status did not correlate with later autoimmune diseases.

The diagnosis of KFD is based on histopathological findings. The histopathological features are cortical or paracortical necrosis with karyorrhectic debris and various histiocytes, plasmacytoid monocytes, lymphoid cells, and absence of neutrophils. Although fine needle aspiration biopsy (FNAB) has been described to be diagnostic, FNAB has a higher false negative rate than excisional biopsy. Resolution of fever usually occurs several days after excisional biopsy of lymph nodes. Early excisional biopsy of lymph node rather than FNAB is suggested to avoid unnecessary investigation and treatment. The differential diagnosis of KFD includes malignant lymphoma, systemic lupus erythematous (SLE), incomplete Kawasaki disease, and hemophagocytic lymphohistiocytosis (HLH). The histopathological findings could differentiate KFD from malignant lymphoma. However, it is difficult to distinguish KFD from lupus lymphadenitis and HLH in histopathological findings. KFD is a disease by exclusion. Concomitant clinical features and laboratory findings could help differentiate the diagnosis. If Kikuchi's lymphadenitis associated with SLE, it should be regarded as lupus lymphadenitis. If patients had persistent fever for more than 1 week after diagnosis of KFD, increased serum ferritin, and cytopenias, HLH should be considered.

There is no specific treatment for KFD. Nonsteroidal anti-inflammatory drugs are recommended for symptomatic treatment. If a patient has protracted clinical course and other diseases has been excluded, steroids may be used. Because steroid usage may mask clinical presentations and delay appropriate treatment for autoimmune diseases and malignancies, steroid is reserved for those with pathological verification of the diagnosis and with severe inflammation unresponsive to other treatments. Pathological recurrence rate of KFD is 4% in adults and children. Clinical recurrence rate is 15% in adults and can be as high as 40% in children. The risk factors associated with recurrent KFD in children are higher absolute lymphocyte count and a past history of other systemic illness. KFD and SLE shared some clinical and pathological features. The development of SLE or other autoimmune diseases in children with KFD is 4%. Complete work-up and follow-up for several years after diagnosis of KFD are suggested.

Further Reading

Kim TY, Ha KS, Kim Y, Lee J, Lee K, Lee J. Characteristics of Kikuchi-Fujimoto disease in children compared with adults. Eur J Pediatr. 2014;173:111-6.

Chuang CH, Yan DC, Chiu CH, Huang YC, Lin PY, Chen CJ, Yen MH, Kuo TT, Lin TY. Clinical and laboratory manifestations of Kikuchi's disease in children and differences between patients with and without prolonged fever. Pediatr Infect Dis J. 2005;24:551-4.

Lin HC, Su CY, Huang SC. Kikuchi's disease in Asian children. Pediatrics. 2005;115:e92-6.

Selvanathan SN, Suhumaran S, Sahu VK, Chong CY, Tan NWH, Thoon KC. Kikuchi-Fujimoto disease in children. J Paediatr Child Health. 2020;56:389-393.

Kuo TT. Cutaneous manifestation of Kikuchi's histiocytic necrotizing lymphadenitis. Am J Surg Pathol. 1990;14:872-6.

Lee BC, Patel R. Kikuchi-Fujimoto disease: a 15-year analysis at a children's hospital in the United States. Clin Pediatr (Phila). 2013;52:92-5.

Kuo TT. Kikuchi's disease (histiocytic necrotizing lymphadenitis). A clinicopathologic study of 79 cases with an analysis of histologic subtypes, immunohistology, and DNA ploidy. Am J Surg Pathol. 1995;19:798-809.

Tong TR, Chan OW, Lee KC. Diagnosing Kikuchi disease on fine needle aspiration biopsy: a retrospective study of 44 cases diagnosed by cytology and 8 by histopathology. Acta Cytol. 2001;45:953-7.

Yoo IH, Na H, Bae EY, Han SB, Lee SY, Jeong DC, Kang JH. Recurrent lymphadenopathy in children with Kikuchi-Fujimoto disease. Eur J Pediatr. 2014;173:1193-9.

Lim GY, Cho B, Chung NG. Hemophagocytic lymphohistiocytosis preceded by Kikuchi disease in children. Pediatr Radiol. 2008;38:756-61.

Case 41. A 2-Year-Old with Fever, Progressive Lethargy and Skin Rash: Kawasaki Disease with Shock Syndrome

Ching-Chia Kuo

Keywords

Kawasaki disease · Kawasaki disease shock syndrome · Intravenous immunoglobulin Multisystem inflammatory syndrome in children

Key Points

- The highest risk for Kawasaki disease lies in younger children of Asian ancestry, especially in Japan, South Korea, and Taiwan.
- No specific diagnostic tests for Kawasaki disease to date; diagnosis requires awareness of physicians.
- Kawasaki disease shock syndrome is a rare complication requiring early recognition and prompt management.
- Identifying high-risk patients of IVIG resistance contributes to the initiation of more effective therapy and reduces severe cardiac complications.
- Multisystem inflammatory syndrome in children associated with SARS-CoV-2 infection has overlapping manifestations with Kawasaki disease; distinguishing the two diseases helps determine the treatment plan.

C.-C. Kuo (✉)
Division of General and Emergency Medicine, Department of Pediatrics, Linkou Chang Gung Memorial Hospital, Taoyuan, Taiwan

Case Report

A 2-year-old boy presented to the emergency department with 5 days of fever and progressive lethargy. Over the few days before visiting the emergency department, he became unwilling to eat, and the urine amount continued to decrease. There were no other specific respiratory or gastrointestinal symptoms besides fever, which could only be temporarily alleviated with oral antipyretics. Two days before the visit, the parents noticed some rash appearing over his torso as faint little pink spots, without pain or itching. Arriving at the emergency department, the boy appeared weak and sleepy, although still responsive. At the triage, the following vital signs were disclosed: temperature 39.8 °C, pulse 196 beats/min, oxygen saturation 91% on room air, respiration 34 breaths/min, and blood pressure 60/48 mmHg. The capillary refilling time was up to 4 seconds. Further physical examination revealed more scattered erythematous macular rash present on his chest, abdomen, and both thighs. Volume depletion complicated with septic

Y.-C. Huang et al. (eds.), *Paediatric Infectious Diseases*,
https://doi.org/10.1007/978-981-19-7276-8_41

shock and toxic shock syndrome was suspected initially; therefore, fluid resuscitation was initiated with 0.9% saline 20 mL/kg, and a mask with oxygen flow at 6 L/min was applied. The boy was started on empiric vancomycin and ceftriaxone antibiotic treatment. His chest radiograph was relatively normal without active lung lesions or cardiomegaly. The hemogram showed an elevated white cell count of 21,200/μL (segment 81%, lymphocyte 10%, band 5%, monocyte 4%), hemoglobin 9.0 g/dL, and a platelet count of 132,000/μL. Serum chemistry showed glucose 68 mg/dL, blood urea nitrogen 28 mg/dL, creatinine 1.25 mg/dL, sodium 131 mEq/L, potassium 3.2 mEq/L, chloride 99 mEq/L, aspartate transaminase 381 U/L, alanine transaminase 258 U/L, albumin 2.28 g/dL, C-reactive protein 195 mg/L, troponin-I 0.03 ng/mL, creatinine kinase MB form 4.1 ng/mL, and lactate 31 mg/dL. Arterial blood gas analysis revealed a pH of 7.30, partial pressure of carbon dioxide 34 mmHg, partial pressure of oxygen 78 mmHg, and bicarbonate of 22 mEq/L. After a total of 60 mL/kg isotonic saline rapid infusion, the boy stayed hypotensive (66/50 mmHg), and his consciousness level worsened. In response to the refractory hypotension, norepinephrine was administered, and the boy was transferred to the pediatric intensive care unit (PICU).

The broad-spectrum antibiotics and the inotropic agent were continued, and the blood pressure gradually stabilized on hospital day 2 while the norepinephrine infusion went on. As a result, the boy started to regain better awareness and had adequate urine output; the urinalysis result revealed mild sterile pyuria. Follow-up blood tests on hospital day 3 showed persistent leukocytosis (24,500/μL) and elevated CRP level (208 mg/L), and there were no positive results for both blood and urine cultures. Besides persistent fever, the boy developed new symptoms in the PICU, including bilaterally injected conjunctivae, swollen and cracked lips, and prominent erythema surrounding his Bacillus Calmette–Guérin scar. Considering Kawasaki disease (KD), a single dose of intravenous immunoglobulin (IVIG) 2 g/kg was given over 12 h along with oral aspirin on hospital day 4. The boy underwent echocardiography on the same day, which disclosed dilated left main coronary artery (*Z*-Score = 2.6). The fever, skin rash, and red eyes subsided after IVIG administration, and the boy's hemodynamics remained stable after discontinuing the inotropic agent; hence he was transferred to the ordinary ward. The boy stayed afebrile for approximately 48 h after IVIG administration, but conjunctival injection recurred, and the fever recurred since hospital day 6, while his fingertips began to peel. Therefore, a second dose of IVIG 2 g/kg was given for suspected refractory KD. The fever and inflammation signs improved following the second course of IVIG, except for preexisting fingertips desquamation. On the tenth day of hospitalization, the boy was discharged and returned to the outpatient clinic 2 and 4 weeks later as instructed. Serially repeated echocardiography showed that the previous coronary artery abnormality regressed to a normal *Z*-score. The oral aspirin was discontinued after 6 weeks, and the boy went on follow-up at the cardiology clinic yearly for reassessment.

Discussion

Kawasaki disease (KD) is one of the most common childhood vasculitis, mainly affecting medium-sized arteries at the systemic level. Clinical manifestations include fever, extremity changes, rash, conjunctivitis, oral changes, and enlarged neck lymph node(s). Most cases occur among infants and young children aged 6 months to 5 years, and ethnicity-wise the disease is especially prevalent among children whose families are of Asian ancestry, with Japanese children having the highest incidence. The etiology is still not fully understood to date. Still, polymorphisms of variant susceptible genes, along with environmental and infectious triggers, probably contribute to the pathogenesis of KD from different aspects. If left untreated, up to 20–30% of the patients with KD develop coronary artery complications.

Albeit the incidence data from underdeveloped countries are insufficient, the applicable epidemiological patterns of KD worldwide demonstrate geographic or ethnic variations. Epidemiology studies have illustrated the occurrence of KD in less than 5-year-olds among the leading Northeast Asian countries, ranging from 308/100,000 in Japan to 82.8/100,000 in Taiwan, which are approximately 10–30 times higher than that in the United States (U.S.) or Europe.

Kawasaki disease shock syndrome (KDSS) is a rare manifestation of KD, characterized by systolic hypotension with clinical signs of inadequate tissue perfusion. Initial presentations might mimic septic shock or toxic shock. KDSS appears to differ from traditional KD with uncommon age, more incomplete features, more severe laboratory inflammation markers, higher unresponsive rates to IVIG therapy, and higher risk to develop coronary complications. The cause of KDSS is undetermined, but there have been several hypothetical pathophysiological mechanisms, including dysregulated cytokines associated with myocardial and endocardial dysfunction, decreased peripheral vascular resistance mediated by endogenous molecules, and increased capillary permeability resulting from the more intense vascular inflammation. From time to time, systemic capillary leak syndrome may also be relevant. The percentage of potential KDSS among KD patients ranges from 1.45% to 6.95% worldwide. Contrary to KD, most western countries have a higher incidence rate of KDSS than Asian countries. The three largest studies applying insurance coding databases seem to support the possible racial difference, showing 1.45–1.51% in Taiwan and 2.8–5.3% in the U.S.

There is no specific diagnostic test for KD at this moment, although techniques utilizing gene expression as a biomarker have been proposed. Therefore, the diagnosis of KD still relies on the vigilance of the physician to discover fever and other clinical features. Based on the 2017 diagnostic guideline published by the American Heart Association (AHA), classic Kawasaki disease is diagnosed in the presence of fever persisting 5 days or more with at least four of the five essential inflammatory signs: changes of extremity (erythema and edema of distal limbs in the acute phase or periungual desquamation in the subacute phase), polymorphous rash, bilateral conjunctival congestion (bulbar conjunctivitis without exudates), changes of the oral mucosa (erythema/cracking/fissure of lips, strawberry tongue, or mucosal erythema), cervical lymphadenopathy over 1.5 cm diameter. In ambiguous cases, laboratory and echocardiographic work-up help the diagnosis of incomplete KD. Compared to the AHA, the Japanese Circulation Society Joint Working Groups made several significant changes in the sixth revised edition of Japanese diagnostic guidelines in 2019. In this latest edition, the count of days of fever is no longer crucial, and the redness of the bacillus Calmette–Guérin (BCG) scar is recognized as a KD feature as well as skin rash.

Since the classic presentations of KD are often more obscure in KDSS, the key to best manage KDSS is early recognition of KD signs to give IVIG timely. Because KDSS can be a distributive, cardiogenic, or mixed form of shock, it appears reasonable to follow the management guideline of septic shock before KD can be diagnosed, for the resemblance of pathophysiological nature between both conditions. Proper fluid management, inotropics and/or vasopressors, and intensive care are essential to achieve hemodynamic stability in the acute stage.

Once the diagnosis of KD is confirmed, the standard initial treatment is a single dose IVIG therapy (2 g/kg) given over 10–12 h, along with aspirin. Timely treatment initiated within 10 days of disease onset helps reduce the risk of coronary aneurysm to less than 5%. However, 6.7–26.8% of patients with KD are reported to be unresponsive to standard treatment or even resistant to a second course of IVIG, hence at increased risk of coronary artery abnormalities. There are two mainstay strategies for IVIG non-responders. The first one is to intensify primary IVIG therapy with adjuvant corticosteroids. The second strategy is considered a salvage therapy: while many experts recommend retreatment with IVIG 2 g/kg, either a high-dose pulse therapy or longer tapering course of corticosteroids, or biologic agent such as infliximab, can also be applied as an alternative for IVIG-resistant patients. Regarding highly inflamed patients who failed to respond to either single or combined salvage therapy, successful resolution of inflammation after administration of cyclosporine, anakinra, cyclophosphamide, or rarely plasma exchange has been reported. However, the optimal treatment for such profoundly unresponsive patients has not been determined.

The COVID-19 pandemic has made a major impact on the pediatric population. As of spring 2020, pediatricians faced a rare new disease of hyper-inflammatory state caused by SARS-CoV-2, so-called multisystem inflammatory syndrome in children (MIS-C). MIS-C seems to be a post-infectious disorder with a broad spectrum of presentations overlapping with KD, including fever, mucocutaneous manifestations, coronary dilatations, and shock. Although only a small percentage of children infected with SARS-CoV-2 progress to MIS-C, it can lead to mortality. The pathogenesis of MIS-C is yet to be elucidated.

Myocardial involvement may be a hallmark of MIS-C, whereas KD is known to involve predominantly coronary arteries. However, a systemic review indicated that the proportion of shock among children presenting with KD-like features might be up to 28%, which was much higher than that of KDSS. In addition, an indispensably high proportion of these children also have coronary dilatation or aneurysms. For the above reason, IVIG was initially adopted to treat MIS-C because of its similarity with KD. The OVERCOMING COVID-19 study team demonstrated evidence of lower cardiovascular risk with IVIG plus glucocorticoids over IVIG alone in the U.S.-based population.

Disparately, the international study from the Best Available Treatment Study Consortium showed no significant difference between IVIG, steroids, and a combination of the two above. Since the current evidence is inconclusive for MIS-C treatment suggestion, it may be reasonable to consider the impact of cost and availability of treatment options on each individual patient. The Lancet COVID-19 Commission Task Force in India had recommended giving steroids as the first-line treatment for MIS-C and saving IVIG and other biologic agents for non-responders, critically ill ones, and those with features more typical of KD.

Although KD and MIS-C resemble each other, reports suggest that MIS-C belongs to a distinct entity. The affected children are older or adolescents, and the data from the U.S. displayed an overrepresentation of Hispanic and non-Hispanic black children. Intriguingly, MIS-C is much less commonly reported in Asia than in Europe and the U.S., so maybe the genetic background which makes Asian communities very much more at risk from KD is different for MIS-C in a reverse pattern. It may be worth mentioning that many Asian countries committed to public health measures to control COVID and proved effective, so there may not have been a high enough level of transmission to see the expected number of MIS-C cases. Whether the low prevalence of MIS-C in Asia results from genetic factors or better public health measures is uncertain, and it needs further analysis.

Over the past few decades, physicians have gotten better insight into KD, but further research is needed for pathogenic mechanisms, diagnostic tools, and optimized treatment. More precise classification of high-risk groups for IVIG resistance and coronary complication remains to be established in non-Asian countries. As an uncommon complication of KD, KDSS can result in unfavorable outcomes and mortality, and early recognition is essential for timely therapy. In the context of the COVID-19 pandemic, MIS-C can masquerade as KD among areas with high COVID-19 burden; raised alertness is required for pediatricians to correctly distinguish the two diseases in order to develop appropriate treatment strategies.

Further Reading

Lin MT, Wu MH. The global epidemiology of Kawasaki disease: Review and future perspectives. Global Cardiol Sci Pract. 2018;2017:e201720.

Kanegaye JT, Wilder MS, Molkara D, Frazer JR, Pancheri J, Tremoulet AH, et al. Recognition of a Kawasaki Disease Shock Syndrome. Pediatrics. 2009;123:e783–9.

Lin MT, Fu CM, Huang SK, Huang SC, Wu MH. Population-based Study of Kawasaki Disease Shock Syndrome in Taiwan. Pediatric Infect Dis J 2013;32:1384–6.

Liang YC, Chang CH, Lin MT, Kao FY, Huang SK, Wu MH. Shock and unresponsiveness to repeated courses of intravenous immunoglobulin in Kawasaki disease: a nationwide database study. Pediatr Res. 2020;87:961–6.

Kuo CC, Lee YS, Lin MR, Hsia SH, Chen CJ, Chiu CH, et al. Characteristics of children with Kawasaki disease requiring intensive care: 10 years' experience at a tertiary pediatric hospital. J Microbiol Immunol Infect. 2018;51(2):184–90.

Maddox RA, Person MK, Kennedy JL, Leung J, Abrams JY, Haberling DL, et al. Kawasaki Disease and Kawasaki Disease Shock Syndrome Hospitalization Rates in the United States, 2006–2018. Pediatr Infect Dis J. 2020;40:284–8.

McCrindle BW, Rowley AH, Newburger JW, Burns JC, Bolger AF, Gewitz M, et al. Diagnosis, Treatment, and Long-Term Management of Kawasaki Disease: A Scientific Statement for Health Professionals From the American Heart Association. Circulation. 2017;135:e927–99.

Fukazawa R, Kobayashi J, Ayusawa M, Hamada H, Miura M, Mitani Y, et al. JCS/JSCS 2020 Guideline on Diagnosis and Management of Cardiovascular Sequelae in Kawasaki Disease. Circ J 2020; 84:1348–407.

Saneeymehri S, Baker K, So TY. Overview of Pharmacological Treatment Options for Pediatric Patients with Refractory Kawasaki Disease. J Pediatric Pharmacol Ther. 2015; 20:163–77.

Halyabar O, Friedman KG, Sundel RP, Baker AL, Chang MH, Gould PW, et al. Cyclophosphamide use in treatment of refractory Kawasaki disease with coronary artery aneurysms. Pediatr Rheumatol 2021; 19:31.

Lee MS, Liu YC, Tsai CC, Hsu JH, Wu JR. Similarities and Differences Between COVID-19-Related Multisystem Inflammatory Syndrome in Children and Kawasaki Disease. Frontiers Pediatrics. 2021; 9:640118.

Yasuhara J, Watanabe K, Takagi H, Sumitomo N, Kuno T. COVID-19 and multisystem inflammatory syndrome in children: A systematic review and meta-analysis. Pediatr Pulmonol 2021; 56:837–48.

Son MBF, Murray N, Friedman K, Young CC, Newhams MM, Feldstein LR, et al. Multisystem Inflammatory Syndrome in Children — Initial Therapy and Outcomes. New Engl J Med. 2021; 385:23–34.

McArdle AJ, Vito O, Patel H, Seaby EG, Shah P, Wilson C, et al. Treatment of Multisystem Inflammatory Syndrome in Children. New Engl J Med. 2021; 385:11–22.

Crosby L, Balasubramanian S, Ramanan AV. Steroids or intravenous immunoglobulin as first line in MIS-C in LMICs. Lancet Rheumatology. 2021; 3:e615–6.

Stierman B, Abrams JY, Godfred-Cato SE, Oster ME, Meng L, Yip L, et al. Racial and Ethnic Disparities in Multisystem Inflammatory Syndrome in Children in the United States, March 2020 to February 2021. Pediatr Infect Dis J 2021;Publish Ahead of Print.

Li W, Tang Y, Shi Y, Chen Y, Liu E. Why multisystem inflammatory syndrome in children has been less commonly described in Asia? Transl Pediatrics. 2020;9:87375–875.

Case 42. A 6-Year-Old Girl with Fever, Sore Throat, Odynophagia, Dysphagia, and Cervical Mass: Lymph-Node-First Presentation Kawasaki Disease

Ming-Ru Lin and Yhu-Chering Huang

Keywords

Kawasaki disease · Deep neck infection
Lymphadenitis

Key Points

- A group of patients with Kawasaki disease (KD) may initially present as cervical lymphadenitis or deep neck infection.
- Patients with Lymph-node-first presentation of KD (LNF-KD) are more likely to develop coronary artery complications than those with classic KD.
- Kawasaki disease should be considered in children, particularly more than 4 years of age, with fever and antimicrobial unresponsive cervical lymphadenitis.

M.-R. Lin (✉)
Division of General and Emergency Medicine, Department of Pediatrics, Linkou Chang Gung Memorial Hospital, Taoyuan, Taiwan

Y.-C. Huang
Pediatrics, Chang Gung Memorial Hospital, Chang Gung University, Taoyuan, Taiwan

Case Report

A previously healthy 6-year-old girl who received scheduled vaccination had fever off and on for 4 days and then was admitted to a hospital. She suffered from sore throat, odynophagia, dysphagia, and there was one progressively enlarged mass over her right sub-auricular area. On physical examination, one 3 × 5 cm palpable mass with local heat, erythematous change, and tenderness was noted. Injected throat without enlargement or exudative change of both tonsils was found. Other physical examinations were essentially negative. Initial laboratory data showed white blood cell (WBC) 16,500/μL (segmented 82%, immature neutrophils 2%, lymphocytes 11%, monocytes 5%), platelet count 177,000/μL, hemoglobin (Hb) 11.7 g/dL, and C-reactive protein (CRP) 112 mg/L (normal, <5 mg/L). Cervical lymphadenitis was impressed tentatively. Computed Tomography (CT) with contrast enhancement of head and neck was done due to suspected deep neck infection and disclosed retropharyngeal edema over oropharyngeal level and multiple cervical lymphadenitis over right side parapharyngeal space without abscess formation. Despite decreasing in size of cervical mass after treatment with amoxycillin-clavulanic acid, her fever remained off and on. Multiple blanchable, non-itchy macular rash developed over whole body on hospital day 3 and bilateral injected conjunctivae were observed on the next

Y.-C. Huang et al. (eds.), *Paediatric Infectious Diseases*,
https://doi.org/10.1007/978-981-19-7276-8_42

day. On hospital day 7, she complained about pain sensation over multiple joints. Swelling, redness, and tenderness over distal and proximal interphalangeal joints were found on physical exam. Kawasaki disease was suspected at this point and an echocardiography was done which revealed dilatation of left main coronary artery (diameter 4.5 mm, *Z* score +4.04) and right coronary artery (diameter 3.5 mm, *Z* score +3.06). Intravenous immunoglobulin (IVIG) 2 g/kg was administered (slowly infused for 12 h) and a high dose of oral aspirin (100 mg/kg/day) was given. Her fever gradually subsided on hospital day 9 and her symptoms were all resolved. She was discharged with low dose aspirin (5 mg/kg/day) for a total of 2 months.

Discussion

Kawasaki disease (KD) is a systemic vasculitis that mainly involves children aged between 6 months and 4 years in Asia. The diagnosis of KD is made on clinical features, including fever lasting for at least 5 days and presence of at least four of the following five principal clinical features: extremity changes (including swelling, erythema, and pain with subsequent periungual desquamation), polymorphic rash, non-purulent bulbar conjunctivitis, oral mucosal changes, and cervical lymphadenopathy. The term "incomplete Kawasaki disease" is used in those infants and children who experienced prolonged and unexplained fever with compatible supplementary laboratory criteria or results of the echocardiographic examination, though they do not fulfill diagnostic criteria (fewer than four of the principal clinical features). The diagnosis can be considered as confirmed when coronary artery aneurysms are identified in such patients by echocardiography. Without intravenous immunoglobulin treatment, 20–30% of the patients with KD would develop coronary artery complications. Of note, the five principal clinical features are usually not seen at the same time (day), but manifest sequentially (day by day). As in the illustrated case, erythematous skin rash might develop several days after antibiotic therapy for the initial diagnosis of acute lymphadenitis and be usually presumed as "probable adverse effect of antibiotic usage." The history-taking should be meticulous and alert. A high index of suspicion is important for the diagnosis of incomplete KD.

Among the five principal features, cervical lymphadenopathy is the least common clinical presentation (50–75%) in patients with classic Kawasaki disease, compared with the other four features (≥90%). Of note, there are a group of patients with Kawasaki disease, in whom predominantly present as cervical lymphadenitis or deep neck infection initially, named as lymph-node-first presentation of KD (LNF-KD). Compared with those with classic KD, the patients with LNF-KD are not within the common age for KD (younger than 6 months old or older than 4 years old). They are usually treated with antibiotics under the impression of bacterial lymphadenitis or deep neck infection initially, but the clinical response is unsatisfactory. The patients tend to experience a longer duration of fever and illness before the diagnosis of KD is made and IVIG is administered. Some studies suggest that patients with LNF-KD had a higher incidence of coronary artery complications, which may result from delayed diagnosis and treatment. Furthermore, these patients had a more severe systemic inflammation and tend to receive additional dose of IVIG or to experience recurrent episode of KD. Therefore, physicians should take Kawasaki disease into consideration in children aged younger than 6 months or older than 4 years who have a fever with an enlarged cervical lymph node which are unresponsive to empiric antibiotics.

Apparently, LNF-KD may confuse physicians with bacterial cervical lymphadenitis and deep neck infection. Compared to those with bacterial cervical lymphadenitis, patients with LNF-KD are at an older age, and more likely to have a higher WBC count, absolute neutrophil counts, aspartate aminotransferase (AST) and C-reactive protein (CRP) levels. These findings may reflect a more severe inflammation in patients with LNF-KD. In addition, the characteristics of LNF-KD on CT scan are multiple clustered solid lymph nodes with limited perinodal inflammation. In contrast, a single enlarged lymph node with suppurative change is usually observed in bacterial cervical lymphadenitis. As regards deep neck infection, CT examination remains the optimal tool to detect abscess formation. Compared to deep neck infection, which shows abscess formation localizing at retropharyngeal, parapharyngeal, and peritonsillar spaces, the inflammatory change of LNF-KD localizes more frequently in retropharyngeal space and presents as edema rather than abscess formation.

Further Reading

Lin MT, Chang CH, Hsieh WC, Chang CE, Chang YM, Chen YC, et al. Coronary Diameters in Taiwanese Children Younger than 6 Years Old: Z-Score Regression Equations Derived from Body Surface Area. Acta Cardiol Sin. 2014 Jul;30(4):266-73.

Huang YC, Lin TY, Su WJ. Unusual manifestations in children with Kawasaki disease. J Formos Med Assoc 1997;96:451-6.

McCrindle BW, Rowley AH, Newburger JW, Burns JC, Bolger AF, Gewitz M, et al. Diagnosis, treatment, and long-term management of Kawasaki disease: a scientific statement for health professionals from the American Heart Association. Circulation. 2017;135: e927-99.

Inagaki K, Blackshear C, Hobbs CV. Deep Neck Space Involvement of Kawasaki Disease in the US: A Population-Based Study. J Pediatr. 2019; 215: 118-122.

Lim S, Lee NY, Han SB, Jeong DC, Kang JH. Deep Neck Inflammation: Probable Kawasaki Disease in Korean Children. Clin Exp Otorhinolaryngol. 2020 Feb;13(1):77-82.

Kao HT, Huang YC, Lin TY. Kawasaki disease presenting as cervical lymphadenitis or deep neck infection. Otolaryngol Head Neck Surg 2001;124: 468-70.

Kim JO, Kim YH, Hyun MC. Comparison between Kawasaki disease with lymph-node-first presentation and Kawasaki disease without cervical lymphadenopathy. Korean J Pediatr. 2016;59:54-8.

Kanegaye JT, Van Cott E, Tremoulet AH, Salgado A, Shimizu C, Kruk P, et al. Lymph-node-first presentation of Kawasaki disease compared with bacterial cervical adenitis and typical Kawasaki disease. J Pediatr 2013;162:1259-63, 1263.e1–2.

Kobayashi T, Inoue Y, Takeuchi K, Okada Y, Tamura K, Tomomasa T, et al. Prediction of intravenous immunoglobulin unresponsiveness in patients with Kawasaki disease. Circulation 2006;113:2606–12.

Nomura Y, Arata M, Koriyama C, Masuda K, Morita Y, Hazeki D, et al. A severe form of Kawasaki disease presenting with only fever and cervical lymphadenopathy at admission. J Pediatr 2010;156: 786–91.

Case 43. An 8-Year-Old with Fever, Headache, Muscle Ache, and Retro-Orbital Pain, Followed by Frequent Vomiting: Dengue Fever with Shock

Tzong-Shiann Ho and Ching-Chuan Liu

Keywords

Dengue · Severe dengue · Dengue shock syndrome · Pediatric

Key Points

- Pediatric dengue patients usually present nonspecific symptoms/signs or viral syndrome, and typical skin rashes appear late in a clinical course.
- The tourniquet test, a marker of capillary fragility, can be used as a triage tool to differentiate dengue patients from those with other viral syndromes.
- According to the revised 2009 WHO case definitions, dengue illness can be classified into dengue without and with warning signs and severe dengue.
- Laboratory confirmation of acute dengue infection includes positive RT-PCR and lateral flow immunoassay for NS1 or anti-DENV IgM results.
- First dengue virus infection, or passively acquired dengue antibodies, may increase the severity of the subsequent dengue virus infection of different serotypes, an immunopathological phenomenon named antibody-dependent enhancement.
- Successful management of dengue vascular permeability syndrome relies on careful manipulation of parenteral fluids and colloids and proactive management of significant bleeding during the critical phase.

T.-S. Ho (✉)
Department of Pediatrics, National Cheng Kung University Hospital, College of Medicine, National Cheng Kung University, Tainan City, Taiwan

Department of Pediatrics, Tainan Hospital, Ministry of Health and Welfare, Taipei, Taiwan
e-mail: tsho@mail.ncku.edu.tw

C.-C. Liu
Department of Pediatrics, National Cheng Kung University Hospital, College of Medicine, National Cheng Kung University, Tainan City, Taiwan

Case Report

An 8-year-old boy without underlying diseases visited his primary care physician due to fever (38.5 °C), headache, muscle ache (neck and back), and retro-orbital pain. There was neither cough, rhinorrhea, nor other respiratory symptoms. No skin rashes were noticed. On the second day of fever, he went to a local hospital for a high fever up to 40 °C, poor appetite, and frequent vomiting. The result of the rapid dengue NS1 antigen test was positive. He was then admitted to the hospital for dengue with warning

Y.-C. Huang et al. (eds.), *Paediatric Infectious Diseases*,
https://doi.org/10.1007/978-981-19-7276-8_43

signs. Initial complete blood count (CBC) showed hemoglobin (Hb) 12.8 g/dL, hematocrit (Hct) 37.3%, and platelet (PLT) 230,000/μL. Blood biochemistry showed creatinine 0.8 mg/dL, aspartate transaminase (AST) 32 U/L, and alanine transaminase (ALT) 38 U/L. Follow-up laboratory tests on the next day showed thrombocytopenia (PLT 80,000/μL) and elevated blood transaminase levels (AST 130 U/L, ALT 77 U/L) but without hemoconcentration (Hb 12.2 g/dL, Hct 35%).

However, decreased urine output, nausea, and frequent upper abdominal pain developed. Gum bleeding and coffee-ground vomitus were also presented. He had no bowel movements during his hospitalization in the local hospital. Hemoconcentration (Hct 40.7%), thrombocytopenia (PLT 143,000/μL), and hypotension (blood pressure (BP) 81/54 mmHg) followed. He was transferred to a medical center PICU for dengue shock syndrome on day 4.

On examination, he complained of upper abdominal pain and tenderness but no muscle guarding. Point-of-care abdominal echography v(POCUS) revealed fluid accumulation at Morison's pouch and cul-de-sac. Proton pump inhibitors were given to prevent upper gastrointestinal bleeding. The result of the tourniquet test was positive (Fig. 1). A chest X-ray (CXR) showed no pulmonary edema or pleural effusion. Fluid resuscitation with crystalloids was started for tachycardia (>120 bpm) and relative hypotension (88/62 mmHg). Laboratory data on admission to PICU revealed hemoconcentration (Hct 51%), thrombocytopenia (PLT 13,000/μL), coagulopathy (activated partial thromboplastin time (aPTT) 75.60 s, prothrombin time (PT) 15.10 s), and significantly elevated transaminase levels (AST/ALT = 5487/1833 U/L). Elevated blood lactate dehydrogenase (LDH, 8768 U/L), hypoalbuminemia (2.9 g/dL), and hyponatremia (126 mmol/L) were also noted. Dengue viral PCR and repeated NS1 rapid test were negative, but anti-DENV IgG/IgM were positive.

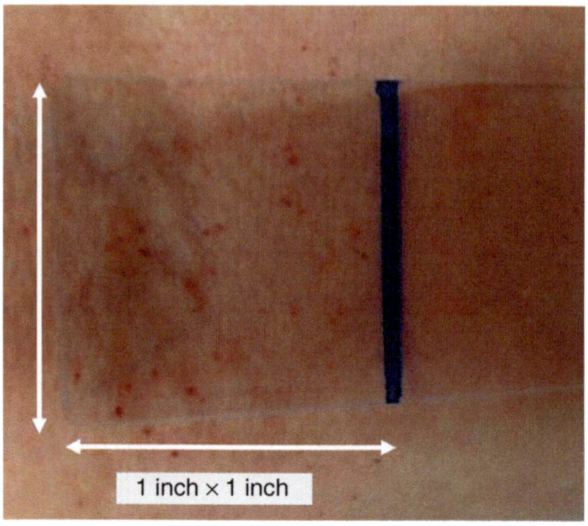

Fig. 1 Tourniquet test on 8-year-old boy on the fifth day of dengue fever. How to do a tourniquet test: Inflate the cuff to a point midway between SBP and DBP and maintain for minutes. Reduce and wait 2 min. Count petechiae below antecubital fossa. See the image above. A positive test is 10 or more petechiae per 1 in^2

His clinical status and laboratory abnormalities (Fig. 2) were corrected and improved after a 48-h careful intravenous crystalloid and colloid fluid management. No blood transfusion was applied during the hospitalization. There was no fever after admitting to PICU on day 4.

Follow-up CXR showed pleural effusion resolved without needle aspiration or tube drainage (Fig. 3). Pleural effusion appeared on day 5 after 1-day fluid resuscitation, but no tachypnea. Oral intake was initiated on day 5. Abdominal echography on day 7 showed no fluid accumulation. Intravenous fluids were discontinued on day 8. He was transferred to the general pediatric ward on day 8 and discharged on day 10.

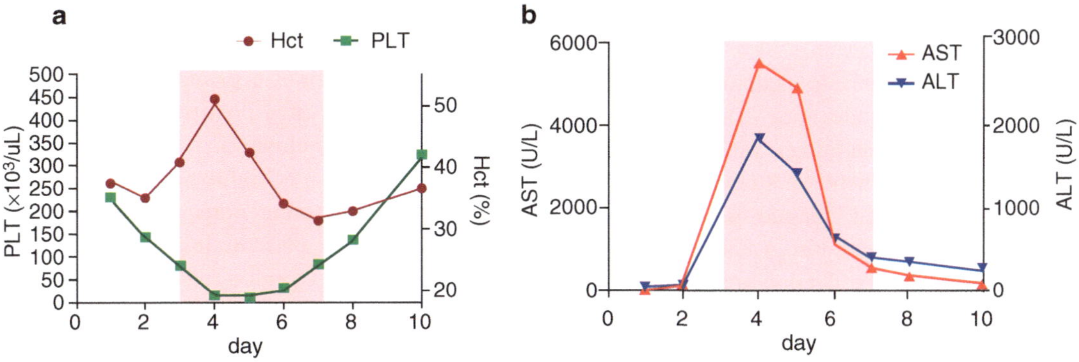

Fig. 2 (**a**) Kinetics of Hct and PLT levels in an 8-year-old boy with dengue shock syndrome. Day 0: first day of fever, Hct: hematocrit, PLT: platelet. The pink rectangle indicates the duration of shock status. (**b**) Kinetics of blood transaminase levels in an 8-year-old boy with dengue shock syndrome. Day 0: first day of fever, AST: aspartate transaminase, ALT: alanine transaminase. The pink rectangle indicates the duration of shock status

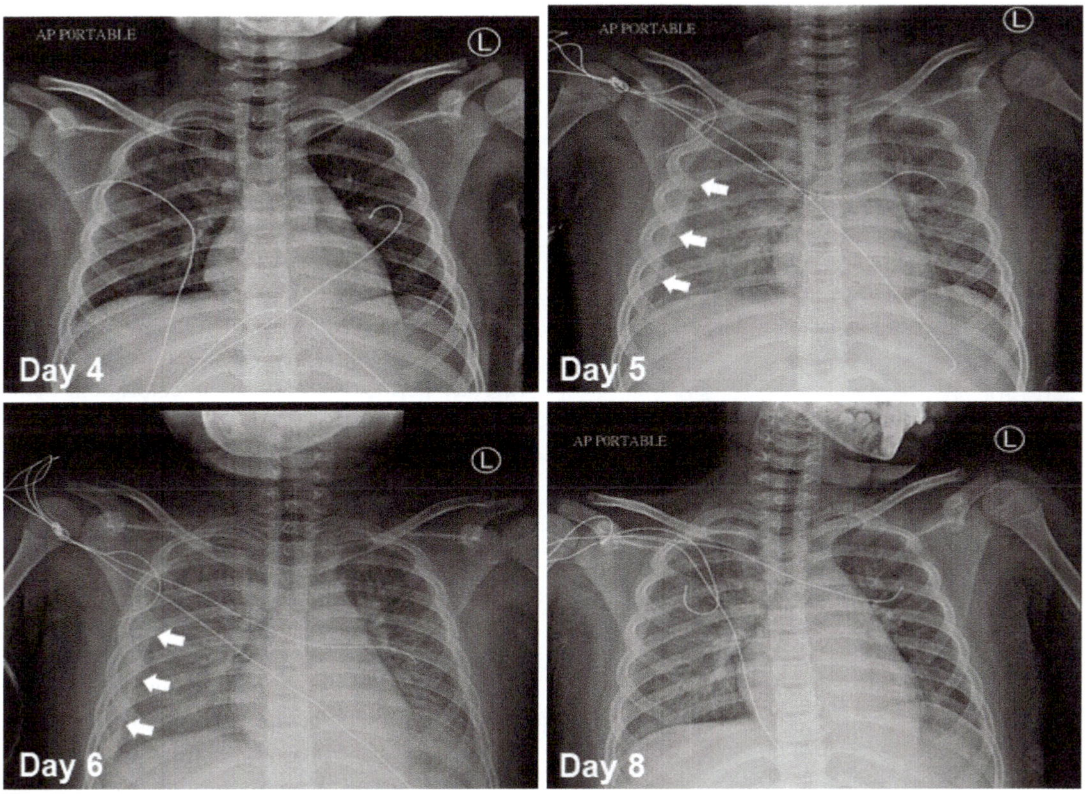

Fig. 3 CXR series in an 8-year-old boy with dengue shock syndrome. Day 0: first day of fever, CXR: Chest X-ray, arrows: pleural lines

Discussion

The incidence of severe pediatric dengue was less than 0.3 episodes per 100 person-years. However, the epidemiology varies significantly among countries. There are 4.6 and 2.9 pediatric laboratory-confirmed dengue per 100 person-years in Asian and Latin American countries, respectively. Besides, dengue episodes requiring hospitalization were 19.1% and 11.1% in Asian and Latin American countries [1]. In a recent dengue outbreak in Taiwan, pediatric patients comprised only 5.91% of the laboratory-confirmed emergency department visits [2]. Pediatric dengue posed significant challenges, especially to pediatricians in non-endemic areas. Symptoms/signs that increase the clinical suspicion of dengue include retro-orbital pain, myalgia, arthralgia/bone pain, bleeding, and rash (Fig. 4) [3].

The natural course of clinical dengue disease can be divided into three phases—febrile (first to third day of illness), critical (fourth to sixth day), and recovery. In the febrile phase, dengue patients usually present nonspecific symptoms/signs or viral syndrome when they first visit primary care pediatricians. In patients with acute febrile illness without a primary site of infection, the presence of a positive tourniquet test (at least 10 petechiae/in.^{2}) and leukopenia ($\leq$5000 WBC/mm^3) is highly suggestive of dengue [4]. Other notable nonspecific laboratory findings in dengue patients include leukopenia, thrombocytopenia, prolonged aPTT, elevated serum levels of aminotransferase, and low CRP [5]. For patients with suspected dengue virus disease, laboratory confirmation can be made by a single acute-phase serum specimen obtained early ($\leq$7 days after fever onset) in the illness by detecting viral genomic sequences with RT-PCR or dengue nonstructural protein 1 (NS1) antigen by immunoassay [6].

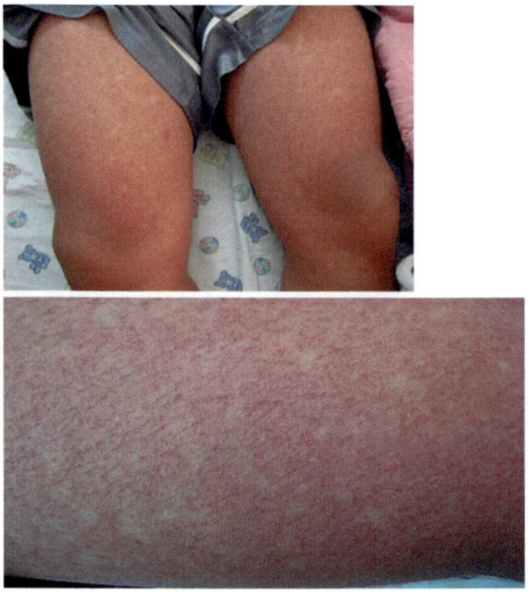

Fig. 4 Dengue rash: white islands in a sea of red. Rash in dengue fever is a maculopapular or macular confluent rash with islands of skin-sparing. The rash typically begins on day 3 and persists for 2–3 days

Dengue patients can be classified into three groups according to 2009 WHO criteria based on levels of clinical severity: (1) group A: dengue without warning signs; (2) group B: dengue with warning signs (abdominal pain, persistent vomiting, fluid accumulation, mucosal bleeding, lethargy, liver enlargement, increasing hematocrit with decreasing platelets); and (3) group C: severe dengue (dengue with severe plasma leakage, severe bleeding, or organ failure) [7]. Severe dengue is commonly characterized by increased vascular permeability, hemoconcentration, hemorrhagic manifestations, and thrombocytopenia [8]. Warning signs of severe dengue usually occur in the late febrile phase around the time of deterioration.

Dengue severity is based mainly on clinical judgment and varies in clinical practice settings. An accurate, efficient, and rapid diagnosis of impending severe dengue is critical for implementing prompt and meticulous care to avoid complications that may lead to a lethal outcome. The host factor composes a significant influence as an immune factor capable of inducing severe infection by antibody-dependent enhancement (ADE) mechanism [9]. In ADE, antibodies from previous different serotype DENV infections bind to viral antigen, making the antibody-antigen complex but unable to neutralize it. It further causes an increase of the Fc-presenting-cell infection, such as monocyte, macrophage, and mature dendritic cells, which the virus can replicate, and results in a higher virus titer in the serum compared to the non-ADE patients [10].

Fluid overload contributes to a substantial proportion of all deaths resulting from dengue vascular permeability syndrome [11]. Successful management of dengue vascular permeability syndrome relies on meticulous regulation of parenteral fluids and colloids during increased vascular leakage, together with proactive management of significant bleeding. Because the fluid lost is approximately equivalent to plasma, isotonic crystalloid solutions are recommended, except in very young infants (<6 months of age), in whom 0.45% sodium chloride can be used. A double-blind, randomized comparison of three fluids for initial resuscitation of Vietnamese children with dengue shock demonstrated that Ringer's lactate is enough to resuscitate children with moderately severe dengue shock syndrome [12].

Prevention of pediatric dengue relied on vector eradication and vaccination. The first live-attenuated chimeric yellow fever/tetravalent dengue vaccine (CYD-TDV), Dengvaxia®, has been licensed in several countries. Low efficacy of this vaccine was observed in children and dengue-naïve individuals. It also increased the risk of severe dengue in persons who had not been exposed to dengue [13].

In conclusion, pediatric dengue infections result in generally mild disease. Severe dengue is commonly characterized by increased vascular permeability, hemoconcentration, hemorrhagic manifestations, and thrombocytopenia. An accurate, efficient, and rapid diagnosis of impending severe dengue is critical for prompt rigorous clinical monitoring and care to avoid complications that could lead to mortality. The keys to successful rescue of pediatric patients with dengue shock syndrome rely on meticulous parenteral fluid regulation and active management of significant bleeding.

References

1. L'Azou M, et al. Symptomatic Dengue in Children in 10 Asian and Latin American Countries. N Engl J Med, 2016; 374: p. 1155-66.
2. Ho TS, et al. Comparing machine learning with case-control models to identify confirmed dengue cases. PLoS Negl Trop Dis 2020; 14: e0008843.
3. Ho TS, et al. Knowledge, attitude, and practice of dengue disease among healthcare professionals in southern Taiwan. J Formos Med Assoc, 2013; 112: p. 18-23.
4. Potts JA, Rothman AL. Clinical and laboratory features that distinguish dengue from other febrile illnesses in endemic populations. Trop Med Int Health 2008; 13: 1328-40.
5. Ho TS, et al. Clinical and laboratory predictive markers for acute dengue infection. J Biomed Sci 2013. 20: 75.
6. Vaughn DW, et al. Dengue in the early febrile phase: viremia and antibody responses. J Infect Dis 1997; 176: 322-30.
7. World Health Organization, Dengue: Guidelines for Diagnosis, Treatment, Prevention and Control: New Edition. 2009: Geneva.
8. Hadinegoro SR. The revised WHO dengue case classification: does the system need to be modified? Paediatr Int Child Health 2012; 32 Suppl 1: 33-8.
9. Goncalvez AP, et al. Monoclonal antibody-mediated enhancement of dengue virus infection in vitro and in vivo and strategies for prevention. Proc Natl Acad Sci USA 2007; 104: 9422-7.
10. Taylor A, et al., Fc receptors in antibody-dependent enhancement of viral infections. Immunol Rev 2015; 268: 340-64.
11. Kalayanarooj S, Rothman AL, Srikiatkhachorn A. Case Management of Dengue: Lessons Learned. J Infect Dis 2017; 215(suppl_2): S79-S88.
12. Wills BA, et al. Comparison of three fluid solutions for resuscitation in dengue shock syndrome. N Engl J Med 2005; 353: 877-89.
13. Tully D, Griffiths CL. Dengvaxia: the world's first vaccine for prevention of secondary dengue. Ther Adv Vaccines Immunother 2021; 9: 25151355211015839.

Case 44. A 4-Year-Old Boy with Fever, Cough, Skin Rash, and Difficulty in Breathing: Streptococcal Toxic Shock Syndrome

Yu-Yu Chuang and Yhu-Chering Huang

Keywords

Group A Streptococcus · Toxic shock syndrome · Intravenous immunoglobulin Contacts

Key Points

- An uncommon, life threatening complication of invasive group A streptococcus (GAS) disease
- May lack evidence of an overt infection or even bacteremia, but may rapidly progress to shock and multi-organ failure
- A severe acute illness characterized by fever, generalized erythroderma, rapid-onset hypotension, and signs of multi-organ involvement is the key clue of this life-threatening disease.
- Management includes immediate aggressive fluid replacement, respiratory and cardiac support, and empiric antimicrobial therapy.
- The risk of subsequent invasive GAS disease among household contacts of patients with invasive GAS infections is higher and postexposure chemoprophylaxis should be considered.

Case 1

A previously healthy 4-year-old boy presented with high fever, cough, generalized skin rash for 6 days and chest pain, difficulty in breathing for 1 day. Chest X-ray taken at local health clinic showed left pneumonia and pleural effusion and he was transferred to our hospital. Growth and development were appropriate for his age. On admission, he was toxic and febrile. His vital signs were body temperature 39.4 °C, heart rate 196 beats/min, respiratory rate 51 breaths/min, and systolic blood pressure (BP) 86 mmHg and diastolic BP 52 mmHg (<5th percentile for age and sex). On physical examination, he was in respiratory distress, tachypnea and retractions were noted. Decreased breath sounds on the left lung and crackles were heard over bilateral lung fields. A general macular rash was noted on the trunk and four extremities. No conjunctival injection and no strawberry tongue were noted.

Y.-Y. Chuang (✉)
Department of Pediatrics, St. Mary's Hospital, Luodong, Yilan, Taiwan

Y.-C. Huang
Pediatrics, Chang Gung Memorial Hospital, Chang Gung University, Taoyuan, Taiwan

Y.-C. Huang et al. (eds.), *Paediatric Infectious Diseases*,
https://doi.org/10.1007/978-981-19-7276-8_44

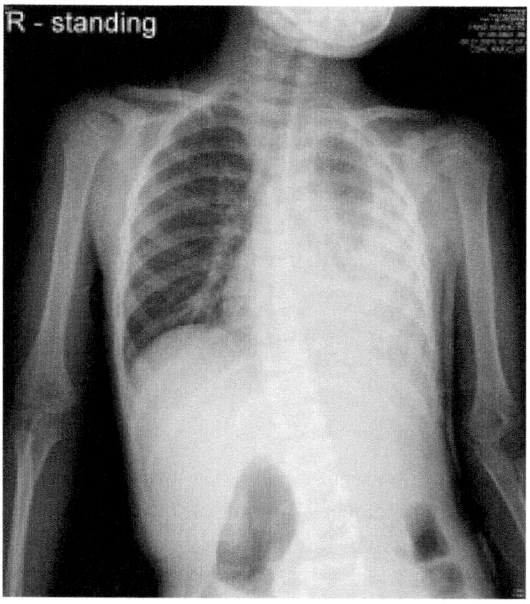

Fig. 1 Chest X-ray on admission showed left lung pneumonia with parapneumonic effusion in Case 1

Initial laboratory data showed a white blood cell count (WBC) 10,800/μL, neutrophils 82%, band 1%, platelet count 202,000/μL, and hemoglobin (Hb) 14.5 g/dL. Blood biochemistries showed elevated blood urea nitrogen (BUN) 67 mg/dL, creatinine 2.1 mg/dL, aspartate transaminase (AST) 37 U/L, alanine transaminase (ALT) 17 U/L, hyponatremia at 126 mEq/L, potassium 4.8 mEq/L, chloride 96 mEq/L, albumin 2.8 g/dL and C-reactive protein (CRP) 491.43 mg/L (normal, <5 mg/L). His prothrombin time 17 s (control value 11) and partial prothromboplastin time 56 s (control 28) were prolonged. Chest X-ray showed left lung pneumonia with parapneumonic effusion (Fig. 1).

He was admitted to the pediatric intensive care unit with a diagnosis of left pneumonia with parapneumonic effusion, impending shock, acute renal failure, and disseminated intravascular coagulation. Initial fluid resuscitation and inotropic agents were given to stabilize BP. He was intubated and left pigtail thoracostomy tube was inserted. Pleural fluid analysis showed turbid appearance, WBC 4000/μL (99% neutrophils), RBC 1225/μL, elevated protein 4.6 g/dL, lactate dehydrogenase (LDH) 9190 U/L and Gram's stain showed positive cocci 3+. Follow-up blood examination showed thrombocytopenia 38,000/μL. Antibiotics with vancomycin, ceftazidime, and clindamycin were given initially, and then changed to ceftriaxone and clindamycin. Chest computed tomography (CT) (Fig. 2) showed necrotizing pneumonia, left lung empyema on the eighth hospital day and video-assisted thoracostomy and decortication was performed on the tenth hospital day. Group A Streptococcus (GAS) was isolated from the pleural fluid and antibiotic was continued with penicillin. He was discharged 25 days after hospitalization and the final diagnosis was pneumonia caused by GAS, complicated with empyema and toxic shock syndrome.

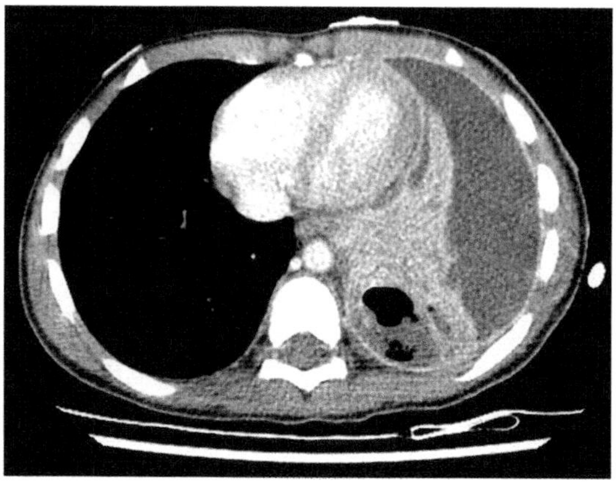

Fig. 2 Chest computed tomography showed necrotizing pneumonia, left lung empyema on the eighth hospital day in Case 1

Case 2

A 6-year-old boy developed fever, vomiting and diarrhea, abdominal pain, and headache for 1 day. His vital signs were body temperature 38.9 °C, heart rate 140 beats/min, respiratory rate 22 breaths/min, and systolic BP 77 mmHg and diastolic BP 44 mmHg (<5th percentile for age and sex). On physical examination, he was toxic and febrile. Injected throat and conjunctivae and no strawberry tongue were noted. An erythematous rash was noted on the trunk. Tenderness over the right upper quadrant of the abdomen was also noted. Laboratory data on admission showed a WBC 7000/μL, neutrophils 55%, band 41%, lymphocytes 3%, platelet count

271,000/μL, and Hb 11.2 g/dL. Blood biochemistries data were BUN 19 mg/dL, creatinine 1.2 mg/dL, AST 40 U/L, ALT 20 U/L, CRP 22 mg/L (normal, <5 mg/L). He was admitted to the pediatric intensive care unit with a diagnosis of acute gastroenteritis and dehydration and shock. Fluid resuscitation and inotropic agents were used to control hypotension. Antibiotics vancomycin, ceftriaxone, and amikacin were used. Intravenous immunoglobulin 2 g/kg single dose was given. Follow-up blood examination showed WBC 8300/μL, neutrophils 87%, band 4%, lymphocytes 5%, thrombocytopenia (platelet count 49,000/μL), and Hb 9.4 g/dL. Blood biochemistries were elevated BUN 24 mg/dL, creatinine 1.7 mg/dL. Prothrombin time 20 s (control 12 s) and partial thromboplastin time 65 s (control 33.7 s) were prolonged, and CRP was elevated to 309 mg/L. Throat swab antigen test on admission was positive for group A streptococcus and blood culture subsequently grew group A Streptococcus. Cerebrospinal fluid culture showed no growth of microorganisms. Antibiotic was continued with aqua penicillin for a total of 14 days. Rifampicin was given for eradication of the carrier state. Immunology studies were normal for age. Recovery was uneventful. The final diagnosis was GAS pharyngitis complicated with bacteremia and toxic shock syndrome.

Discussion

Streptococcal toxic shock syndrome (STSS) is an uncommon, life-threatening complication of invasive group A streptococcus (GAS) disease. GAS infections are common and can lead to a range of diseases from pharyngitis and cellulitis to severe invasive disease, such as necrotizing fasciitis or myositis, bacteremia, pneumonia, and STSS.

The incidence of invasive GAS infections was stable in the 1990s and subsequently increased. Reported incidence rates range from 3.8 to 10.24 invasive GAS cases per 100,000 persons per year and death rates vary from 4.2% to 56% for STSS. STSS develops in one third of patients with invasive disease. STSS can occur at any age. The incidence of invasive group A streptococcal infection in children younger than 10 years of age was 3.5 per 100,000 per year. Among the children with severe streptococcal infection, 4.6% developed STSS and a 7.2% case fatality rate. In children, STSS has been reported with focal infections, varicella, trauma, osteomyelitis, pneumonia, and bacteremia without a defined focus. Mortality rates are lower for children than adults with STSS.

Risk factors for invasive GAS infection are young and old age, diabetes and alcoholism, surgical procedures, trauma, varicella, and nonsteroidal anti-inflammatory drugs. The pathogenesis of invasive GAS infections have been found to be linked to some streptococcal virulence factors, including M-protein and the pyrogenic exotoxins A and B, which were implicated as superantigens mediating the systemic effects of streptococcal TSS.

Typical manifestation of STSS is characterized by fever, generalized erythroderma, sudden onset of shock, and multi-organ failure. STSS begins with an influenza-like prodrome characterized by fever, chills, myalgias, nausea, vomiting, and diarrhea that precedes hypotension by 24–48 h. Local soft tissue infections such as cellulitis, myositis, or necrotizing fasciitis, if present, are associated with rapidly increasing pain. In both children and adults, soft tissues are the most common primary site of infection. STSS has been reported among children with varicella, cellulitis, pneumonia, empyema, osteomyelitis, and bacteremia without any identifiable focus of infection.

In patients who have necrotizing fasciitis, fever and severe pain are the early clinical symptoms. CT and magnetic resonance imaging (MRI) are helpful. Laboratory test serum creatinine is useful because renal impairment is apparent before hypotension. Serum creatine phosphokinase are markedly elevated in those with necrotizing fasciitis and myonecrosis. WBC count may be normal or leukocytosis. Shock and multiple organ failure may occur rapidly in 4–8 h and many patients die within 24–48 h of admission despite aggressive treatment.

The Working Group on Severe Streptococcal Infections proposed a consensus definition for streptococcal TSS based on clinical criteria in 1993 and updated these criteria in 2010. Briefly, the clinical criteria included hypotension (defined by a systolic blood pressure less than the fifth percentile by age for children aged less than 16 years), and multi-organ involvement characterized by two or more of the following: renal involvement, coagulopathy, liver involvement, acute respiratory distress syndrome, a generalized erythematous macular rash, and soft tissue necrosis (including necrotizing fasciitis or myositis or gangrene). In addition to satisfying the clinical criteria, for a confirmed case, isolation of group A *Streptococcus* from a normally sterile site should be met; isolation of group A *Streptococcus* from a non-sterile site can meet for a probable case.

Management of STSS includes immediate aggressive fluid replacement, respiratory and cardiac support, and aggressive surgical debridement of any deep-seated infection, antimicrobial therapy, and administration of intravenous immunoglobulin (IVIG).

Initial antimicrobial therapy of TSS should include coverage with vancomycin and clindamycin for similarities of streptococcal and staphylococcal TSS. The addition of clindamycin is beneficial for serious GAS infections, because the antimicrobial activity of clindamycin is not affected by inoculum size, has a long post-antimicrobial effect and acts on bacteria by inhibiting protein synthesis. Inhibition of protein synthesis results in suppression of synthesis of the *S. pyogenes* antiphagocytic M-protein and bacterial toxins.

Penicillin and clindamycin remained the treatment of choice for confirmed GAS cases. The duration of therapy depends on the primary site of infection. If necrotizing fasciitis is suspected, immediate surgical exploration is needed for early debridement and pathogen identification. If patient is severely ill, intravenous immunoglobulin may be considered as adjunctive therapy for STSS or necrotizing fasciitis. The proposed mechanism of action of IVIG in IGAS is multifactorial and includes toxin neutralization, opsonization and improved phagocytic killing, and suppression of the massive inflammatory response through Fc-receptor interactions. An IVIG regimen of 1 g/kg on day 1, followed by 0.5/kg on 1–2 subsequent days is recommended, but the optimal regimen is unknown.

STSS is most common as community-acquired and sporadic. Transmission occurs through direct person-to-person contact. The risk of subsequent invasive GAS disease among household contacts of patients with invasive GAS infections is higher (200- to 2000-fold) than the risk among the general population. The benefits and optimal regimen of antibiotic prophylaxis in close contacts of patients for prevention of invasive GAS infection remain uncertain and differ among regions of the world. In the United Kingdom, prophylaxis is recommended for both mother and baby if either developed an invasive GAS infection in the neonatal period due to an increased risk of disease in this subpopulation, and to the entire household if ≥2 invasive GAS cases occur in a 30-day period. In Canada, prophylaxis is recommended for close contacts of confirmed severe cases who were exposed to the index patient during the period from 7 days prior to symptom onset to 24 h after the index patient initiates antibiotics. Recommended antibiotic regimens include penicillin and rifampin, azithromycin, clindamycin, and first-generation cephalosporins.

Further Reading

Stevens DL. Streptococcal toxic-shock syndrome: spectrum of disease, pathogenesis, and new concepts in treatment. Emerg Infect Dis. 1995;1:69-78.

Nelson GE, Pondo T, Toews KA, Farley MM, Lindegren ML, Lynfield R, et al. Epidemiology of invasive group A streptococcal infections in the United States, 2005–2012. Clin Infect Dis. 2016;63:478–86.

Tyrrell GJ, Fathima S, Kakulphimp J, Bell C. Increasing rates of invasive group A streptococcal disease in Alberta, Canada; 2003–2017. Open Forum Infect Dis. 2018;5:ofy177.

Chuang YY, Huang YC. Toxic shock syndrome in children (chapter 32). In Wheeler DS et al edi. Pediatric Critical Care Medicine, 2014, 2nd edi., Springer-Nature.

American Academy of Pediatrics. Group A Streptococcal Infections. In:Kimberlin DW, Brady MT, Jackson MA, Long SS, eds. Red Book:2018 Report of the Committee on Infectious Diseases. 31st ed. Itasca, IL: American Academy of Pediatrics;2018:748-762

Bryant AE, Stevens DL. Streptococcus pyogenes. In Mandell, Douglas, and Bennett's Principles and Practice of Infectious Diseases;2019:2446-2461.e5

Javouhey E, Bolze P-A, Jamen C, et al. Similarities and Differences between Staphylococcal and Streptococcal Toxic Shock Syndromes in Children: Results from a 30-Case Cohort. Front. Pediatr. 2018;6:360.

Cook A, Janse S, Watson JR, Erdem G. Manifestations of Toxic Shock Syndrome in Children, Columbus, Ohio, USA, 2010–2017. Emerg Infect Dis 2020; 26: 1077-1083.

Lamagni TL, Oliver I, Stuart JM. Global assessment of invasive group A streptococcus infection risk in household contacts. Clin Infect Dis 2015;60:166.

Health Protection Agency, Group A *Streptococcus* Working Group. Interim UK guidelines for management of close community contacts of invasive group A streptococcal disease. Commun Dis Public Health 2004; 7:354–61.

Moore DL, Allen UD. Invasive group A streptococcal disease: management and chemoprophylaxis. Paediatr Child Health 2019; 24:128-9.

Adebanjo T, Apostol M, Alden N, et al. Evaluating Household Transmission of Invasive Group A *Streptococcus* Disease in the United States Using Population-based Surveillance Data, 2013–2016, *Clin Infect Dis 2020;*70: 1478–1481.

Case 45. A 4-Year-Old Boy with Fever, General Skin Rash, Vomiting, and Diarrhea, Following an Operation for Bone Fracture: Staphylococcal Toxic Shock Syndrome

Yu-Yu Chuang and Yhu-Chering Huang

Keywords

Staphylococcus aureus · Toxic shock syndrome · Intravenous immunoglobulin Myocarditis · Coagulopathy

Key Points

- A toxin-mediated disease characterized by acute onset of fever, hypotension, and signs of multisystem dysfunction, diffuse erythroderma, late desquamation of the palms and soles, and conjunctival and pharyngeal hyperemia
- May lack evidence of an overt infection or even bacteremia, but may rapidly progress to shock and multi-organ failure
- Early recognition of disease, source control, adequate antimicrobial agents capable of suppressing toxin production are essential to optimize the effectiveness of treatment
- The signs of bone infections may be masked by the critical symptoms of toxic shock

Case Scenario

A previously healthy 4-year-8-month-old boy presented with high fever, general skin rash, vomiting, and diarrhea for 3 days. One month ago, he had a fall while riding the bicycle and sustained a supracondylar closed fracture of left distal humerus, Gartland type III, and underwent closed reduction with K wire fixation (post-operation day 33). Growth and development were appropriate for his age.

On admission, he was toxic, drowsy, and febrile. His vital signs were body temperature 39 °C, heart rate 128 beats/min, respiratory rate 32 breaths/min, and systolic blood pressure (BP) 66 mmHg and diastolic BP 69 mmHg (<5th percentile for age and sex). On physical examination, his left elbow was swollen with erythema and local heat and tenderness. A general macular rash on the face and trunk was noted. No conjunctival injection and no strawberry tongue were noted.

Y.-Y. Chuang (✉)
Department of Pediatrics, St. Mary's Hospital, Luodong, Yilan, Taiwan

Y.-C. Huang
Pediatrics, Chang Gung Memorial Hospital, Chang Gung University, Taoyuan, Taiwan

Y.-C. Huang et al. (eds.), *Paediatric Infectious Diseases*,
https://doi.org/10.1007/978-981-19-7276-8_45

Initial laboratory data showed a white blood cell count (WBC) 10,600/μL, neutrophils 80%, band 8%. Blood biochemistry data showed blood urea nitrogen (BUN) 62.7 mg/dL, creatinine 1.84 mg/dL, aspartate transaminase (AST) 104 U/L, alanine transaminase (ALT) 68 U/L, and C-reactive protein (CRP) 326.2 mg/L (normal, <5 mg/L).

He was admitted to the pediatric intensive care unit with a diagnosis of toxic shock syndrome. Initial fluid resuscitation and inotropic agents with dopamine and levophed were given to stabilize BP. Antibiotics with vancomycin, cefotaxime, and clindamycin were given. Fever subsided after admission, and BP stabilized after 2 days. Wound culture showed *Pseudomonas aeruginosa* and *Staphylococcus aureus*. On the fourth hospital day, he was transferred to pediatric ward and antibiotics deescalated to oxacillin and ceftazidime according to susceptibility report. Clindamycin was continued. Follow-up laboratory data showed a WBC 14,800/μL, neutrophils 61%, band 4%. Blood biochemistries showed improvement, BUN 49.4 mg/dL, creatinine 0.95 mg/dL, AST 69 U/L, ALT 53 U/L, and CRP 151.69 mg/L.

He developed desquamation of the palms and soles after the first week of illness (Fig. 1). Intravenous antibiotics were continued to the 14th day and follow up X-ray of the elbow showed poor bone healing with periosteal abscess formation, suspect osteomyelitis. Soft tissue echo showed local edema over periosteal tissue, a low echogenic lesion (1.5 × 1.3 × 0.8 cm) adjacent to the joint space and no osteal plane disruption. Antibiotics therapy was continued for 6 weeks.

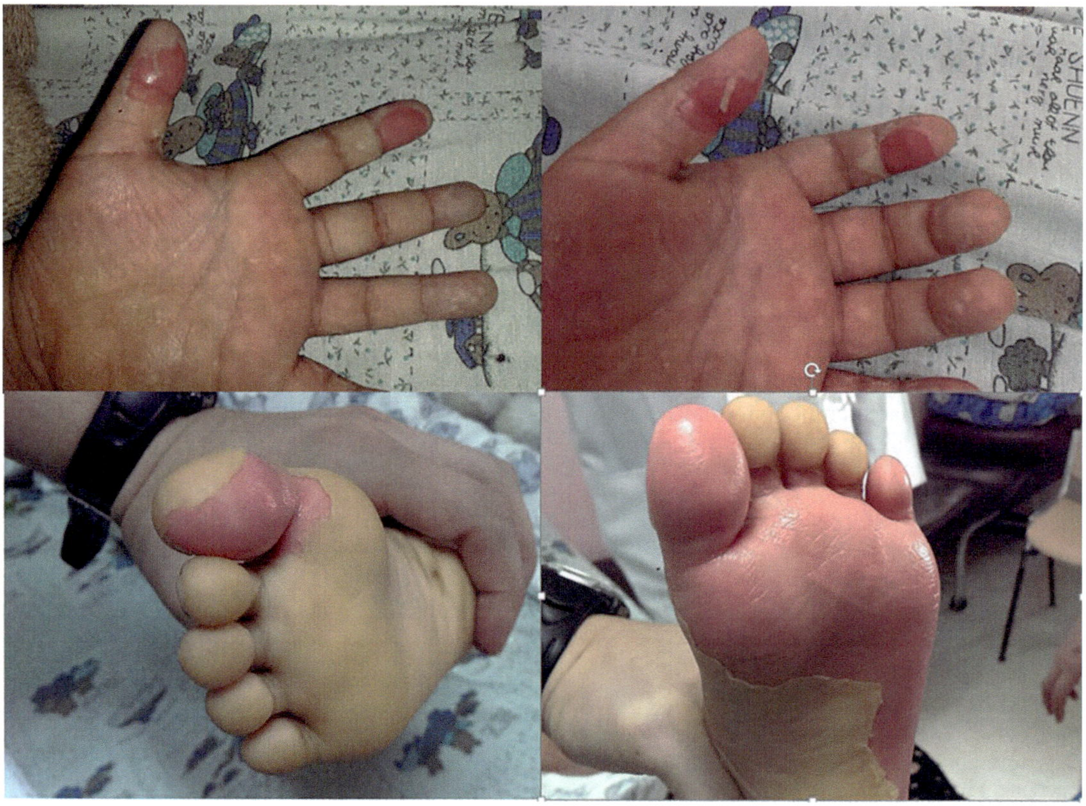

Fig. 1 Desquamation of the palms and soles after the first week of illness

Discussion

Toxic shock syndrome (TSS) is a toxin-mediated disease, characterized by acute onset of fever, hypotension, and signs of multisystem organ dysfunction. It has unique clinical findings not noted in septic shock, including diffuse erythroderma, late desquamation of the palms and soles, and conjunctival and pharyngeal hyperemia. Toxic shock syndrome (TSS) is mainly caused by *Staphylococcus aureus and Streptococcus pyogenes*. Staphylococcal TSS can be menstrual and non-menstrual.

TSS accounts for an estimate of 11.1% of the pediatric septic shock, and staphylococcal TSS represented 83% of TSS cases and occurred more commonly in females and at a higher median age than streptococcal TSS (14 years vs. 9.5 years).

Staphylococcal TSS was first described by Todd et al. in 1978 in a series of healthy children. Early reports of TSS were mostly menstrual associated with the use of high absorbency tampons in young women and cases declined after public awareness and the withdrawal of some tampon brands.

Non-menstrual TSS now accounts for approximately one-half of the reported TSS cases. The overall case-fatality rate in children was 4.1% and the mortality rates were 3% for menstrual and 5% for non-menstrual cases. Non-menstrual TSS occur after surgical and postpartum wound infections, cutaneous and subcutaneous lesions, osteomyelitis, arthritis, burns, and respiratory infections following influenza. The incidence of postoperative cases of TSS was 3/100,000 population after all types of surgeries and 16.5/100,000 population following ear, nose, and throat surgery.

TSS is caused by certain strains of *S. aureus* that produce one or more exotoxins, TSS toxin 1 (TSST-1) and staphylococcal enterotoxin. These toxins act as superantigens that stimulate lymphocytes and endothelial cells to produce endogenous mediators, tumor necrosis factor (TNF), and interleukin 1 (IL-1). Massive cytokine release causes extensive capillary leakage, loss of intravascular volume and hypotension, shock and multiple organ system dysfunction. TSST-1 production is enhanced in specific growth conditions such as increased level of protein, aerobic PO_2, neutral pH, increased level of CO_2, which are conditions found in abscesses and the vagina with tampon use during menstruation. Individuals who have previously been exposed to lesser concentrations of TSS toxins from nasal carriage may develop antibody that protects from overt disease. Ninety percent of healthy adults have antibodies to TSST-1. TSST-1 antibody was 78.6% in infant under 6 months old and 21.3% in the age group from 6 to 12 months old. Risk factors necessary for TSS include colonization of a toxin-producing strain of *S. aureus*, absence of protective antitoxin antibody, and an infected site with or without a foreign body.

The onset is abrupt, with fever, vomiting, and diarrhea, accompanied by sore throat, headache, and myalgia. Confusion, somnolence, irritability, and agitation may occur due to cerebral edema. Oliguria, hypotension may progress to shock. Diffuse erythematous rash develops within 24–48 h, and accompanied by pharyngeal, conjunctival, and mucous membranes hyperemia. Desquamation of the palms and soles occurs in 1–3 weeks after onset of illness. The clinical features of menstrual and non-menstrual TSS are similar in most cases. The onset of illness in menstrual TSS is 2–3 days of menstruation and 2–4 days in post-surgical cases, but can be as short as 12 h or as long as 35 days. Non-menstrual TSS was associated with earlier onset of rash and fever, more frequent renal and central nervous system complications, and less musculoskeletal involvement.

Laboratory findings consistent with toxic shock syndrome were leukocytosis, thrombocytopenia, and anemia. Blood urea nitrogen and creatinine, liver function tests, creatine phosphokinases were elevated. Hypocalcemia and hypoproteinemia and disseminated intravascular coagulation may be present. Blood cultures are positive in less than 5% of patients, and cultures from sites of infection are usually positive.

Recurrent TSS tends to occur in those who received inadequate antibiotic treatment and who fail to develop antibody response to staphylococcal toxins and recurrent tampon use. Recurrent menstrual TSS is generally milder than the initial disease. Recurrence can occur days to months after the initial episode. Unfortunately, there is no single diagnostic test available to clearly identify patients with staphylococcal TSS. The diagnosis of staphylococcal TSS is based on clinical presentation using the Centers for Disease Control and Prevention (CDC) case definition. Briefly, five clinical criteria included fever (≥38.9 °C), rash (diffuse macular erythroderma), desquamation (1–2 weeks after onset of rash), hypotension, and multisystem involvement (three or more organ systems). The organ systems include gastrointestinal, muscular, mucous membranes, renal, hepatic, hematologic (platelets count <100,000/mm^3), and central nervous system. Laboratory criteria included negative results for blood (may be positive for *S. aureus*), throat or CSF cultures and serologic tests for Rocky Mountain spotted fever, leptospirosis, or measles. A case which meets the laboratory criteria and all five of the clinical criteria is categorized as a confirmed case, while as a probable case, if it meets four of the five clinical criteria.

Management of TSS includes treatment of shock, surgical debridement, and antibiotic therapy. Rapid extensive fluid resuscitation and vasopressors are frequently needed to maintain perfusion because of hypotension and diffuse capillary leak. Focus of infection must be drained and, if packing or tampons are present, should be removed. Initial parenteral antibiotic for both *S. aureus* and *S. pyogenes* should be started because of similarity in the clinical appearances of streptococcal and staphylococcal TSS.

We recommend empiric therapy with vancomycin (40–60 mg/kg/day IV in four divided doses) plus clindamycin (25–40 mg/kg/day in three divided doses) for patients with suspected TSS. Regimen for methicillin-susceptible *S. aureus* is oxacillin (150–200 mg/kg/day IV in 4 divided doses) or cefazolin (100–150 mg/kg/day in three divided doses) plus clindamycin. Regimen for methicillin-resistant *S. aureus* is vancomycin plus clindamycin. Clindamycin is added for treatment of TSS because it inhibits protein synthesis to suppress ongoing toxin production. Antimicrobial treatment should be continued for at least 10–14 days to eradicate the organism and prevent recurrences by eliminating the carrier state. The total duration depends on the underlying etiology.

Linezolid is active against a broad range of gram-positive pathogens, has been used successfully to treat staphylococcal TSS by reducing TSST-1 production. Linezolid and clindamycin are both protein synthesis inhibitors that suppressed toxin synthesis. They are more efficacious than the cell-wall active agents in TSS. Intravenous immunoglobulin may neutralize circulating toxin, and may be beneficial when administered in addition to antibiotic therapy. IVIG may be considered for infection refractory to several hours of aggressive therapy or in the presence of an undrainable focus or persistent oliguria with pulmonary edema. Regimens are 150–400 mg/kg/day for 5 days or a single dose of 1–2 g/kg has been used.

In summary, staphylococcal TSS is a severe pediatric illness that early recognition and directed treatment are important to reduce morbidity. Staphylococcal TSS treatment should be included in pediatric septic shock treatment protocol to keep awareness of this diagnosis particularly in a severely ill child with erythroderma, conjunctival hyperemia, strawberry tongue, laboratory findings (elevated BUN and creatinine, elevated liver enzymes, and thrombocytopenia), and menstruation or tampon use or other focus of infection.

Further Reading

Gaensbauer JT, Birkholz M, Smit MA, et al. Epidemiology and clinical relevance of toxic shock syndrome in US children. Pediatr Infect Dis 2018;37:1223-26.

Chuang YY, Huang YC, Lin TY. Toxic shock syndrome in children: epidemiology, pathogenesis and management. Pediatr Drug 2005; 7:11-25.

Centers for Disease Control (CDC). Reduced incidence of menstrual toxic-shock syndrome--United States, 1980-1990. MMWR Morb Mortal Wkly Rep. 1990;39(25):421.

DeVries AS, Lesher L, Schlievert PM, Rogers T, Villaume LG, et al. Staphylococcal Toxic Shock Syndrome 2000–2006: Epidemiology, Clinical Features, and Molecular Characteristics. PLoS ONE 2011; 6(8): e22997.

Graham DR, O'Brien M, Hayes JM, et al. Postoperative toxic shock syndrome. Clin Infect Dis. 1995;20(4):895-899

Llewelyn M, Cohen J. Superantigens: microbial agents that corrupt immunity. Lancet Infect Dis. 2002;2(3):156-62.

Chen KYH, Cheung M, Burgner DP, et al. Arch Dis Child 2016;101:736–740.

Quan L, Morita R, Kawakami S. Toxic shock syndrome toxin-1 (TSST-1) antibody levels in Japanese children. Burns. 2010 Aug;36(5):716-21.

Chuang YY, Huang YC. Toxic shock syndrome in children (chapter 32). In Wheeler DS et al eds. Pediatric Critical Care Medicine, 2014, 2nd edi, Springer-Nature.

Case 46. A 3-Year-Old Girl with Fever and Pancytopenia: Hemophagocytic Lymphohistiocytosis Associated with Epstein-Barr Virus Infection

Chih-Jung Chen and Yhu-Chering Huang

Keywords

Hemophagocytic lymphohistiocytosis
Epstein-Barr virus

Key Points

- If symptomatic, acute primary EBV infection is commonly associated with classic infectious mononucleosis and occasionally with pneumonia (0–5%).
- Hemophagocytic lymphohistiocytosis (HLH), a hyperinflammation syndrome, is a rare but potentially life-threatening disease.
- Most of HLH cases are sporadic, and secondary form, which can be caused by a wide array of diseases, including various infections, autoimmune disorders, and malignant diseases. EBV is the common viral trigger.
- Treatment of EBV-associated HLH includes antineoplastic agents (e.g., cyclosporine and etoposide), corticosteroids, and immunomodulators.
- Intravenous immunoglobulin and antiviral therapy can be provided in cases with ongoing viral infection.

Case Report

A 3-year-10-month-old girl presented with fever for 6 days before being admitted to a regional hospital. Upon admission, the workup disclosed leukocytosis with a peripheral white blood cell count of 13,900/μL (neutrophils 63%, lymphocytes 28%, monocytes 9%), hemoglobin 10.8 g/dL, platelet count 205,000/μL, and elevated C-reactive protein level with a value of 169.3 mg/L. The consolidation of left lower lobe and bilateral pleural effusion was revealed by chest roentgenography, which was later confirmed on computed tomography scan on day 20 of fever (Fig. 1).

She was initially on amoxicillin/clavulanate, gentamicin, and azithromycin treatment under the impression of pneumonia and was later escalated to vancomycin and ceftriaxone due to clinical deterioration (transferred to a medical center). She was found hypotensive on day 16 of fever.

C.-J. Chen (✉)
Division of Pediatric Infectious Diseases, Department of Pediatrics, Chang Gung Memorial Hospital, Chang Gung University College of Medicine, Taoyuan, Taiwan

Molecular Infectious Diseases Research Center, Chang Gung Memorial Hospital, Taoyuan, Taiwan
e-mail: chinjung@cgmh.org.tw

Y.-C. Huang
Pediatrics, Chang Gung Memorial Hospital, Chang Gung University, Taoyuan, Taiwan

Y.-C. Huang et al. (eds.), *Paediatric Infectious Diseases*,
https://doi.org/10.1007/978-981-19-7276-8_46

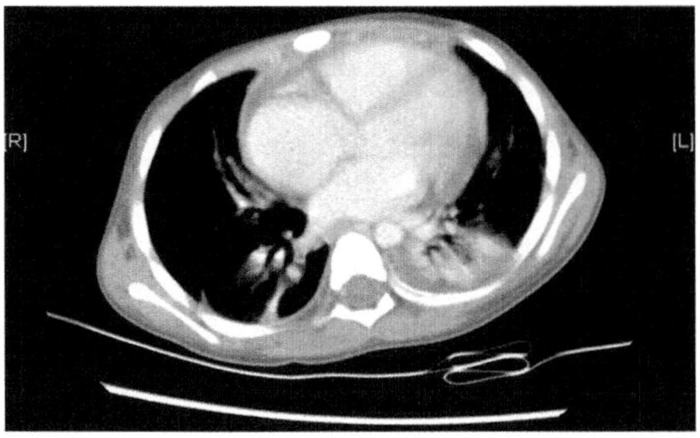

Fig. 1 Consolidation of left lower lobe and pleural effusion was noted on chest computed tomography scan on day 20 of fever

The echocardiography disclosed cardiomegaly and presence of a mild to moderate amount of pericardial effusions (10 mm). Pericardiocentesis was performed, 50 mL foamy red fluid was aspirated out, and disclosed a WBC count of 2030/μL, supporting the diagnosis of pericarditis. Biochemistry studies showed high levels of lactate dehydrogenase (LDH, 1146 U/L), ferritin (8642.8 ng/mL), and hypoalbuminemia (2.3 g/dL). The studies on common viral and bacterial etiology of pneumonia were mostly negative. The only relevant findings were the serologic study of Epstein-Barr virus (EBV), which disclosed positive IgG and IgM to viral capsid antigen and negative IgG antibody to early antigen and nuclear antigen, suggesting acute primary EBV infection. To determine if the EBV was actually the organism accounting for the pneumonia and pericarditis, biopsy of lung and pericardium was performed on day 26 of fever. EBV was detected, while negative for *Mycoplasma pneumoniae* and *Mycobacterium tuberculosis*, by polymerase chain reaction (PCR) in both tissue specimens.

On day 30 of fever, the hemogram started to show leukopenia (WBC count of 4100/μL), anemia (6.2 g/dL), and thrombocytopenia (61,000/μL). Extremely high levels of aspartate transaminase (AST, 2438 U/L), alanine aminotransferase (ALT, 854 U/L), LDH (2567 U/L) and ferritin (81,892 ng/mL) was identified in the biochemistry study. The diagnosis of hemophagocytic lymphohistiocytosis (HLH) was suspected and later confirmed by the bone marrow study. The clinical condition was improved dramatically after administration of intravenous immunoglobulin. The patient recovered uneventfully and was discharged on day 40 of hospitalization. The final diagnosis was acute primary EBV infection associated with pneumonia, pericarditis, and hemophagocytic lymphohistiocytosis.

Discussion

EBV is a ubiquitous virus belonging to the *Lymphocryptovirus* genus of *Gammaherpesvirinae* subfamily. The virus was transmitted by close contact between persons through saliva. There was a marked variation of the ages when primary (initial) EBV infection occurred. Approximately 80–100% of individuals acquired the infection in early childhood at 3–6 years old in the developing countries, whereas most of the infections occurred at the age of 10–30 years in the developed countries. The seropositive rate of EBV was universally high at the range of 80–95% throughout the world. In Taiwan, a seroepidemiologic survey showed that the seropositive rate of EBV reached 52.8% (95% CI, 44.0–61.6%) in children aged 2 years, rapidly rose to 88.7% (95% CI, 79.0–95.1%) in those aged 5–7 years, and 93.0% (95%CI, 83.0–98.1%) for those aged 14–16 years.

Primary infection of EBV is usually asymptomatic in young children and, if symptomatic, is commonly associated with classic infectious mononucleosis (IM). The other reported clinical syndromes include acute neurologic disease, aplastic anemia, pharyngotonsillitis, and pneumonia. The lymphoproliferative diseases in immunocompromised hosts, Burkitt lymphoma, nasopharyngeal carcinoma, HLH, and chronic fatigue syndrome can be encountered during chronic infections or reactivation from latent infections of EBV.

The classic manifestations of EBV-associated IM are fever, malaise, fatigue, sore throat, cervical lymphadenopathy, pharyngotonsillitis, hepatosplenomegaly, puffy eyelid, and skin rash. The lymph nodes are usually diffusedly involved, with characteristics of slight tenderness and moderate enlargement. The IM symptoms usually resolve within several days to 3–4 weeks and most of immunocompetent patients recover uneventfully. However, fatigue-like syndromes could occasionally persist for several months. Upper airway obstruction following severe pharyngotonsillitis is a common complication of IM. However, the lower respiratory tract is usually spared and radiographic evidence suggesting pulmonary infiltration is identified only in a small proportion (0–5%) of patients with IM. In such patients, the pleural effusion can present as shown in the illustrated case. It remained not conclusive if the uncommon pulmonary infiltration in IM was caused by EBV itself or other coinfected organisms.

Hemophagocytic lymphohistiocytosis (HLH) is a rare but potentially life-threatening disease. HLH can be primary and secondary. Primary HLH (i.e., familial erythrophagocytic lymphohistiocytosis [FEL]), an inherited form, is a heterogeneous autosomal recessive disorder found to be more prevalent with parental consanguinity. Most of the HLH cases are sporadic, of secondary form, and are triggered by a wide array of infection (viral, bacterial, and parasitic infections, etc.), malignancy and collagen vascular diseases. Macrophage activation syndrome is used to describe the HLH-like illness induced by autoimmune disorders. Of infection-associated HLH, EBV is the most common viral trigger and the EBV-associated HLH is usually of poor prognosis.

HLH is a hyperinflammation syndrome and elevated interferon-gamma (INF-gamma) is thought to be part of the pathogenesis that causes the hyperinflammation associated with HLH. It is characterized by prolonged fever (7 or more days), cytopenia (at least two of three cell linages), splenomegaly, hypertriglyceridemia or hypofibrinogenemia (or hyperferritinemia), and hemophagocytosis demonstrated in bone marrow, spleen, or lymph nodes. All these five criteria must be met to establish the diagnosis. Skin can be involved, and as many as 65% of the cases may have nonspecific skin rash. Central nervous system can also be involved and showed neurologic symptoms including seizures, ataxia, hemiplegia, mental status changes, or simply irritability. Liver damage has also been reported as evidenced by hyperbilirubinemia, hypoalbuminemia, and elevated AST and ALT.

Rapid diagnosis and early therapy can be pivotal. A pediatric hematology-oncology specialist is best equipped to manage HLH. Generally, treatment regimens include antineoplastic agents (interfere with cell reproduction), corticosteroids (as anti-inflammation drugs), and immunomodulators (e.g., intravenous immunoglobulin). According to the HLH 2004 protocol, the management of HLH should include induction therapy with dexamethasone, cyclosporine, etoposide (VP-16) and intrathecal methotrexate in cases with central nervous system involvement. Continuation therapy with pulses of dexamethasone and VP-16 for up to 1 year was suggested for those with active disease after induction therapy. In addition, antiviral therapy and intravenous immunoglobulin (0.5 g/kg IV) once every 4 weeks can be administered to patients with ongoing viral infections. Emapalumab, a monoclonal antibody that binds and neutralizes INF-gamma, was approved by the FDA in 2018. It is indicated for primary HLH in adults and children with refractory, recurrent, or progressive disease, or who are intolerant to conventional HLH therapy. Emapalumab was found beneficial for primary HLH.

Further Reading

Henter, J. *et al.* HLH-2004: Diagnostic and therapeutic guidelines for hemophagocytic lymphohistiocytosis. file:///Users/jameschen/Desktop/henter2007.pdf (2007).

Castagnini LA, Leach CT. In Feigin and Cherry's Textbook of Pediatric Infectious Diseases, 18th ED, Chapter 160 Epstein-Barr virus, P. 1450-1474

Kogawa K, *et al.* Prognostic factors of Epstein–Barr virus-associated hemophagocytic lymphohistiocytosis in children: Report of the Japan Histiocytosis Study Group. *Pediatr Blood Cancer* 2014; 61: 1257–1262.

Locatelli F, Jordan MB, Allen C, et al. Emapalumab in children with primary hemophagocytic lymphohistiocytosis. N Engl J Med 2020;382:1811-1822.

Lee WI, Chen SH, Hung IJ, Yang CP, Jaing TH, Chen CJ, *et al.* **Clinical aspects, immunologic assessment, and genetic analysis in Taiwanese children with hemophagocytic lymphohistiocytosis.** Pediatr Infect Dis J 2009; 28: 30-34

Chen CY, Huang KY, Shen JH, Tsao KC, Huang YC. A large-scale seroprevalence of Epstein-Barr virus in Taiwan. PLoS One. 2015;10:e0115836.

Zhao Y, Lu D, Ma S, Li L, Zhu J, Zhou, *et al.* Risk factors of early death in adult patients with secondary hemophagocytic lymphohistiocytosis: a single-institution study of 171 Chinese patients. Hematology 2019; 24:606-612

Xu XJ, Wang HS, Ju XL, Xiao PF, Xiao Y, Xue HM, *et al.* Clinical presentation and outcome of pediatric patients with hemophagocytic lymphohistiocytosis in China: a retrospective multicenter study. Pediatr Blood Cancer, 2017;64(4), https://doi.org/10.1002/pbc.26264

Chen TY, Hsu MH, Kuo HC, Sheen JM, Cheng MC, Lin YJ. Outcome analysis of pediatric hemophagocytic lymphohistiocytosis. J Formos Med Assoc 2021; 120:172-179

Yu TY, Lu MY, Lin KH, Chang HH, Chou SW, Lin DT, et al. Outcomes and prognostic factors associated with 180-day mortality in Taiwanese pediatric patients with Hemophagocytic Lymphohistiocytosis. J Formos Med Assoc 2021;120:1061-8

Case 47. A 2-Month-Old Infant with Fever, Progressive Skin Rash and Eosinophilia: Drug-Induced Fever and Skin Rash in Children

Chun-Bing Chen, Hsi Yen, and Wen-Hung Chung

Keywords

Drug reaction with eosinophilia and systemic symptoms (DRESS) · Drug-induced hypersensitivity syndrome (DIHS) · Adverse drug eruption · Skin rash · Antibiotics · Allergy

Key Points

- Drug reaction with eosinophilia and systemic symptoms (DRESS) is a syndrome characterized clinically as an extensive infiltrative maculopapular exanthem accompanied by fever, lymphadenopathy, internal organ involvement, and hematological abnormalities.
- Generalized, infiltrated papuloplaques with purpuric change, facial edema, and desquamation are suggestive dermatological features.
- Manifestations of DRESS range from mild disease to severe internal organ involvement with potential life-threatening consequences.
- Early recognition and withdrawal of the offending drug are key to managing for patients with this severe cutaneous adverse drug reaction.
- Systemic corticosteroid remains the first-line treatment for DRESS; cyclosporine or tofacitinib have been used for recalcitrant cases.

C.-B. Chen (✉)
Drug Hypersensitivity Clinical and Research Center, Department of Dermatology, Chang Gung Memorial Hospital, Linkou, Taipei and Keelung, Taiwan

School of Medicine, National Tsing Hua University, Hsinchu, Taiwan

Department of Dermatology, Chang Gung Memorial Hospital, Linkou, Taipei and Keelung, Taiwan

College of Medicine, Chang Gung University, Taoyuan, Taiwan

H. Yen · W.-H. Chung
Drug Hypersensitivity Clinical and Research Center, Department of Dermatology, Chang Gung Memorial Hospital, Linkou, Taipei and Keelung, Taiwan

Department of Dermatology, Chang Gung Memorial Hospital, Linkou, Taipei and Keelung, Taiwan

College of Medicine, Chang Gung University, Taoyuan, Taiwan

Y.-C. Huang et al. (eds.), *Paediatric Infectious Diseases*,
https://doi.org/10.1007/978-981-19-7276-8_47

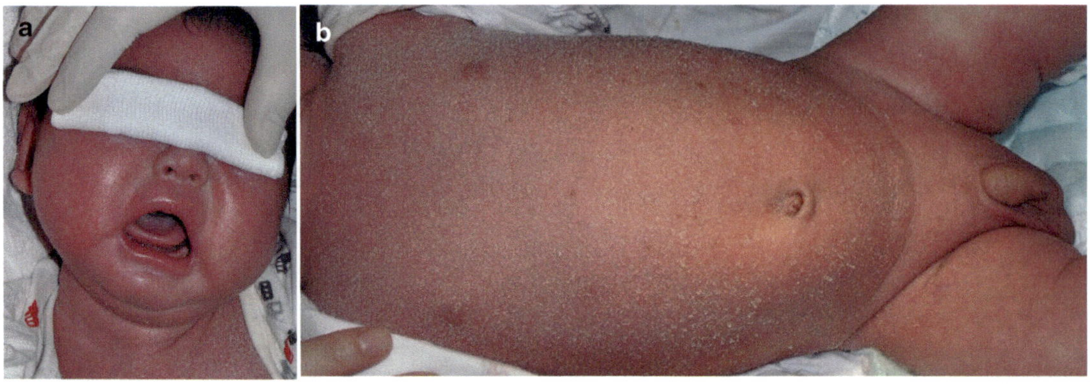

Fig. 1 Clinical picture of the 2-month-old boy with DRESS. Skin examination showed facial swelling with generalized infiltrative erythema on the face (**a**), and trunk, and lower extremities. Scaling on the erythrodermic skin (**b**) was also noticed days later

Case Report

A 2-month-old male infant was admitted to the neonatal unit due to progressive skin rash and fever with decreased appetite and activity for 3 days. Skin examination showed generalized, infiltrative erythematous maculopapular rash with areas of confluent erythema. Facial swelling (Fig. 1a) and bilateral cervical lymphadenopathy were also noted. Laboratory data demonstrated leukocytosis and eosinophilia (white blood cell count 25,100/μL with 0.5% bands, 51.5% segmented cells, 27.5% lymphocytes, 5.5% monocytes, 6% eosinophils, and 9% atypical lymphocytes), platelet count 307,000/μL, and hemoglobin 10.5 g/dL. Blood biochemistry data showed elevated liver enzymes (aspartate transaminase 395 U/L, alanine transaminase 677 U/L), gamma-glutamyl transferase 600 U/L, alkaline phosphatase 233 U/L, serum bilirubin direct/total 0.2/0.3 mg/dL, blood urea nitrogen 10.1 mg/dL, serum creatinine 0.24 mg/dL, and C-reactive protein 25.28 mg/L. Based on the clinical impression of drug reaction with eosinophilia and systemic symptoms (DRESS), skin biopsy was performed on an infiltrated plaque lesion of the abdomen. The histopathology revealed basket weave hyperkeratosis, scattered dyskeratotic cells in the epidermis with necrotic keratinocytes of basal layer, mild vacuolar interface change, and perivascular lymphocytic infiltrates. The pathological finding was consistent with DRESS. Further serological tests for hepatitis B virus, hepatitis C virus, Epstein-Barr virus (EBV), cytomegalovirus (CMV), *Mycoplasma pneumonia*, anti-nuclear antibody, and blood culture were all negative. Based on the Registry of Severe Cutaneous Adverse Reactions (RegiSCAR) criteria, a definite case of DRESS was diagnosed (Kardaun et al. 2013).

Under the diagnosis of DRESS syndrome, systemic corticosteroid with intravenous methylprednisolone (1 mg/kg/day) was administered for 2 weeks. However, due to the progression of skin lesions with persistent fever, eosinophilia, and elevated liver enzymes, treatment with cyclosporine (1 mg/kg/day) was added. The skin eruption, hematological abnormalities and elevated hepatic enzymes gradually improved after 2 months of treatment. Scaling on the erythrodermic skin (Fig. 1b) was also noticed days later.

According to the boy's drug history, he was given amoxicillin for about 10 days for respiratory tract infection before the onset of skin eruption. Further lymphocyte activation test confirmed the culprit drug as amoxicillin.

Discussion

DRESS is potentially life-threatening severe cutaneous adverse drug reactions (SCARs) that can occur in both adults and children. DRESS, also known as drug induced hypersensitivity syndrome (DIHS), presents clinically as an extensive maculopapular exanthem accompanied by fever, lymphadenopathy, internal organ involvement (such as hepatitis and nephritis), and hematological abnormalities, including eosinophilia and elevated atypical lymphocytes. Drugs such as aromatic antiepileptics and antibiotics have been most commonly associated with DRESS in children.

In most patients, the reaction begins 2–6 weeks after the initiation of the offending medication (Afiouni et al. 2021), with an average latency of 18.9 days in one review of pediatric DRESS cases. This latency between drug exposure and onset of symptoms in DRESS is considerably longer than in most other drug eruptions. However, asymptomatic changes in lymphocyte blood count or liver function tests may begin earlier.

The skin eruption usually starts as a morbilliform eruption that progresses to become diffuse, confluent, infiltrated papuloplaques. The eruption becomes suggestive of DRESS when it involves more than 50% of the body surface area and includes two or more of the followings: edema (especially facial edema), infiltrated skin lesions, scaling/desquamation, or purpura. The face, upper part of the trunk, and extremities are often involved initially. DRESS in children most often presents as diffuse maculopapular exanthem, with facial edema and oral mucosal involvement in 30% and 20%, respectively. Systemic organ involvement is common, especially involving the liver, kidneys, and lungs. Other severe cutaneous drug eruptions, viral or bacterial infections, Kawasaki disease, hypereosinophilic syndrome, lymphoma, febrile mucocutaneous syndrome, and autoimmune connective tissue diseases may also present with clinical symptoms that mimic DRESS. Exclusion of these other etiologies can help validate a diagnosis of DRESS.

A drug-specific immune response contributes to the pathogenesis of DRESS. During the acute phase of disease, there is an expansion of activated T lymphocytes in the blood, including both CD8 and CD4 cells, and an expansion of regulatory T cells. The frequent peripheral blood eosinophil activation and high serum levels of interleukin-4, interleukin-5, interleukin-13, and thymus and activation-regulated chemokine/chemokine ligand 17 in DRESS patients indicate that the Th2-type immune response also plays a major role. Reactivation of several viruses of the herpes group (human herpesvirus [HHV]-6, HHV-7, EBV, and CMV) is frequent in DRESS and can contribute to clinical symptoms or complications.

Identification and prompt withdrawal of the offending drug is crucial for patients with DRESS. New medications should be introduced carefully during the course of DRESS and in patients in whom DRESS is suspected. Of note, selection of structurally different alternative drugs is important to prevent recurrence. Systemic corticosteroids are usually the first-line treatment for DRESS with extensive rash and severe organ involvement in both adults and children. Though the efficacy and side effect of corticosteroids have not been evaluated in randomized trials to our knowledge, there is general consensus among experts on the use of systemic corticosteroids for the treatment of DRESS with severe organ involvement. There have been cases reports of rapid resolution of DRESS using oral cyclosporine, which can be considered for patients who do not respond well to systemic corticosteroids or when corticosteroids are contraindicated (Su et al 2021). A recent study reported satisfactory control of a recalcitrant and refractory DRESS after 2 weeks of tofacitinib, an inhibitor of the Janus kinase-signal transducer and activator of transcription (JAK-STAT) pathway. Finally, because viral reactivation can cause severe complications such as encephalitis, hemophagocytosis, or severe erosive colitis, antiviral agents active against HHV-6 or CMV may be warranted.

Most patients with DRESS recover completely in weeks to months after drug withdrawal and appropriate treatment. The prognosis of DRESS in children tends to be better with lower mortality compared to adults. However, sequelae with autoimmune diseases have been reported in some patients months or years after the resolution of the drug reaction, including vitiligo, Graves' disease, type 1 diabetes mellitus, and autoimmune hemolytic anemia. One systematic review of DRESS in pediatric patients found a death rate of 3%, with 8% reporting autoimmune sequelae. In the same review, almost 5% of the children with DRESS had a recurrent or relapsing course, which was associated with more comorbidities such as renal and pulmonary involvement. In this group of relapsing pediatric DRESS, initial presentation with erythroderma, facial edema, fever, lymphadenopathy, and prolonged leukocytosis were more frequently detected.

Further Reading

Kardaun SH, Sekula P, Valeyrie-Allanore L, et al. Drug reaction with eosinophilia and systemic symptoms (DRESS): an original multisystem adverse drug reaction. Results from the prospective RegiSCAR study. Br J Dermatol 2013;169:1071-80.

Afiouni R, Zeinaty P, Kechichian E, et al. Pediatric drug reaction with eosinophilia and systemic symptoms: A systematic review of the literature, with a focus on relapsing cases. Pediatr Dermatol 2021;38:125-31.

Ann Allergy Asthma Immunol. 2021;127(6):674-81. https://doi.org/10.1016/j.anai.2021.08.012.

Kim GY, Anderson KR, Davis DMR, Hand JL, Tollefson MM. Drug reaction with eosinophilia and systemic symptoms (DRESS) in the pediatric population: A systematic review of the literature. J Am Acad Dermatol 2020;83:1323-30.

Miyagawa F, Asada H. Current Perspective Regarding the Immunopathogenesis of Drug-Induced Hypersensitivity Syndrome/Drug Reaction with Eosinophilia and Systemic Symptoms (DIHS/DRESS). Int J Mol Sci 2021;22:2147.

Copaescu A, Gibson A, Li Y, Trubiano JA, Phillips EJ. An Updated Review of the Diagnostic Methods in Delayed Drug Hypersensitivity. Front Pharmacol 2020;11:573573.

Rive CM, Bourke J, Phillips EJ. Testing for drug hypersensitivity syndromes. Clin Biochem Rev. 2013;34:15-38.

Teraki Y, Fukuda T. Skin-Homing IL-13-Producing T Cells Expand in the Circulation of Patients with Drug Rash with Eosinophilia and Systemic Symptoms. Dermatology 2017;233:242-9.

Husain Z, Reddy BY, Schwartz RA. DRESS syndrome: Part II. Management and therapeutics. J Am Acad Dermatol 2013;68:709.e701-709; quiz 718-720.

Lin YF, Yang CH, Sindy H, et al. Severe cutaneous adverse reactions related to systemic antibiotics. Clin Infect Dis 2014;58:1377-85.

Chiou CC, Yang LC, Hung SI, et al. Clinicopathological features and prognosis of drug rash with eosinophilia and systemic symptoms: a study of 30 cases in Taiwan. J Eur Acad Dermatol Venereol 2008;22:1044-9.

Nguyen E, Yanes D, Imadojemu S, Kroshinsky D. Evaluation of Cyclosporine for the Treatment of DRESS Syndrome. JAMA Dermatol 2020;156:704-6.

Kim D, Kobayashi T, Voisin B, et al. Targeted therapy guided by single-cell transcriptomic analysis in drug-induced hypersensitivity syndrome: a case report. Nat Med. 2020;26(2):236-243.

Eshki M, Allanore L, Musette P, et al. Twelve-year analysis of severe cases of drug reaction with eosinophilia and systemic symptoms: a cause of unpredictable multiorgan failure. Arch Dermatol 2009;145:67-72.

Chen YC, Chang CY, Cho YT, Chiu HC, Chu CY. Long-term sequelae of drug reaction with eosinophilia and systemic symptoms: a retrospective cohort study from Taiwan. J Am Acad Dermatol 2013;68:459-65.

Su H-J, Chen C-B, Yeh T-Y, Chung W-H. Successful treatment of corticosteroid-dependent drug reaction with eosinophilia and systemic symptoms with cyclosporine. Ann Allergy Asthma Immunol. 2021;127(6):674–681. https://doi.org/10.1016/j.anai.2021.08.012.

Case 48. A 4-Month-Old Infant with Fever, Diarrhea, Followed by Abdominal Distention and an Ulcer-Like Skin Lesion: Community-Acquired *Pseudomonas aeruginosa* Sepsis (Shanghai Fever)

Chih-Hsien Chuang

Keywords

Pseudomonas aeruginosa · Sepsis · Diarrhea Children · Community-acquired

Key Points

- *Pseudomonas aeruginosa* can cause enteric infection. The disease severity ranges from self-limited diarrhea to sepsis (Shanghai fever).
- Shanghai fever and other *P. aeruginosa* associated diarrheal diseases can be distinguished by clinical features and laboratory findings.
- Early appropriate antibiotic treatment can reduce mortality.
- No common primary immune deficiency was found.

Case Report

A 4-month-old boy infant was admitted because of fever with hepatomegaly and massive ascites. The patient was a full-term baby with a birth body weight of 2850 g. He was a well-nourished and developed infant. His body weight was 7 kg (25–50th percentile) and body height was 65 cm (50–75th percentile). He was well until 4 days before admission when he had fever and diarrhea. The characteristic of stool was watery with scanty mucus and blood in green appearance. A carbuncle-like lesion was found over right shoulder 2 days after fever developed. Progressive abdominal distension was found. His appetite and activity became poor. He was admitted to a local hospital and received antibiotic treatment with vancomycin and ceftriaxone for suspicion of methicillin-resistant *Staphylococcus aureus* infection and salmonella enterocolitis. Computed tomography of abdomen revealed hepatomegaly with massive ascites. Respiratory distress developed on the next day. He was transferred to a tertiary care medical center.

On physical examinations, he was lethargic. Vital signs were temperature 39.2 °C, respiratory rate 56/min, pulse 160 beats/min, and blood pressure 76/32 mmHg. His respiratory pattern was rapid with suprasternal and intercostal retraction. His abdomen was severe distension with hepatomegaly and hypoactive bowel sounds. Erythematous swelling with pus formation and gangrenous change was noted over right shoul-

C.-H. Chuang (✉)
Department of Pediatrics, Saint Paul's Hospital, Taoyuan, Taiwan
e-mail: doc1860@mail.sph.org.tw

Y.-C. Huang et al. (eds.), *Paediatric Infectious Diseases*,
https://doi.org/10.1007/978-981-19-7276-8_48

der. Other physical findings were unremarkable. Blood test showed leukopenia (WBC 1600/μL, immature neutrophils 13%, segmented 5%, lymphocytes 55%, monocytes 15%, eosinophil 7% and atypical lymphocyte 5%), anemia (hemoglobin 7.3 g/dL), thrombocytopenia (platelet 90,000/μL), and disseminated intravascular coagulation (Prothrombin time/Activated partial thromboplastin time 18.6/33.7 s, fibrinogen 190 mg/dL, fibrin degradation product >80 μg/mL and D-dimer >10,000 mg/L). Blood biochemistry data were sugar 67 mg/dL, blood urea nitrogen (BUN) 11.4 mg/dL, creatinine 0.4 mg/dL, bilirubin (direct/total) 0.9/0.6, aspartate transaminase (AST) 13 U/L, alanine transaminase (ALT) 9 U/L, sodium 128 mEq/L, potassium 4.6 mEq/L, chloride 96 mEq/L, C-reactive protein (CRP) 202 mg/L (normal, <5 mg/L), procalcitonin 19.8 ng/mL, albumin 2.1 g/dL, total protein 3.5 g/dL, and ferritin 322 ng/mL. Arterial blood gas showed mild metabolic acidosis (pH 7.32, HCO_3 18 mm/L). Under the impression of sepsis and ecthyma gangrenosum, he was treated with vancomycin and piperacillin-tazobactam. Blood components were transfused for anemia, thrombocytopenia, and coagulopathy. Blood, pus, stool, and sputum cultures all revealed *Pseudomonas aeruginosa*, which was susceptible to all anti-pseudomonal antibiotics. Antibiotics were shifted to piperacillin-tazobactam and amikacin. Immunological studies revealed IgG: 241 mg/dL (normal 196–558), IgA: 9.9 mg/dL (normal 4.4–73), IgM: 21.4 mg/dL (normal 4.4–73) and IgE: <17.3 IU/mL. IgG subclass level were IgG1: 186 mg/dL (normal 190–620), IgG2 49 mg/dL (normal 30–140), and IgG3 31 mg/dL (normal 9–62). Lymphocyte subpopulation study showed negative finding. WBC count increased to 25,000/μL (immature neutrophils 5%, segmented 65%, lymphocytes 13%, monocytes 5% and atypical lymphocyte 6%) 1 week after admission. Series plain film of abdomen did not find bowel perforation despite persistent abdominal distension for 2 weeks.

The ecthyma gangrenosum extended from right shoulder to right arm, accounting for 7% of total body surface area (Fig. 1). He received debridement 2 weeks after admission and skin graft was performed 4 weeks after admission. After 55 days of hospitalization, he was discharged with the diagnosis of community-acquired *Pseudomonas aeruginosa* sepsis, enteritis, and extended ecthyma gangrenosum. Follow-up was uneventful for this patient and no more severe infection occurred.

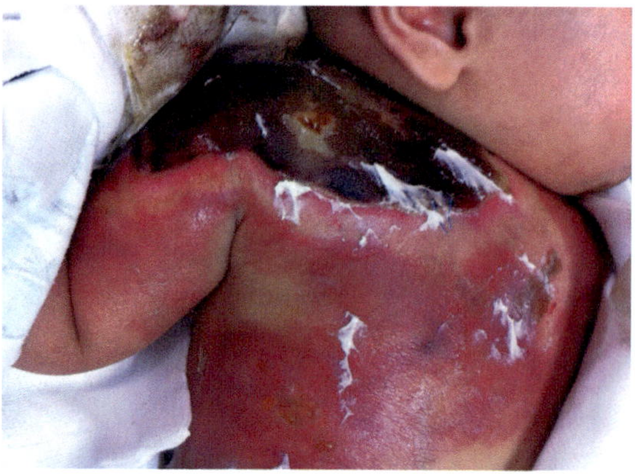

Fig. 1 Ecthyma gangrenosum extended from right shoulder to right arm, accounting for 7% of total body surface area, in an infant with Shanghai fever

Discussion

Pseudomonas aeruginosa is an aerobic, gram-negative bacillus. The morphological characteristics of *P. aeruginosa* on laboratory media are production of bluish-green phenazine pigment. *P. aeruginosa* can metabolize a wide range of organic substances that make it a ubiquitous microorganism living in soil, water, plants, and hospital environment. *P. aeruginosa* possesses multiple virulence factors, including flagella, type IV pilus, protease, exotoxin A, neuraminidase and type III secretion system toxins, etc. Virulence factors are expressed under specific environment and host immune response. Due to intrinsic resistance of *P. aeruginosa* to many classes of antibiotics and acquisition of resistant genes from other microorganisms, infection of *P. aeruginosa* could cause severe therapeutic problems.

P. aeruginosa is an important opportunistic pathogen causing infections in patients with compromised immunity, hematological malignancy, and cystic fibrosis. *P. aeruginosa* can be isolated from mucosal sites such as respiratory, urinary, and gastrointestinal tracts. It is a major pathogen of hospital-acquired pneumonia and catheter-related urinary tract infection. The diseases associated with *P. aeruginosa* in gastrointestinal tract are usually mild. Antibiotic-associated diarrhea caused by *P. aeruginosa* is self-limited. However, in immunocompromised patients, *P. aeruginosa* could result in typhlitis or rectal abscess in neutropenic patients due to chemotherapy, and necrotizing enterocolitis in premature infants. The carriage rate of *P. aeruginosa* in stool in healthy children is about 2% and 1% in hospitalized adult patients. In diarrheal children, *P. aeruginosa* represents 1% in stool cultures and accounts for 6% of positive stool cultures.

Diarrheal diseases caused by *P. aeruginosa* could range from self-limiting diarrhea to severe necrotizing enteritis with sepsis. In a study from Taiwan, the investigators classified *P. aeruginosa* associated diarrheal diseases into four groups: Shanghai fever (community-acquired *P. aeruginosa* sepsis), *P. aeruginosa* enterocolitis, *P. aeruginosa*-related diarrhea, and antibiotic-associated diarrhea. Enteric disease with sepsis caused by *P. aeruginosa* had been reported in Shanghai in 1918. Community-acquired *P. aeruginosa* sepsis in previously healthy children was subsequently reported in East Asia, mainly from Taiwan, Hong Kong, and China. Nearly 90% of Shanghai fever patients are infants with male predominance. The disease usually occurred during the summer season. Fever and diarrhea were the initial clinical symptoms. The stool pattern is watery, some with little mucus, blood tinged, and green in appearance. The median time from first symptom to sepsis was 4 days. Dyspnea developed in 40% of patients. Approximately 80% of patients had septic shock and necrotizing enteritis. Bowel perforation was observed in one-third of patients. Multiple patchy necrosis with fibrin coating of small intestine or colon was the major operative finding. Ecthyma gangrenosum is a characteristic skin manifestation of *P. aeruginosa* septicemia. The cutaneous lesion occurred in 1.3–2.8% of patients with *P. aeruginosa* bacteremia. However, ecthyma gangrenosum was seen in 60% of patients with Shanghai fever. More than half of them had multiple sites involvement. Seizure occurred in one-fourth of patients. Most of them were induced by hyponatremia. Meningitis was infrequently seen (<10%) but it led to a devastating complication. Patients with meningitis resulted in severe neurological sequelae such as brain atrophy and hydrocephalus. The characteristic laboratory findings of Shanghai fever were leukopenia (WBC <4000/μL), anemia (hemoglobin <10 g/dL), thrombocytopenia (platelet <100,000/μL), coagulopathy, high CRP level (>100 mg/L), hyponatremia (<130 mEq/L), and hyperglycemia (>150 mg/L). Community-acquired *P. aeruginosa* sepsis can be the initial presentation of underlying immunodeficiency, and hypogammaglobulinemia is reported as the most common underlying primary immune deficiency. Almost none of patients with Shanghai fever had hypogammaglobulinemia. No common humoral or cellular immune deficiency was found through lymphocyte subpopulation study. No severe or recurrent infection was observed among surviving patients. Microbiological studies revealed Shanghai fever was caused by high virulent strains of *P. aeruginosa*. Both host (infant) and microbial factors play a role in the pathogenesis. *P. aeruginosa* isolated from Shanghai fever were susceptible to all anti-pseudomonal antibiotics. The mortality rate of Shanghai fever ranged from 10% to 90%. Prompt administration of antipseudomonal antibiotics within 24 h is associated with favorable outcome.

The clinical manifestation of *P. aeruginosa* enterocolitis is similar to that seen in other bacterial enterocolitis. More than 80% of patients with *P. aeruginosa* enterocolitis had fever for more than 3 days. The stool pattern was bloody and mucoid. Laboratory findings included high CRP. Antibiotic-associated diarrhea is the most common *P. aeruginosa*-associated diarrheal diseases (43%). The clinical features of *P. aeruginosa*-related diarrhea and antibiotic-associated diarrhea mimics viral or toxin-mediated enteritis. Their stool pattern was watery, without blood or mucus. Most of them did not have prolonged fever. Laboratory data were non-specific. Antibiotics therapy is not recommended for *P. aeruginosa*-related diarrhea or antibiotic-associated diarrhea. Shanghai fever and other *P. aeruginosa* diarrheal diseases could be differentiated by clinical features and laboratory findings. Early recognition of *P. aeruginosa* sepsis and prompt administration of anti-pseudomonal antibiotics are the key factors for reducing mortality.

Further Reading

Paul J. Planet. Principles and Practice of Pediatric Infectious Diseases, 5th ed. Philadelphia, PA: Elsevier. 2017: 155, 866-870.e1.

Quartin AA, Scerpella EG, Puttagunta S, Kett DH. A comparison of microbiology and demographics among patients with healthcare-associated, hospital-acquired, and ventilator-associated pneumonia: a retrospective analysis of 1184 patients from a large, international study. *BMC Infect Dis*. 2013;13:561.

Ortega M, Marco F, Soriano A, et al. Epidemiology and prognostic determinants of bacteraemic catheter-acquired urinary tract infection in a single institution from 1991 to 2010. *J Infect*. 2013;67:282-287.

Speert DP, Campbell ME, Davidson AG, Wong LT. *Pseudomonas aeruginosa* colonization of the gastrointestinal tract in patients with cystic fibrosis. *J Infect Dis*. 1993;167:226-229.

Chuang CH, Janapatla RP, Wang YH, Chang HJ, Huang YC, Lin TY, Chiu CH. *Pseudomonas aeruginosa*-associated Diarrheal Diseases in Children. *Pediatr Infect Dis J* 2017;36:1119-1123.

Dold H. On pyocyaneus sepsis and intestinal infections in Shanghai due to *Bacillus pyocyaneus*. *Chin Med J* 1918;32:435.

Huang YC, Lin TY, Wang CH. Community-acquired *Pseudomonas aeruginosa* sepsis in previously healthy infants and children: analysis of forty-three episodes. *Pediatr Infect Dis J*. 2002;21:1049-1052.

Chuang CH, Wang YS, Chang HJ, et al. Shanghai fever: a distinct *Pseudomonas aeruginosa* enteric disease. *Gut*. 2014;63:736-743.

Zhang Q, Smith JC, Zhu Q, Guo Z, MacDonald NE. A five-year review of *Pseudomonas aeruginosa* bacteremia in children hospitalized at a single center in southern China. *Int J Infect Dis*. 2012;16:e628-632.

Zomorrodi A, Wald ER. Ecthyma gangrenosum: considerations in previously healthy child. *Pediatr Infect Dis J* 2002;21:1161-4.

Case 49. A 2-Year-Old Girl with Erythematous Swelling in the Left Thigh Following DTaP-Hib-IPV Vaccination: Extensive Limb Swelling Following Vaccination

Hsin Chi

Keywords

Cellulitis · Delayed hypersensitivity
Extensive limb swelling · Prophylaxis
Vaccination

Key Points

- Extensive limb swelling (ELS) can occur after any vaccination in an individual of any age.
- The common vaccines that cause ELS are polyvalent pneumococcal vaccine, diphtheria and tetanus toxoids and acellular pertussis vaccine (DTap), Td, DTP, and influenza vaccine
- Defined as a swelling of the vaccinated extremity extending at least to the elbow or knee, or extending from the joint proximal, to the joint distal to the injection site, or to the entire circumference.
- Develops 24–48 h after vaccination and mostly resolves spontaneously within several days
- There is no specific therapy.

Case 1

A 2-year-6-month-old girl received the fourth dose of DTaP-Hib-IPV in her left thigh and the third dose of *Japanese encephalitis vaccine in her right thigh*. Erythematous swelling with heat and pain developed in the left thigh on the same day following vaccination (Fig. 1), accompanied with decreased appetite and activity. Symptoms did not subside after local ice packing. She was brought to the outpatient department of a hospital on the second day and hospitalized for antibiotic treatment under the impression of cellulitis in the left thigh. Blood culture was negative for bacteria. The erythematous swelling improved gradually. She was then discharged 2 days later. The final diagnosis was extensive limb swelling following DTaP-Hib-IPV vaccination.

H. Chi (✉)
Division of Pediatric Infectious Diseases, Department of Pediatrics, MacKay Children's Hospital, Taipei, Taiwan

MacKay College of Medicine, Taipei, Taiwan
e-mail: chi.4531@mmh.org.tw

Y.-C. Huang et al. (eds.), *Paediatric Infectious Diseases*,
https://doi.org/10.1007/978-981-19-7276-8_49

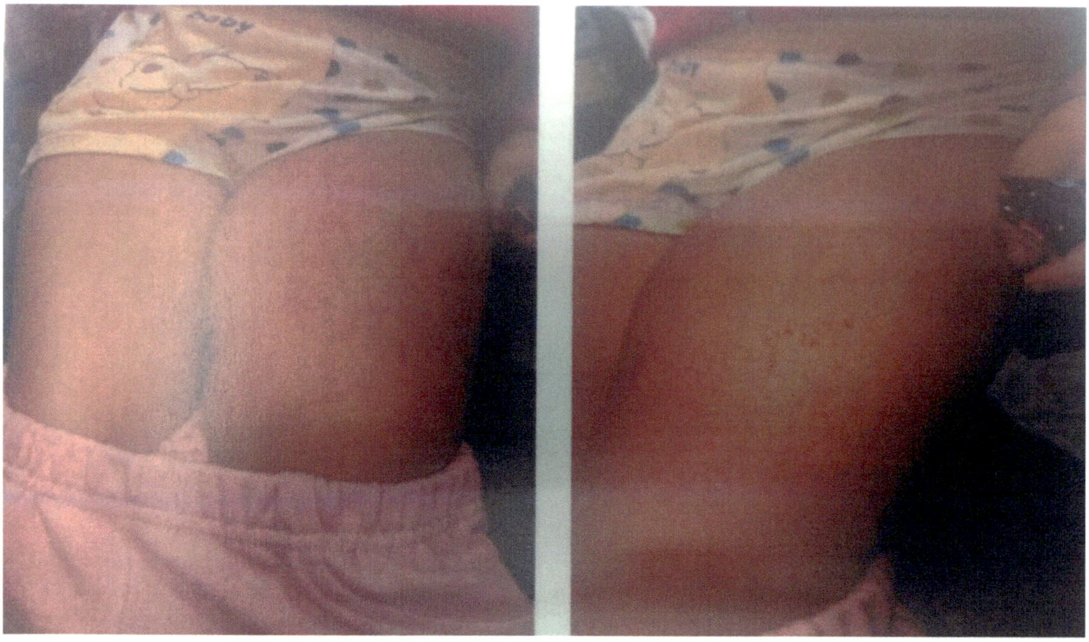

Fig. 1 Erythema and swelling in the left thigh following DTaP-Hib-IPV vaccination in a 2-year-old girl (Case 1)

Case 2

A previously healthy 1-year-3-month-old girl received the third dose of pneumococcal conjugate vaccine (PCV)-13 in the left thigh. Mild erythematous swelling and tenderness were noted at the injection site later on the same day. She was brought to the emergency department of a local hospital. Vaccination-induced local injection site reaction was diagnosed and anti-inflammatory drugs were prescribed. However, the symptoms persisted despite medications. She was brought to our outpatient department 2 days later. Then she was hospitalized for intravenous empiric antibiotic with the tentative diagnosis of cellulitis in the left thigh. On admission, physical examination revealed an erythematous swelling measuring 18–20 × 15 cm in the left thigh (Fig. 2). Laboratory examinations showed leukocytosis (12.28 × 10^9 cells/L) and mildly elevated C-reactive protein (23.3 mg/L). Blood culture was negative for bacteria. The erythematous swelling and tenderness subsided gradually. She was discharged on the fourth day of hospitalization with a final diagnosis of extensive limb swelling following vaccination of PCV-13.

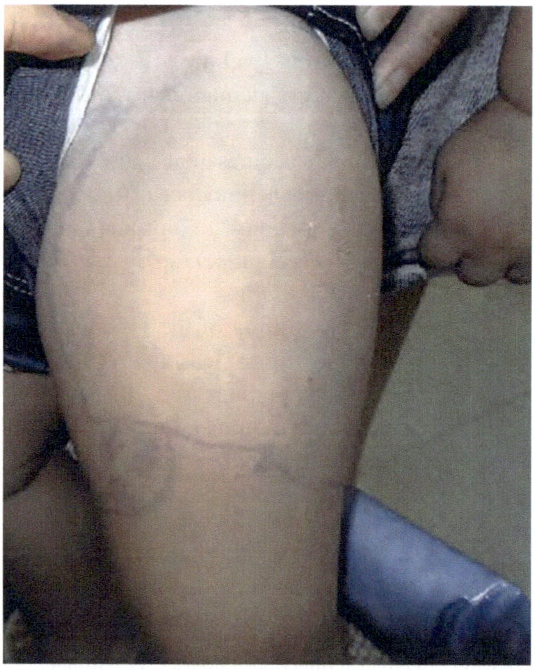

Fig. 2 Extensive limb swelling in the left thigh 2 days following PCV13 vaccination in a 1-year-3-month-old girl (Case 2)

Discussion

Extensive limb swelling (ELS) can occur with any vaccine in an individual of any age. According to the largest study on ELS so far, the common vaccines that cause ELS are polyvalent pneumococcal vaccine (PPV), diphtheria and tetanus toxoids and acellular pertussis vaccine (D-Tap), tetanus and diphtheria toxoids (adsorbed adult; Td), diphtheria and tetanus toxoids and pertussis vaccine (adsorbed pediatric; DTP), and influenza vaccine (FLU). In Australia, by 2016 annual surveillance vaccine adverse events report, the incidence of ELS is 8%, of which 65% occur in individuals younger than 7 years of age and 35% in those older than 7 years of age. In the group younger than 18 years of age, 40% are girls, while in the group older than 18 years of age, 75.4% are women. The incidence of ELS caused by DTaP boosters is about 1–4% in all. In the population under 8 years of age, DTaP accounts for 75% of all ELS. And the incidence of ELS positively correlates with the doses of DTaP, especially with the fourth and fifth doses. Interestingly, ELS, in terms of "coronavirus disease 2019 (COVID-19) arm" has been reported in adults receiving severe acute respiratory syndrome coronavirus 2 (SARS-CoV-2) vaccines. In the study of SARS-CoV-2 mRNA vaccine, the incidence of ELS in the second dose is greater than in the first dose. In a study of Pfizer-BioNTech vaccine, the probability of ELS in the first dose was 4.6%, while the second dose was 6.5%. In a study of Moderna mRNA vaccine, the probability of ELS in the first dose was 3.1%, while the second dose was 11.9%.

The exact pathophysiological mechanism of ELS has not been thoroughly clarified. Recher et al. proposed that type IV delayed hypersensitivity reaction may cause extensive limb swelling, with skin biopsy showing a dense dermal and subdermal perivascular-intensified infiltration dominated by CD4+ T cells and CD68+ macrophages. But Liese JG et al. reported that the probable cause of large local reactions may be type III hypersensitivity reaction with existing IgG antibodies previously induced by circulating immune complexes of vaccine antigen. Some researchers found that humoral immunity responses and prior sensitization to antigens or excipients may have some influence on ELS. In summary, ELS is a local inflammatory reaction rather than an allergic reaction.

Extensive limb swelling (ELS) is a known side effect specific to vaccination and is defined as a swelling of the vaccinated extremity extending at least to the elbow or knee, or extending from the joint proximal to the joint distal to the injection site, or extending the entire circumference around the extremity. Sometimes this covers more than half of the vaccinated limb. The types of ELS could be classified into three groups. First, "whole-limb swelling" is defined as swelling of the entire limb (i.e., from the hip to the foot or from the shoulder to the hand). Second, "more-than-proximal (MTP) limb swelling" involves the entire proximal segment of the limb (i.e., from the hip to the knee or the shoulder to the elbow) and the swelling in the distal segment which does not extend all the way to the foot or hand. The last type of ELS is called "proximal limb swelling," in which swelling extends only from the hip to the knee or from the shoulder to the elbow. In most cases, extensive swelling is limited to the proximal half of the upper extremity. The reaction develops 24–48 h after vaccination and mostly resolves spontaneously within several days. The symptoms often develop in the first day after the injection, sometimes it can occur as early as a few hours after vaccination. Other inflammation symptoms, such as erythema, warmth, or pain have also been reported. The pain is usually mild, and movement of the extremity is usually not restricted. Concomitant symptoms include fever, influenza-like symptoms, and agitation/crying. However, most patients appear well with no bacterial infection or allergic hypersensitivity.

Post-vaccinated extensive limb swelling is benign and self-limiting and ameliorates gradually without sequelae. There are no specific management recommendations, and no antibiotics and surgical intervention are needed. Besides, these vaccination-induced reactions do not respond to antibiotics. Hence, we separate symptomatic treatment into two parts. The first part is local reaction relieving, the second one is fever management. Cold pack, pain-relieving medication, and topical steroids cream. For example, 1% hydrocortisone cream may be effective for local reaction of ELS. It is locally used once or twice per day. Besides, if needed, we could give acetaminophen or ibuprofen every 4–6 h for fever management. Most importantly, we should timely inform the Vaccine Adverse Event Reporting System (VAERS) for the vaccination injury evaluation if the local reactions get worse.

Further Reading

Woo EJ, et al. Extensive limb swelling after immunization: reports to the Vaccine Adverse Event Reporting System. Clin Infect Dis 2003; 37: 351-8.

Dey A, et al. Surveillance of adverse events following immunisation in Australia annual report, 2016. Commun Dis Intell 2018; 2018: 42.

Huber BM, GoetschelP. Extensive limb swelling after vaccination. J Pediatr 2011; 158: 1033.

Rennels MB. Extensive swelling reactions occurring after booster doses of diphtheria-tetanus-acellular pertussis vaccines. Semin Pediatr Infect Dis 2003; 14: 196-8.

Lindgren AL, Austin AH, Welsh KM. COVID Arm: Delayed Hypersensitivity Reactions to SARS-CoV-2 Vaccines Misdiagnosed as Cellulitis. J Prim Care Community Health 2021; 12: 21501327211024431.

Recher M, et al. Immune system correlates of extensive limb swelling in response to conjugated pneumococcal vaccination. NPJ Vaccines 2018; 3: 17.

Liese JG, et al. Safety and immunogenicity of Biken acellular pertussis vaccine in combination with diphtheria and tetanus toxoid as a fifth dose at four to six years of age. Munich Vaccine Study Group. Pediatr Infect Dis J 2001; 20: 981-8.

Cohen E, Tahri S, Lukkassen I. Two cases of extensive limb swelling after influenza vaccination. Pediatr Infect Dis J 2015; 34: 114.

Huang DT, et al. Protracted fever with cellulitis-like reaction in pneumococcal polysaccharide-vaccinated children. Pediatr Infect Dis J 2008; 27: 937-9.

Case 50. A 9-Year-Old Girl with a Right Lateral Chest Wall Mass: Thoracic Actinomycosis

Po-Yen Chen

Keywords

Child · Asymptomatic · Chest wall mass
Excisional biopsy · Sulfur granule · Penicillin

Key Points

- Thoracic actinomycosis is not uncommon and sporadic cases occur.
- Attacks individuals of all age and any site of human body
- Symptoms depend on the body site being involved, and afebrile infection can occur.
- CT scan may show invasive infection of multiple body sites, including lung, bone, chest wall, and abdominal psoas muscle.
- Diagnosis is based on clinical manifestations, isolation of *Actinomyces* species, and/or pathologic findings of granulomatous change and sulfur granules in the lesion
- Penicillin is the drug of choice, and long duration of therapy is needed.
- Prognosis is generally good.

P.-Y. Chen (✉)
Pediatrics, Taichung Veterans General Hospital,
National Chung Hsing University,
Taichung City, Taiwan
e-mail: pychen@vghtc.gov.tw

Case Report

A 9-year-old girl was in good health before. Two months ago, she complained of right flank pain for 2–3 days and it subsided without medication. She seemed well until 2 weeks ago, when productive cough developed, accompanied with fever for 5 days. She also had decreased appetite and activity. She firstly visited LMD, common cold was suspected, and medication for symptom control was prescribed. Although her fever subsided, a soft mass protruding from her right lower chest wall (Fig. 1) was accidentally discovered during bathing. She was taken to the hospital again where a chest X-ray film also revealed right lower lung consolidation with pleural effusion (Fig. 2). She was then transferred to our hospital.

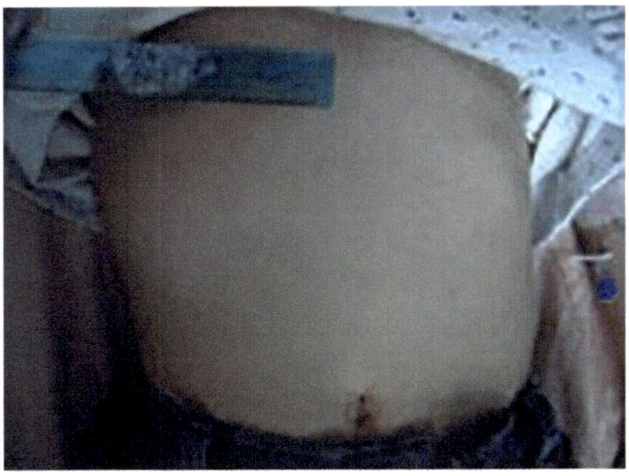

Fig. 1 Image of right lower chest mass at admission

Y.-C. Huang et al. (eds.), *Paediatric Infectious Diseases*,
https://doi.org/10.1007/978-981-19-7276-8_50

When arriving at our hospital, she was fairly well without respiratory distress. Her vital signs were stable. Physical examination revealed a soft, skin-colored nontender mass in her right lower chest. Laboratory evaluation showed leukocytosis (white blood cell 21,900/μL, neutrophils 69.8%, lymphocytes 24.8%, eosinophils 0.7%, hemoglobin 12.2 g/dL), thrombocytosis (914,000/μL), and an elevated erythrocyte sedimentation rate (118 mm/h) and C-reactive protein (65 mg/L). Chest computed tomography (CT) scan showed subphrenic abscess, pleural effusion, and a subcutaneous mass over right chest area (Fig. 3).

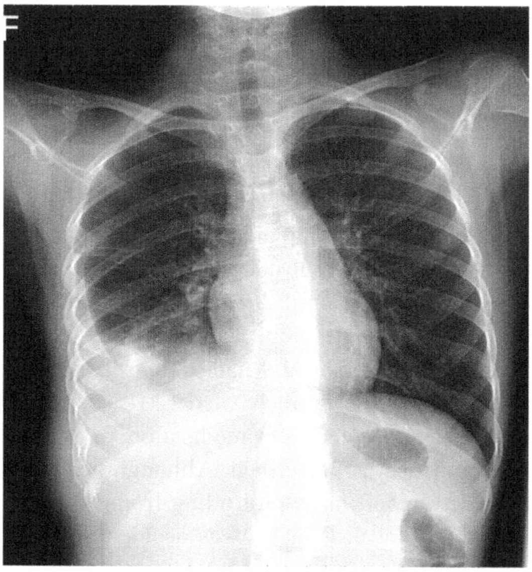

Fig. 2 Chest X-ray film in a local hospital showed right lower lung consolidation with pleural effusion

She reported no chronic illnesses and no history of foreign or rural travel within 14 days before the onset of symptoms. She had two domestic dogs and three birds. During hospitalization, she initially received empirical treatment with intravenous ceftriaxone. Three days after admission, CT-guided biopsy was performed and the culture yielded no growth. After a further 2 days, excisional biopsy and drainage surgery were performed. Excisional biopsy revealed acute and chronic xanthomatous inflammation with actinomycosis sulfur granules (Fig. 4), showing the invasion of the lung, diaphragm, chest wall, and abdomen. Tuberculosis workup was carried out and showed negative findings.

She began to receive intravenous penicillin treatment once when thoracic actinomycosis was diagnosed. After 5 weeks of antibiotic treatment, she was discharged from the hospital (Fig. 5). Upon discharge, her chest X-ray showed residual right effusion. She received sequential treatment with oral penicillin and amoxicillin for additional 4 months with complete resolution achieved.

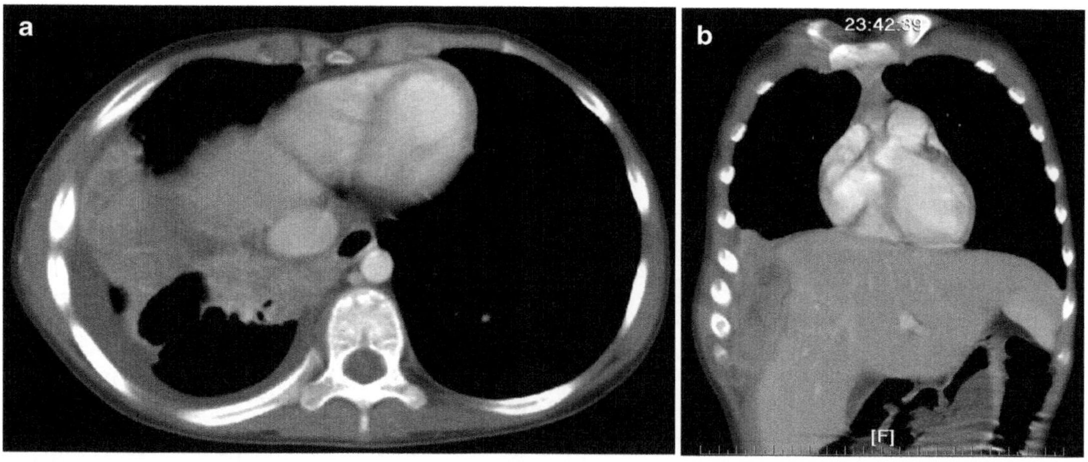

Fig. 3 Chest CT at admission showed subphrenic abscess, pleural effusion, and a subcutaneous mass over right chest area in axial (**a**) and coronal (**b**) views

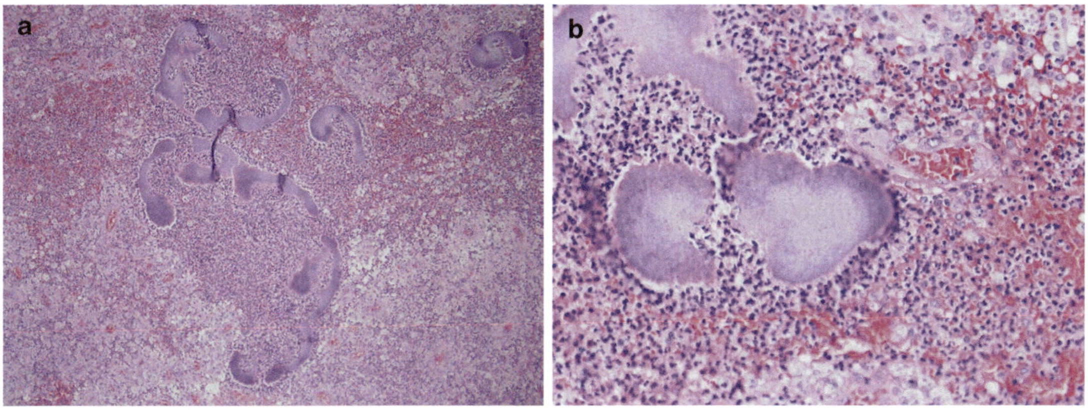

Fig. 4 Histological image of the excisional biopsy showed acute and chronic xanthomatous inflammation (**a**) with actinomycosis sulfur granules (**b**)

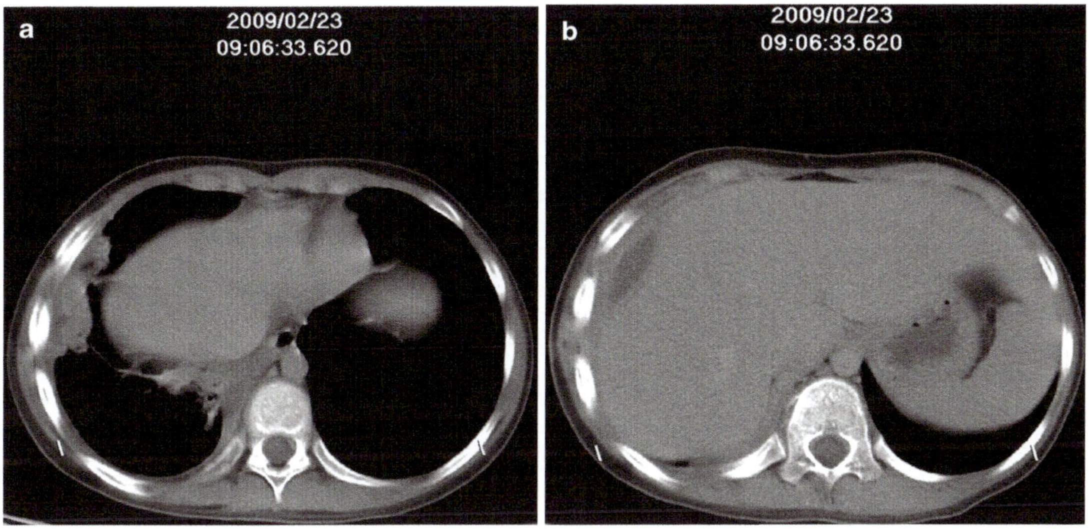

Fig. 5 Chest CT during hospitalization, 1 month after antibiotic treatment and drainage surgery in axial (**a**) and coronal (**b**) views

Discussion

Actinomyces species is a facultative anaerobe. It can be normal flora of the oropharynx, gastrointestinal tract, and female genital tract, but it can also cause indolent, invasive infection of any part of human body. Risk factors for invasive actinomycosis in children include dental caries, trauma, debilitation, and poorly controlled diabetes mellitus.

Pulmonary actinomycosis is difficult to diagnose and delayed diagnosis or misdiagnosis as tuberculosis or cancer are common. A literature review of 55 pediatric patients with thoracic actinomycosis from 1950 to 2006 showed that their average age was 10 years and the most common clinical manifestations were chest wall mass (49%), cough (40%), pain (back, chest, shoulder, or axillary) (36%), weight loss and fever (35%), a draining sinus (15%), and hemoptysis (9%).

Bone involvement was also found in over 40% of these pediatric patients.

The classic radiographic triad of thoracic actinomycosis consists of chronic lower lobe pulmonary consolidation, empyema, and wavy periostitis of the ribs. The lesion may cross anatomic boundaries from the lung through interlobar fissures to adjacent soft tissue and bone structure. The diagnosis of thoracic actinomycosis usually relies on invasive procedures (i.e., fine needle aspiration, incision and drainage, or thoracentesis), bronchoscopy, open procedure, or thoracotomy. The Isolation of *Actinomyces* species is found in nearly 60% of the patients. Typical pathology findings include granulomatous change, sulfur granules, and ray fungus.

Combination of surgical and medical treatment is the best option for management. *Actinomyces* species are susceptible to penicillin, amoxicillin, and other beta-lactam antibiotics. Alternative agents include clindamycin, doxycycline, and erythromycin. There is no optimal duration of antibiotic therapy. The average duration of treatment was 5.9 months in a study of 38 cases of thoracic actinomycosis. Most experts would recommend intravenous penicillin for 4–6 weeks followed by 6–12 months of oral antibiotic therapy.

Further Reading

Bartlett AH, Rivera AL, Krishnamurthy R, Baker CJ. Thoracic actinomycosis in children: case report and review of the literature. Pediatr Infect Dis J 2008;27(2):165-9.

Lin TP, Fu LS, Peng HC, Lee T, Chen JT, Chi CS. Intra-abdominal actinomycosis with hepatic pseudotumor and xanthogranulomatous pyelonephritis in a 6-y-old boy. Scand J Infect Dis 2001 33: 551–553.

Goussard P, Eber E, Rabie H, Nel P, Schubert P. Paediatric pulmonary actinomycosis: A forgotten disease. Paediatr Respir Rev 2021; 10: S1526-0542(21)00089-0.

GPSR Compliance

The European Union's (EU) General Product Safety Regulation (GPSR) is a set of rules that requires consumer products to be safe and our obligations to ensure this.

If you have any concerns about our products, you can contact us on ProductSafety@springernature.com

In case Publisher is established outside the EU, the EU authorized representative is:

Springer Nature Customer Service Center GmbH
Europaplatz 3
69115 Heidelberg, Germany

Batch number: 09336741

Printed by Printforce, the Netherlands